Rheumatoid Arthritis: The Infection Connection

Targeting and Treating the Cause of Chronic Illness

Katherine M. Poehlmann, Ph.D

satori press

Rheumatoid Arthritis: The Infection Connection

Targeting and Treating the Cause of Chronic Illness

by Katherine M. Poehlmann, Ph.D.

Published by: satori press
904 Silver Spur Road #323
Rolling Hills Estates, CA 90274

Cover design and illustrations (unless otherwise cited): KEPI studios
Author photo: Jim Beavers
Editors: Paula Larich, Judy Sunderland
Printing: One2One Direct, 27460 Avenue Scott, Valencia, CA 91355

First Printing 1997, doctoral dissertation
Second Printing 2002, completely revised

Printed in the United States of America

Library of Congress Cataloging-in-Publication Data

Poehlmann, Katherine M.

Rheumatoid arthritis: the infection connection—targeting and treating the cause of chronic illness / by Katherine M. Poehlmann, Ph.D. — 2nd ed.
Includes bibliographical references and index.
ISBN: 0-9617268-6-5 (pbk.)

1. Rheumatoid Arthritis—Cause and treatment. 2. Bacterial infection—Identification and eradication. 3.Chronic disease—Nutritional aspects. 4. Immune system—Improvement. 5. Chronic disease—Cause and treatment. 6. Allergies—Identification and eradication.

"Bacteria are cleverer than men."

—Dr. Harold Neu,
Columbia University, 1992

"Bugs are always figuring out ways to get around the antibiotics we throw at them. They adapt; they come roaring back."

—Dr. George Jacoby,
Harvard Medical School, 1992

"All warfare is based on deception."

—Sun Tzu, *The Art of War*, 500 B.C.

"Rheumatism *is a common name for many aches and pains which have yet got no peculiar appellation, though owing to very different causes. It is besides often hard to be distinguished from some which have a certain name and class assigned them."*

—Dr. William Heberden, *Commentarii de morborum historia et curatione*, 1802

"No major disease has ever been cured before science has first developed an understanding of how it works"

—Dr. Thomas McPherson Brown, 1988

"So, Nat'ralists observe, a Flea
Hath smaller Fleas that on him prey,
And these have smaller Fleas to bite 'em,
And so proceed ad infinitum."

—Jonathan Swift, Irish author
and satirist, 1720

About

the

Author

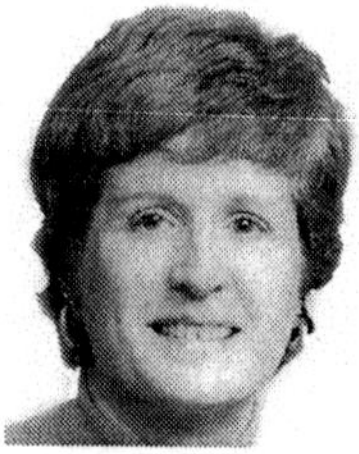

Dr. Katherine Poehlmann
is a professional researcher and a systems engineer with a magna cum laude degree in mathematics and an MBA with a specialty in technology management. She has authored more than a dozen scientific reports on space technology, defense policy analysis, and aircraft logistics.

She used her research skills, honed at the RAND Corporation as a senior analyst from 1984-1994, to obtain a Ph.D. in health counseling in 1997. The goal was to find the cause of a debilitating case of rheumatoid arthritis (RA) which developed in both ankles soon after a fall down stairs. She saw that the usual course of treatment involved using powerful drugs with harmful side effects. These medications only masked the painful RA symptoms but did not target the root cause of the RA condition.

Dr. Poehlmann has progressed from being "25% disabled," as determined by several physicians and rheumatologists in 1993, to being completely ambulatory and pain-free, using the techniques described in this book. She became a certified hypnotherapist in order to learn techniques for stress control and pain management and teach them to others.

Since recovery from RA, she has hiked in Tibet, Chile, and over sections of the Great Wall of China.

FOREWORD *by DR. HAROLD W. CLARK*

This book offers both patients and health care providers an unabridged encyclopedia of information on the infectious cause and effective treatments of rheumatoid arthritis and other related chronic illnesses. Hundreds of books about arthritis have been written but few are more extensively referenced in support of both cause and treatment than this one.

The introduction of antibiotic therapy in rheumatoid and related chronic diseases by my colleague, the late Dr Thomas McPherson Brown, was based on a mechanistic approach to an infectious cause rather than the typical symptomatic control of broad systemic illnesses. I believe that the treatment was successful because under our multi-disciplinary team approach the patient was educated and became part of the team. These patients encouraged us to document their success stories in *The Road Back* and *Why Arthritis?*.

Prior to our experiments, research was aimed at the typical viral and bacterial responses that do not fit the premise of an Infection Connection. The diverse therapeutic agents for RA, such as gold salts, hydroxyquinoline, bee venom, and the tetracycline antibiotics all inhibited *Mycoplasma*. These are uniquely different microbes being noncytopathic *in vitro* but are persisting viable allergens in the host.

Our target was narrowed to filterable and pleomorphic microbes that were difficult to isolate and identify. These served as the key allergens in a chronic and progressive hypersensitivity reaction. They elicit antibody responses with the formation of more pathogenic immune complexes that activate the proteolytic complement system.

The tetracyclines have several actions in the host as a result of their chelation and electron scavenging properties. These actions include: anti-inflammatory; inhibiting the proteinases; antioxidant; immunosuppressing, blocking the immune complex formation; nucleophilic, inhibiting protein synthesis; and inhibiting the metalloenzymes such as collagenase. Pulse therapy (taking a tetracycline dose between meals on alternate days) can be beneficial with minimum toxicity; it limits the development of resistance while allowing cellular renewal.

The complex and ever-changing environment of infectious microbes, in turn resulting in a variety and location of symptoms, blurs the identification of these organisms as the cause of RA in their human hosts.

When these pathogenic microbes incorporate basic proteins from a variety of tissues (IgG cells, pancreas, myelin, kidney, etc.) the alteration (conformation) of attached basic cell proteins is recognized as non-self (i.e., a foreign allergen). As a result, mycoplasmas acquire the role of auto-antigens. With their insoluble lipoprotein membrane, mycoplasmas can also act as an adjuvant required in experimental autoimmune reactions. The several common strains of human mycoplasmas each have their characteristic properties that are dependent on the host tissue composition and the resulting systemic reactions.

It took me ten years after my retirement to publish *Why Arthritis?*, which perhaps in retrospect should have been titled *Why Do You Still Have Arthritis?*! I can't wait another 30 years for the medical and scientific community to remove their self-imposed cataracts to see what's on the horizon.

My hope is that this book will raise their curiosity to complete the untold story of the cause of rheumatoid disease.

H.W.C.

Dedication

To the late Carl Builder—friend, colleague, mentor, and hero—who convinced me that one person can indeed make a difference. His genius touched countless minds and hearts.

The world is a better place for his having been here.

ACKNOWLEDGMENTS

The author relied upon a variety of essential resources during the development of this book.

Human Resources

The author thanks family members, friends, and colleagues who encouraged and supported this research project and writing effort, directly or indirectly, especially John Medvetz, Robert Zwirn, Mary Lyn Miller, Paula Larich, Judy Sunderland, Judy Brigham, Dana Johnson, Varda Murrell, Rachel Fintzy, Laurie Rennie, Audrey Porter, Bernadette Shih, Stephen Mette, John Giroux, Hilary Hogan, Laura and Tony Ponter, Joseph and Catherine Miller, Hannah Sampson, and the late Dr. Stefan T. Possony.

Particular appreciation goes to Karl F. Poehlmann, Jr., whose perceptive comments, assistance with Internet research, spirited discussion, analytical critique, probing questions, thoughtful suggestions, unflagging support, and husbandly encouragement during the course of the research were invaluable.

Text References

Sincere kudos go to Dr. Thomas McPherson Brown, whose theories on mycoplasmal infection started me on my own "Road Back" to recovery. His prescient scientific observations and rigorous testing methods make him one of the as-yet unheralded giants of medical research. The Arthritis Institute of the National Hospital in Arlington, VA, has been renamed the Thomas McPherson Brown Arthritis Institute in memory of its founder and former director.

Harold W. Clark, Ph.D., gifted scientist and author, was a colleague of Dr. Brown's at George Washington University since the 1950s. Recently, Dr. Clark has lectured and written extensively on his 45-year experience developing techniques for mycoplasma detection and treatment during a period when the popular view of arthritis actively excluded support for the infectious mycoplasmal causes. Dr. Clark established the Mycoplasma Research Institute in Beverly Hills, FL, as a nonprofit corporation committed to the promotion of research and education toward understanding mycoplasma diseases.

Laurie Garrett's *The Coming Plague* was found to be a scholarly, well-documented text that provided historical and statistical data of great utility supporting the hypotheses presented in this book. It is understandable why this talented analyst and author won the Pulitzer Prize in 1996 for her reporting on the Ebola virus.

Electronic Media

The author recognizes the wealth of data and discussion obtained via the Internet to support this research project. The excellent scientific data provided electronically by Dr. Garth Nicolson's Institute for Molecular Medicine and also through MEDLINE's Medscape by Dr. Joel B. Baseman, University of Texas Health Science Center at San Antonio, and Dr. Joseph G. Tully, recently retired head of the Mycoplasma Chapter of the National Institute of Allergy and Infectious Diseases demonstrate the Internet's power to educate and inform on a global scale.

The reader is cautioned that websites cited in the endnotes and in Appendix IV are correct and active as of this writing but may change or become inactive over time.

Medical Reviewers

Dr. Joseph Mercola's website and electronic newsletter offer timely, practical, and valuable information addressing a wide variety of health issues. At this writing, his website, www.mercola.com, is among the top three most-visited health sites on the Internet. The site is linked to over 20,000 medical pages and includes an improved version of Dr. Brown's protocol, which he has used successfully to treat thousands of arthritis patients. Dr. Mercola has generously given permission to reprint this protocol as Appendix II of this book.

Dr. Garth Nicolson is currently the President, Chief Scientific Officer and Research Professor at the Institute for Molecular Medicine in Huntington Beach, California. He was formally the David Bruton Jr. Chair in Cancer Research, Professor and Chairman at the University of Texas M. D. Anderson Cancer Center in Houston, and Professor of Internal Medicine and Professor of Pathology and Laboratory Medicine at the University of Texas Medical School at Houston.

Dr. Nicolson was also Adjunct Professor of Comparative Medicine at Texas A & M University. Among the most cited scientists in the world, having published over 520 medical and scientific papers, edited 14 books, served on the Editorial Boards of 20 medical and scientific journals, including the *Journal of Chronic Fatigue Syndrome*, and currently serving as Editor of two (*Clinical & Experimental Metastasis* and the *Journal of Cellular Bio-chemistry*), Professor Nicolson has held numerous peer-reviewed research grants. He is a recipient of the Burroughs Wellcome Medal of the Royal Society of Medicine, Stephen Paget Award of the Metastasis Research Society and the U. S. National Cancer Institute Outstanding Investigator Award.

Dr. Nicolson has been nominated for the Nobel Prize in cell microbiology. His Institute's dietary considerations for chronic illness patients are reprinted in Appendix III of this book.

Dr. Tsuyoshi Okada, M.D., F.A.C.P., maintains a private practice in Southern California. He is the author of several publications in the areas of Geriatric Medicine and Internal Medicine. He is a member of the active staff of the Gardena Community Hospital and has been Chief of Staff and Chief of Medicine at that facility. Dr. Okada is also on the courtesy staff of Little Company of Mary Hospital in Torrance. Dr. Okada's observations on interactions between prescription drugs and herbal/vitamin supplements are much appreciated.

The work of these dedicated professionals is quoted and referenced throughout this book. I thank each of them sincerely for their contributions and for reviewing draft versions of the text.

Warning—Disclaimer

The advice in this book is based on the research available to, and experiences of, the author. It is not intended to be a substitute for consultation with the reader's own physician or other qualified health care provider. Because each individual's physiology is unique, the reader is urged to check with a qualified health care professional whenever there is a question regarding appropriateness or applicability of any treatment, substance, or regimen.

While significant beneficial effects of the tetracycline family of antibiotics, as well as particular vitamins and supplements mentioned in this book, may be realized, the author does not endorse any medical benefits that may be claimed by commercial distributors of these products. The reader should be aware of risks involved in any course of health treatment. Seeking a second opinion is always prudent in matters of health.

The purpose of this book is to educate and inform. To that end, every effort has been taken to assure accuracy. However, there may be errors both typographical and in content. Therefore, the reader should use this text as a general guide and not the ultimate authority on chronic disease information. Material presented is current only up to the printing date.

Neither the publisher nor the author takes responsibility for any adverse effects or consequences resulting from the use of any of the procedures or substances described in this book.

CONTENTS

FIGURES AND TABLES

Figures

Tables

DEFINITIONS

Adaptogenic: pertaining to the natural selection of the offspring of a mutant organism better adapted to a new or changed environment, particularly applicable to drug resistant microbes.

Adjuvant: a substance which, administered with a drug or antigen, enhances its pharmacological effect or its antigenicity.

Absorption: the uptake of substances into or across tissues.

Adsorption: the action of a substance in attracting and holding other materials or particles on its surface.

Allergen: a substance capable of triggering an allergic state when introduced into the body. Major categories of allergens are cellular, viral, bacterial, food, chemical, and mycoplasmal. An incoming allergen produces a histamine reaction that prompts the body to generate hydrogen peroxide, which initiates the body's cell-destruction process, leading to inflammation at the site of the invasion.

Anaerobe: an organism that lives and grows in very low levels of molecular oxygen.

Antibody: a soluble protein molecule with disease-fighting properties. Antibodies are produced and secreted by B-cells in response to antigenic stimulus. These molecules are capable of binding to a specific antigen, so they are shape-related to the sugar coat of the cells or microorganisms they are intended to attack.

Antigen: a substance consisting mainly of proteins (but which can also consist of carbohydrates, lipids, and sometimes nucleic acids) that is recognized as foreign and gives rise to an immune reaction, i.e., production of antibodies or immune cells. It can also be the toxin secreted by mycoplasmas.

Apoptosis: programmed cell death.

Arbovirus: a viral disease spread by the bite of an arthropod. E.g., mosquito-transmitted Dengue Fever.

Ayurvedic: pertaining to Ayurveda, a holistic system of medicine indigenous to and widely practiced in India for more than 5,000 years. Ayurveda was first recorded in the *Vedas*, said to be the world's oldest extant literature.

Bacteria: any of numerous widely distributed unicellular, pleomorphic microorganisms that exhibit both animal and plant characteristics. Their three main varieties (*bacillus*, *coccus*, and *spirillum*) range from the harmless and beneficial to the intensely virulent and lethal.

Basophil: a granular leukocyte with an irregularly shaped nucleus. A basophil is also considered to be any structure, cell or histologic element staining readily with basic dyes. A high number could be an indicator of malignancy such as cancer or leukemia.

Blood/brain barrier: the biochemical partition that separates the brain and central nervous system from the blood stream so that only certain biochemicals can cross over. This complex physiologic filtering mechanism keeps many of the large molecules that circulate in the blood out of the central nervous system

B-lymphocyte or B-cell: small white blood cells crucial to immune system defenses. B-cells originate in the bone marrow and develop into plasma cells, which produce antibodies.

Bone marrow: soft tissue located in the cavities of the bones. Bone marrow is the source of all blood cells in the healthy adult.

Budding: the process by which microbes pull a portion of invaded cell membrane around their inner envelope and chromosomes, creating an outer protective coating and tethering the new "bud" to the parent cell.

Bursa: a pouch or sac-like cavity containing synovia and located at the points of friction in the bodies of vertebrates.

Carcinogen: any cancer-causing agent or substance.

Cartilage: a fibrous connective tissue forming most of the temporary skeleton of the embryo, providing a model for development of bones; also denotes a mass of such tissue, composed of collagen fibers and proteoglycans, at any particular site in the body.

Chemotactic: acting in response to chemical stimulation by initiating the inflammatory reaction, attracting leukocytes to the site of tissue damage.

Chemotherapeutic: pertains to the treatment of certain malignant diseases (e.g., cancer) by the disinfection of affected tissues through the use of chemically synthesized drugs having a specific action against certain pathogenic microorganisms.

Cholesterol: an alcohol compound ($C_{27}H_{45}O$) found in animal fats and oils, bile, blood, brain tissue, milk, egg yolk, myelin sheaths of nerve fibers, liver, kidneys, and adrenal glands.

Chondrocytes: cells that can produce cartilage by increasing the synthesis of proteoglycans.

Cofactor: an element or principle, e.g., a coenzyme, with which another element must unite in order to function.

Collagen: a protein substance of the white fibers of skin, tendon, bone, cartilage, and nails.

Complement: a complex series of blood proteins whose action "complements" the work of antibodies. Complement destroys antibody-coated cells, produces inflammation, and regulates immune reactions.

Conjugation: the mating process in bacteria by which genetic information is exchanged between two genetically distinct organisms.

Cytokines: chemical messengers that help regulate the immune response by mobilizing white blood cells as necessary.

Cytopathic: pertaining to pathologic (unhealthy or diseased) changes in cells.

Cytotoxic T-cells: a special category of T-cells (lymphocytes) that kill other cells infected by viruses, fungi, or certain bacteria, or cells transformed by cancer.

DNA: genetic material deoxyribonucleaic acid that carries the directions a cell uses to perform a specific function, such as making a given protein.

Edema: excessive fluid retention in intercellular spaces of the body.

ELISA (Enzyme Linked Immuno-Sorbant Assay): a highly accurate testing and diagnostic protocol used to identify specific antigens using IgG or IgE antibodies in a person's blood sample.

Endemic: a disease of usual low morbidity present in a human community at all times but clinically recognizable in only a few individuals. Dengue fever is an example.

Enzyme: an organic compound that acts as a catalyst to the change in chemical composition of a material. Certain types of enzymes are required for the proper digestion and metabolism of food in the body. Enzymes break down the agent causing inflammation.

Eosinophil: a granular leukocyte having a nucleus with two lobes connected by a thread of chromatin, and cytoplasm containing coarse, round granules of uniform size. An increase is usually associated with an allergic condition such as asthma or intestinal worms.

Epidemic: a disease of high morbidity only occasionally present in a human community, attacking many in a region at the same time and spreading rapidly. Hepatitis C is an example.

Etiology: a theory of the cause(s) of a disease.

Etiopathogenesis: the origin of the cause(s), development of cellular events, reactions and other pathologic mechanisms occurring during the development of disease.

Eucaryotes: organisms made up of complex cells that have organelles and a membrane-bounded nucleus. These organisms comprise four of the five Kingdoms of species taxonomy—Protista, Plantae, Fungi and Animalia. The remaining and most primitive is Kingdom Monera, which includes bacteria and other prokaryotic cells.

Exanthematic: pertaining to an eruptive disease or fever.

Exudates: materials that have escaped from blood vessels and been deposited in tissue or on tissue surfaces, usually the result of trauma or inflammation. The product is usually fluid, cells, or cellular debris.

Gram-negative: bacteria that lose the primary Gram stain (a violet colored chemical) and pick up a counterstain, usually carbolfuchsin or safranine.

Gram-positive: retaining the color of the gentian violet stain in Gram's method of staining.

Gram stain (Gram's method): a process developed by Danish physician Hans Gram (1853-1938) for staining bacteria; the stain used to identify broad classes of bacteria based on their cell coat or capsule's ability to pick up specific dyes.

Helper T-cells: a subset of T-cells that typically carry the CD4 marker and are essential for turning on antibody production, activating cytotoxic T-cells, and initiating many other immune system responses.

Hematopoietic: pertaining to the formation of blood cells.

Histamine: an active chemical, released from mast cells, that causes smooth muscle contraction of human bronchioles and small blood vessels, increased permeability of capillaries, and increased secretion by nasal and bronchial mucous glands.

Hydrogen Peroxide (H_2O_2): a natural chemical compound that can be generated by the histamine reaction, or by certain microorganisms when they are attacked, or by leukocytes in the process of developing killer T-cells.

In vitro: observable in a test tube or other artificial environment.

In vivo: within the living body.

Iatrogenic: Caused or precipitated by physician intervention.

Immunoglobulins (Ig): These antibodies are Y-shaped protein molecules produced by the B-cells. There are five classes of immunoglobulins: IgA, IgD, IgE, IgG, and IgM.

Immunosuppressive: capable of reducing normal immune responses, e.g., drugs given to prevent transplant rejection

Interferon: a molecule produced by cells (most often white blood cells) that can inhibit cell division and which has a variety of effects on the immune system.

Interstice: a small interval, space, or gap in a tissue or structure.

Jarisch-Herxheimer reaction: a short-term hypersensitivity response that is often mistakenly interpreted as antibiotic sensitivity.

Killer T-cells: see Cytotoxic.

L-Form: also called the L-phase variant; a bacterium that has partially or entirely lost its cell walls. The "L" is for the Lister Institute in France where it was first discovered. Mycobacteria and other bacteria transform to the L-form when attacked by penicillin and related antibiotics. L-forms and mycoplasmas are of similar size and usually reproduce more slowly than bacteria. L-forms can regrow their cell walls, and therefore have a means to escape attack by antibiotics and emerge later.

Leukocyte: a white or colorless blood corpuscle, constituting an important agent in protection against infectious diseases.

Lipid: any of a group of organic substances, including fatty acids, neutral fats, waxes, steroids, and phosphatides, which are insoluble in water but soluble in alcohol, ether, chloroform, and other fat solvents; lipids are a source of body fuel and an important constituent of cells.

Lipoprotein: a combination of a lipid and a protein, having the general solubility property of proteins.

Lymphatic system: a bodily system composed of channels whose principal function is to maintain blood volume by returning to the general circulation those fluid and protein molecules that leak from the capillaries into interstitial spaces. The lymphatic system includes circulating lymphocytes and lymphoid organs, which are important in defense against infection and tumor growth as well as removal of wastes from the body.

Lymphocyte: white blood cells that are the smallest of the leukocytes, producing cytokines in the bone marrow and thymus, and that are essential for immune defense.

Macrophages: enlarged, amoeba-like cells that entrap microorganisms and particles of foreign matter by phagocytosis. They usually arrive after the neutrophils to clean up the debris of dead cells and bacteria.

Mast cells: specialized immune cells found in the skin and nasal passages and in the gastrointestinal (GI) and respiratory tracts.

Metabolism: the sum of all the chemical and physical processes by which elements of a living organism are produced and maintained; also the transformation by which energy is made available to the organism.

Metalloenzyme: any enzyme that contains tightly bound metal atoms, e.g., the cytochromes, a class of hemoproteins that are widely distributed in plant and animal tissues and whose main function is electron transport.

Microbe: a microscopic organism, especially one of the disease-causing bacteria or viruses.

Microorganism: a general term for protozoa, fungi, bacteria, and viruses.

Mollicutes: from the Latin for "soft" and "skin," the class of cell wall-less prokaryotes to which mycoplasmas belong.

Motility: the ability to move spontaneously.

Mutagen: an agent that induces genetic mutation.

Mutate: to change a gene or unit of hereditary material that results in a new inheritable characteristic.

Mycobacteria: a slender, typically aerobic bacterium difficult to stain. Examples are tuberculosis and leprosy.

Mycoplasma: from the Latin base words for "fungus" and "fluid"; of intermediate size between bacteria and viruses, are characterized by the absence of a cell wall and pleomorphism; the smallest and simplest self-replicating organisms phylogenetically related to gram-positive bacteria, especially to mycobacteria, which have affinity for synovial tissue and cholesterol.

Myelin: the lipid substance surrounding the axis of a group of nerve fibers.

Neurogenic: originating in the nervous system, to form nervous tissue or to stimulate nervous energy.

Neuropeptide: a peptide synthesized within the body that influences neural activity or functioning.

Neutrophils: cells that migrate to the site of an injury and stick to the interior walls of the blood vessels. They then form projections that enable them to push their way into the infected tissues where they engulf and devour (phagocytize) microorganisms and other foreign particles.

Nucleophilic: having an affinity for the nucleus of a cell.

Palliative: affording relief; also a drug that acts to do so.

Pandemic: occurring over a wide geographic area and affecting an exceptionally high proportion of the population; e.g., malaria.

Parasite: a plant or animal that lives on or within another organism, from which it derives sustenance or protection without making compensation; applies to all infectious microbes, from viruses to ringworms. Parasites can be symbiotic, i.e., adapting and providing beneficial effects on the host. Some parasites can kill the host but others evolve into forms that do not.

Pareto Chart: a method used by economists to show allocation of resources in an economic system; a histogram to illustrate comparative values in a bar chart format.

Parvovirus: a group of extremely small, morphologically similar DNA viruses resistant to fungicides and sporicides.

Peptide: any of various amides derived from two or more amino acids by combination of the amino group of one acid with the carboxyl group of another; usually obtained by partial hydrolysis of proteins.

Peyer's patches: a collection of lymphoid tissues in the intestinal tract.

Phagocyte: any cell that engulfs and ingests microorganisms or other cells and foreign particles.

Pharmacodynamic: pertaining to the action of drugs on living systems.

Pharmacokinetic: pertaining to the study of drug activity or effectiveness for a certain purpose.

Physiology: the sum of all basic processes underlying the functioning of a species or class of organism.

Phytochemicals: plant-derived chemical extracts. There are tens of thousands of these, with varying bioactivity. Some have protective and antibiotic effects, e.g., allicin obtained from garlic

Plasmids: extrachromosomal circular DNA molecules capable of independent replication and carrying genetic information for a variety of different functions, such as drug resistance.

Pleomorphism: exhibiting a variety of shapes.

Polymerase Chain Reaction (PCR): an extremely sensitive means of amplifying small quantities of DNA to detect low-level bacterial infections or rapid changes in transcription at the single cell level. It can also be used in DNA sequencing, screening for genetic disorders, site-specific mutation of DNA, cloning (or sub-cloning), and forensic science applications.

Prokaryote: an organism without a true nucleus, the nuclear material being scattered in the cytoplasm of the cell, and which reproduces by cell division. A bacterium is an example.

Prophylaxis: preventive treatment of disease.

Prostaglandins: naturally occurring fatty acids found in various tissues that work to stimulate the contraction ability of smooth muscle, to lower blood pressure, and to affect the action of certain hormones.

Proteinase: any enzyme that catalyzes the splitting of interior peptide bonds in a protein.

Proteoglycans: the component of cartilage that gives it elasticity.

Proteolysis: the splitting of proteins by hydrolysis of the peptide bonds with formation of smaller polypeptides.

Retrovirus: an RNA virus that gains entry into cells, making mirror-image copies of their RNA to produce a DNA version of their genes, then exploiting vulnerable locations along the host's DNA to insert themselves, like a transposon, into the cell's genetic material.

R-factors: genetically coded Resistance Factors possessed by an organism to withstand chemical assaults by one or more chemotherapeutic agents. An example is a transferable plasmid found in many bacteria in the small intestine.

Salmonella: a gram-negative bacterium causing mild to severe gastroenteritis, occasionally leading to death, e.g. in the case of *S. typhus*.

Streptococcus: the genus of gram-positive bacteria, usually occurring in chains, that includes species pathogenic to humans, especially children. A typical chain would include one or more of the following: *S. pneumonia, S. synovium, S. aureus, S. hemophilia,* scarlet fever, and/or rheumatic heart disease. This initial bacterial infection could lead to production of mycoplasmal microorganisms and L-forms and in turn to rheumatic diseases.

Streptomyces: a genus of bacteria, usually soil forms, but occasionally parasitic on plants and animals.

Subacute: a condition between acute and chronic.

Synovia: pertaining to the transparent, albuminous fluid secreted by the inner layer of the synovial membrane and found in the joint cavities, bursae, and tendon sheaths where lubrication is necessary. This fluid provides nourishment to the cartilage covering the bone and contains white blood cells that battle infection.

Synovial joint: a freely moveable joint where cartilage covers the ends of the bones and the entire joint is encapsulated in a double layer of connective tissue with the joint cavity and its synovial fluid lying in-between the two layers. The outer layer of the capsule is made up of dense connective tissue holding the bones of the joint together. Some of these tissues are bundled together as ligaments. Tendons join muscles to bone. The inner layer of the capsule is made up of loose connective tissue including elastic fibers and fat.

T-cells: disease-fighting, thymus-derived ("T") lymphocytes (white blood cells) of the immune system that have the ability to recognize foreign substances (antigens).

Teratogen: an agent or influence causing a physical defect or deformity in a developing embryo.

Tetracyclines: a family of broad-spectrum antibiotics that inhibit bacterial protein synthesis; tetracycline ($C_{22}H_{24}N_2O_8$) is derived from certain species of the bacteria genus *Streptomyces*; the base and hydrochloride salt are used as an antiamoebic, antibacterial, and antirickettsial.

Thymus: one of the primary lymphatic system organs, located high in the chest, where T-cells proliferate and mature.

Transposons: genes which move from one position to another on chromosomes; at the bacterial level, movable bits of DNA that generate helpful/harmful chemicals, enzymes, or other substances that confer the ability to resist chemotherapeutic agents.

Vector: a carrier, usually a biting insect (tick, flea, fly, spider, chigger, mosquito) that transfers an infectious agent from one host to another.

Virulence: the capacity to injure an organism and/or produce disease by invasion of tissue and generation of internal toxins. Invasiveness and toxigenicity are measured with reference to a particular host.

Virus: any of a class of filterable, submicroscopic pathogenic agents, chiefly protein and nucleic acid in composition but often reducible to crystalline form, and typically inert except when in contact with certain living cells.

PREFACE

My goal in writing this book is to help sufferers of rheumatoid arthritis to understand the underlying causes of the disease so that they may better combat it and find relief from its effects. It is written for intelligent and well-educated non-medical individuals, with enough scientific terminology to foster effective communication and informed dialog between doctor and patient.

In my view, the fragmented and distinct specialties within the framework of medical science often become so focused on a particular course of study that they ignore salient findings along another track. This book brings together research findings from a wide variety of sources, posing significant questions that should be investigated further by the medical and scientific community. I wish to stimulate thinking across these traditional boundaries and to suggest new research directions.

The naturopathic methods described are intended to help *all* individuals with chronic illnesses—not just RA victims—who seek to improve their health and well being by bolstering their immune systems. In particular, I have suggested specific tests and potential treatments that do not have deleterious side effects.

In this book there is no pretense to suggest a one-size-fits-all approach or magic bullet to combat rheumatoid arthritis. However, the evidence of decades of proven success with Dr. Thomas McPherson Brown's regimen centered on a low-dose, long-term course of tetracycline-type antibiotics is remarkable. This regimen, if diligently followed and coupled with lifestyle modifications, will train the body's immune system to combat the microbial infection that is the root cause of the disease.

Allergies play an important part in chronic illness. Knowing which tests to request and what indicators to look for helps the individual work with the doctor to obtain a definitive diagnosis. If further tests reveal mycoplasmal infection, the next step should be a request to try Dr. Brown's approach.

It's a shame that we Americans have trained ourselves to reach for a pill to get quick relief for our aches and pains. Treating symptoms has not just become acceptable and commonplace; it has become big business worth billions of dollars. In this book there are many approaches suggested to achieve pain relief without harmful or expensive drugs.

Confrontation with the frightening prospect of being permanently disabled by rheumatoid arthritis was the impetus for writing this book, which is based on my 1997 doctoral dissertation. I am no longer an arthritis sufferer, thanks in large part to Dr. Brown's insights.

My intent is that others may benefit from what I have learned. My hope is that the proposed hypotheses regarding the insidious actions of pathogenic microorganisms as a growing public health hazard will be investigated further by concerned scientists.

To that end, I am donating a percentage of the profits from the sale of this book to enable research directed toward the etiology, testing, and treatment of mycoplasmas and other parasitic infections.

K.M.P.

INTRODUCTION

Dr. Homer F. Swift theorized in 1928 that rheumatic fever was caused by hypersensitivity to a bacterium after isolating streptococcal bacteria from a patient with tonsillitis. At that time, tonsillitis was a precursor to rheumatic fever. This beta-hemolytic streptococcus is a common cause of "strep throat" but not all cases lead to rheumatic fever. Dr. Thomas McPherson Brown, as a young resident physician in 1937, studied with Swift to find the allergic response link to this bacterium that seemed to cause rheumatic fever.[1]

In the 1940s, Dr. Brown first proposed his theory that bacterial infection was the primary cause of rheumatoid arthritis. He described the effectiveness of tetracycline in RA in 1949 at the 7th International Rheumatology Congress and in the *Journal of Laboratory and Clinical Medicine*. Over the next two decades at the Rockefeller Institute, Johns Hopkins Hospital, and the George Washington University School of Medicine in Washington, D.C., Dr. Brown conducted detailed, fully documented scientific tests to prove this assertion. Early use of tetracycline-family antibiotics for connective tissue diseases was also endorsed by Dr. Albert Sabin, discoverer of the polio vaccine.

What has become of Dr. Brown's work? For decades it has been largely ignored by the medical community because physicians have not assiduously sought to test for the mysterious microorganisms Dr. Brown identified. There are a few noteworthy exceptions.

In 1993, the Road Back Foundation, a nonprofit corporation run by volunteers who found relief using Dr. Brown's methods, began a campaign of information sharing regarding long-term antibiotic treatment. They established a website at www.roadback.org.

In the late 1990s, an improved website was established which provided more detailed information on a wide range of rheumatic diseases, a suggested regimen based on Dr. Brown's findings, with links to other credible and helpful Internet resources. This site is www.rheumatic.org.

Dr. Joseph Mercola has successfully treated over 2,000 RA patients using his modified version of Dr. Brown's protocol, which can be found at www.mercola.com. A reprint appears in Appendix II.

Dr. Harold Clark, a former colleague of Dr. Brown, continues to educate through the Mycoplasma Research Institute. His 1997 book *Why Arthritis*? is an excellent overview of the manner in which controlled antibiotic therapy combats pathogenic microbes.[2]

The Institute for Molecular Medicine under the direction of Dr. Garth Nicolson has recently begun innovative mycoplasma research programs and unique testing methods.[3]

Terminology is difficult when referring to mycoplasmas. Dr. Brown described them as "somewhere between a bacteria and a virus." Some medical researchers call them "microbes" while others call them "microorganisms," but mycoplasmas are included within the current classification of bacteria (or prokaryotes) in a separate class (Mollicutes). Their actions are unique since they borrow from other cells in a dynamically evolving manner. Their distinction from most other bacteria is that they have lost the ability to develop a cell wall. In this text, when mycoplasmas are discussed, they will be referred to as microbes or microorganisms.

Chronic infections linked to causes other than mycoplasmas present their own set of problems for diagnosis, testing, and treatment. A separate chapter is devoted to this serious and growing public health concern. Vector-borne infections are discussed in detail, using Lyme Disease as an example.

The extraordinary complexity of the human immune system has not been well understood until very recently. Noteworthy, credible research only began in the early 1980s, with the definitive work on virology written in 1985.[4] A decade ago there was no discipline of microbial ecology dedicated to studies of the behavior of microbes in the human body. At that time, investigation into the causes of disease, particularly AIDS, in immunosuppressed people became highly politicized on moral rather than medical grounds and as a result was seriously under-funded. Today AIDS is finally recognized as a growing threat with global implications. However, funding has been diverted to AIDS research at the expense of scientific investigation into the causes of other widespread infections.

We need to design better research tools to culture, test, investigate and diagnose infectious diseases before they emerge as global threats. Sadly, sufficient funding to develop these tools is not being allocated in the United States for a variety of reasons, some involving petty academic turf battles and others associated with bottom-line cost considerations by government agencies, pharmaceutical companies, and insurance firms. Although significant research is being done abroad, national rivalries sometimes lead to the suppression of valid foreign results and ideas.

In the mid-1990s, after the Gulf War (1991), serious attention was drawn to returning U.S. military personnel's complaints, many of which mimicked those of arthritis sufferers. When these veterans by chance belonged to a family group that included physicians, personal and vested interests sparked investigation into the mysterious cause of Gulf War Illness.

The number of grassroots advocates for more research funding for vector-borne chronic diseases such as Lyme Disease is growing. Media attention is increasingly focusing on these infections. It is no longer acceptable for our government and the scientific and medical community to downplay or ignore what may be the most serious global scourge after AIDS.

Those medical professionals who embark on privately funded research, unwilling to wait for government action, are producing startling test results. Rather than being lauded as pioneers, their unpopular findings often lead to their being branded as "mavericks" and working at cross purposes to "mainstream medicine."

As a result of the efforts of a few highly motivated and superbly qualified individuals, a new era of infection research may be underway at last.

---

[1] Clark (1997) p. 15.

[2] See http://arthritistrust.org/topics/mycoplasmal.html and Dr. Clark's website at www.digitalusa.net/~hwcmri.

[3] See www.immed.org.

[4] Fields, B.N. , Knipe, D.M., Chanock, R.M., et al. *Virology.* Raven Press: New York, 1985.

1. WHAT IS ARTHRITIS?

The word arthritis originates from the Greek *arth*, meaning "joint" and *itis*, meaning "inflammation." Arthritis has been found in the bones of mammals since prehistoric times. Egyptian mummies show evidence of treatment for the disease. Hippocrates offered the first description of arthritis in the fourth century B.C. using the term *rheums*, meaning "migrating between joints."[1] Although there are claimed to be over one hundred various kinds of arthritis, this may just reflect the complexity and severity of combinations of categories of symptoms. Yet it was only comparatively recently, within the last century, that other factors besides the joints were considered to play a role in arthritis.

Two main categories of the disease afflict millions of Americans: rheumatoid arthritis and osteoarthritis. Medical texts identify several subforms of rheumatoid arthritis, but they all seem to be basically the result of inflammation. The difference seems to be the location in the body and severity of the symptoms. For example, Ankylosing Spondylitis occurs when inflammation afflicts areas where ligament attaches to bone. Tendonitis, bursitis, Carpal Tunnel Syndrome and low back pain are examples of inflammation involving synovial tissue interfaces with musculoskeletal elements. The chronic fatigue experienced by arthritics is the sign of a body weakened by a persistent battle with the cause of the disease.

Although physicians admit that one type of arthritis—reactive arthritis—is linked to an infection of the joints caused by bacteria, virus, or fungus, the hallmarks of this type are the same as other arthritis forms. Two processes characterized by inflammation can cause cell destruction: either trauma or bacterial allergy.

Dr. Gabe Mirkin lists the following causes of reactive arthritis[2]:

- Salmonella intestinal infection
- Mononucleosis
- Parvovirus
- Chronic hepatitis B and C
- Retroviruses
- Venereal diseases such as Chlamydia, Ureaplasma, Mycoplasma, Gonorrhea, and Gardnerella
- Mycoplasma
- Human T-cell leukemia virus-1
- Chlamydia
- Urinary tract infections such as Chlamydia, Ureaplasma, and Mycoplasma
- Lyme Disease
- Salmonella diarrhea
- Parvovirus B19
- Cytomegalovirus
- Streptococcal sore throat
- Cat scratch disease
- Human Herpes Virus-6 (HHV-6)
- Hemophilus influenza bacteria
- AIDS (HIV)
- Staphylococcus aureus bacterial infections
- Many different intestinal infections

In rheumatoid arthritis, infection leads to a buildup of calcium nodules that wall off and surround the infecting organism. The same process occurs with cancer cells. This may be the result of the body's attempt to keep the organism from spreading. If these nodules are present in the feet, they may be mistaken for the needle-shaped uric acid crystals that characterize gout. These RA nodules are painless, hard round or oval masses that appear under the skin, usually on pressure points such as the elbow or Achilles tendon. Nodules are present in about 20% of RA cases.[3] Occasionally they are found in the eye where they can cause inflammation. Inflammation of the lung lining (pleurisy) may cause shortness of breath.

When used in this book, the word "arthritis" is intended to refer to rheumatoid arthritis, although inflammation associated with other categories may also be the result of some bacterial infection and a rheumatoid component.

TWO MAIN TYPES OF ARTHRITIS

Although physicians like to categorize arthritis, and different types of arthritis have different characteristics in general, at least one of the following symptoms are experienced by all arthritis sufferers:

- swelling, redness, warmth, pain/tenderness or irritation in one or more joints;
- stiffness around the joints, usually upon awakening and lasting about an hour; or
- difficulty or pain in normal movement of the joint(s).

At this writing, some form of arthritis afflicts an estimated 40 million Americans of all ages. The Centers for Disease Control (CDC) in Atlanta, GA, estimates that by 2020, sixty million persons in the United States may be afflicted with arthritis, and the activities of 11.6 million persons may be limited by arthritis symptoms.[4]

Rheumatoid Arthritis (RA)

Many rheumatoid diseases are assumed to be the result of aging or wear and tear, so there has been little motivation to find a cause or cure. However, chronic disease afflicts both the young and old, male and female, and all races. Rheumatoid diseases can affect one or more tissues and organs and not just the joints, so it is understandable why investigation into the causes and cures have baffled medical researchers. With hundreds of symptomatic variations and various stages, zeroing in on a probable cause is a daunting prospect. Compounding the problem are each individual's unique biochemical makeup, particular environmental influences, and possible co-infections.

The health of every tissue and organ depends on thousands of delicately balanced chemical reactions that occur continuously within our bodies. Rheumatic diseases exhibit inflammatory destruction of collagen proteins that hold cells together as connective synovial tissue, blood vessels, and skin.

Every cell in the body uses substances supplied by the blood and surrounding cells. These substances are either acquired topically or ingested. To say we "are what we eat" is not completely true; we are what we *assimilate.*

Rheumatoid arthritis is actually a family of related diseases characterized by persistent or cyclic bouts of inflammation of the joint membrane. In general, localized, short-term inflammation is a good thing, because it shows that the body is actively dealing with the problem, as the white blood cells (leukocytes) fight the infection. In RA, however, inflammation is not short-term nor does it have any known beneficial effect. The inflammation occurs in the layers of tissue (the synovium) lining the joint, causing pain, swelling, and stiffness when the joint is moved. There may be an accompanying excessive production of the synovial fluid that lubricates the joint, building up pressure on the joint and causing pain.

Inflamed tissues surrounding a particular joint are referred to as tendonitis (tendon), bursitis (bursa), myositis (muscle), neuritis (nerve), and vasculitis (blood vessel). Inflammation around a joint space that looks and feels normal can be detected using a highly sensitive radioisotopic scan or magnetic resonance imaging (MRI).[5]

The characteristic early morning joint and muscle stiffness reported by individuals with rheumatic disease does not necessarily indicate a lack of lubricating oils in the joints. In fact, there may be an excessive amount of fluid in the joints that inhibits flexibility.[6] The temporary stiffness indicates inadequate blood supply circulating through the tendons and muscle tissue surrounding the joints.

Morning joint stiffness correlates with overnight body temperature drop caused by lower blood pressure and decreased circulation. Joint fluid becomes more viscous and stiff until increased activity through exercise or applied warmth (water, heating pad, massage, topical creams containing stimulants) raises body temperature. In addition, the supply of nutrients and metabolites normally carried by the blood to the joints may be diverted and depleted as the body attends to the gastrointestinal problems sometimes associated with RA.

Whether the bulk is fluid or inflamed tissue, the effect is the same: painful pressure on the joint. Tendons, connecting the muscles that supply force to operate joints, may also be affected as the sheath containing the tendons becomes inflamed. This sheath is the same type of tissue as the synovium. Scar tissue may form between the tendon and its sheath, causing tendon operation to become stiff. Damage to the tendon itself may result, with the loss of the use of the hands or limbs. Deformities may be seen in the sideways displacement of fingers or toes. A representative drawing of a joint capsule and surrounding tissue is shown in Figure 1.

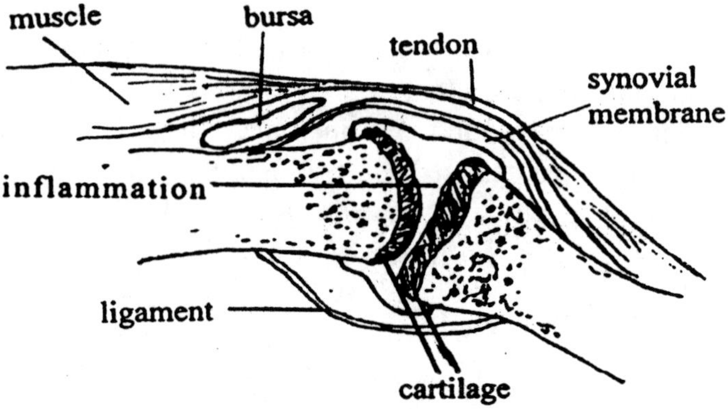

Figure 1. Joint Capsule

Although any joint can be affected, RA is first noticed in the small peripheral joints, such as those in the fingers or wrist. Figure 2 shows the weblike pattern of synovial membranes in the hand. These tissues are thin layers between bone surfaces that would otherwise rub together.

The synovial membrane of the knee joint is the largest and most extensive in the body. Joints are often affected symmetrically, so arthritis sufferers will usually have pain in knees, elbows, shoulders, or hands. Other symptoms of RA include the presence in the blood of a protein called the Rheumatoid Factor or R-factor, found by tests that measure the ratio of antibody to gamma globulin. After several months, pits or erosions in the joints can be observed using x-rays.

RA can occur at any age, even in young children, but it usually begins to affect people in their forties and older as the immune system begins to deteriorate as part of the aging process. A contributing factor is the malfunctioning of the immune system after years of stress, poor diet, allergies, and indiscriminate medication with immunosuppressing drugs.

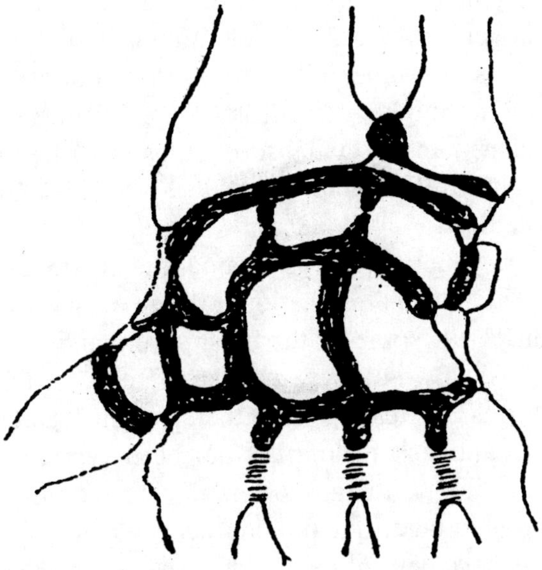

Figure 2. Synovial Tissue (shaded) in the Hand

According to the Arthritis Foundation, RA afflicts nearly 2.1 million Americans. RA occurs three times as often in women as in men, but during the first four years after diagnosis, 47 percent of men develop joint erosion, compared to 33% of women.[7] RA is called a multifactorial disease, with a variety of causes particular to each sufferer. In all cases, however, there is a component of the immune system perpetuating the disease rather than working to suppress and dispel it as a transient problem.

RA should not be considered a disease of the elderly. It can strike at any age, although it commonly affects those between 30 and 50. For the most part, it strikes when people are active and vigorous. However, the elderly have a wide range of other disorders not seen in young patients, including endocrine, metabolic, neurologic and vascular disorders that can lead to degenerative joint disease. Thus researchers are faced with the difficult task of determining which started first, the arthritis or some other disorder(s). For example, arthritis symptoms might result from a pre-existing thyroid dysfunction[8] or perhaps by malabsorption as part of a gastro-intestinal condition. The latter could be brought about by prescription medications.

No race or genetic type is spared rheumatic disease. Despite the United States' reputation for high quality medical care, our country has some of the most severe and crippling forms of arthritis. Dr. Clark laments that, "Except for the new and exotic forms of testing and therapy, the search for possible causes and risk factors has not been very active or productive."[9] Antibiotic therapy offers documented evidence for a very probable cure, but funding agencies, foundations, and institutions have control over which research projects are worthy of support. The politics, hidden motives for suppression of research, and infighting among various groups controlling funds for serious arthritis research are detailed in Dr. Clark's perceptive book *Why Arthritis?*.

Rheumatic disease itself is not contagious, but as this text will assert, there are linkages to an initial infection with the onset of RA and the persistence of symptoms. This assertion runs counter to the prevailing medical establishment's stance that the body's own defense systems attack "healthy cells" in the synovial membrane by mistake. They call this process an "autoimmune reaction."[10] A list of autoimmune diseases appears in Table 1[11].

Table 1. Recognized Autoimmune Diseases

1	Alopecia Areata
2	Ankylosing Spondylitis
3	Antiphospholipid Syndrome
4	Autoimmune Addison's Disease
5	Autoimmune Hemolytic Anemia
6	Autoimmune Hepatitis
7	Behcet's Disease
8	Bullous Pemphigoid
9	Cardiomyopathy
10	Celiac Sprue-Dermatitis
11	Chronic Fatigue Syndrome (CFS) [also called Chronic Fatigue Immune Dysfunction Syndrome (CFIDS)]
12	Chronic Inflammatory Demyelinating Polyneuropathy
13	Churg-Strauss Syndrome
14	Cicatricial Pemphigoid
15	CREST Syndrome
16	Cold Agglutinin Disease
17	Crohn's Disease
18	Discoid Lupus
19	Essential Mixed Cryoglobulinemia
20	Fibromyalgia - Fibromyositis
21	Graves' Disease
22	Guillain-Barré
23	Hashimoto's Thyroiditis
24	Idiopathic Pulmonary Fibrosis
25	Idiopathic Thrombocytopenia Purpura (ITP)
26	IgA Nephropathy
27	Insulin-dependent Diabetes
28	Juvenile Arthritis
29	Lichen Planus
30	Lupus (Systemic Lupus Erthematosus)
31	Ménière's Disease

Table 1. Recognized Autoimmune Diseases, cont'd

33	Multiple Sclerosis
34	Myasthenia Gravis
35	Pemphigus Vulgaris
36	Pernicious Anemia
37	Polyarteritis Nodosa
38	Polychondritis
39	Polyglandular Syndromes
40	Polymyalgia Rheumatica
41	Polymyositis and Dermatomyositis
42	Primary Agammag-lobulinemia
43	Primary Biliary Cirrhosis
44	Psoriasis
45	Raynaud's Phenomenon
46	Reiter's Syndrome
47	Rheumatic Fever
48	Rheumatoid Arthritis
49	Sarcoidosis
50	Scleroderma
51	Sjögren's Syndrome
52	Stiff-Man Syndrome
53	Takayasu Arteritis
54	Temporal Arteritis/Giant Cell Arteritis
55	Ulcerative Colitis
56	Uveitis
57	Vasculitis
58	Vitiligo
59	Wegener's Granulomatosis

Carpal Tunnel Syndrome (CTS) is curiously absent from this list, but it bears the hallmarks of a possible mycoplasmal infection.[12] It is estimated that more than 2% of the population (5.5 million) are affected by CTS, and this number is growing. CTS surgery has become the most common operation performed on the hand. Over 200,000 Americans undergo CTS correction surgery each year.[13]

Surgical treatment for CTS has been part of mainstream medicine since 1947. Its pioneer, Dr. George S. Phalen, now retired, admits that more than half of his patients did not need surgery. Dr. Phalen notes that 85% of his CTS patients were older, female homemakers who did not perform repetitive motions. He predicts that simple vitamin B_6 therapy may be the best option in most cases.[14]

One may ask why surgery is still being performed for CTS. The answer is simple: money. A bottle of Vitamin B_6 costs $3. The surgery brings a $3,000 fee to doctors and the HMOs to which they belong. Attorneys charge that CTS is an "industrial disease" in lawsuits against corporations for abusive work conditions.

In the early 1970s, Dr. John Ellis discovered that CTS was caused by a vitamin deficiency. Mainstream medical theory still maintains that repetitive motion is the cause of CTS. While repeated action certainly exacerbates CTS, severe B_6 (riboflavin) deficiency has been shown to be a major cofactor in the disease.

In a series of studies and carefully documented experiments, Dr. Ellis detected very low levels of the enzyme erythrocyte glutamic oxaloacetic transminase (EGOT) that reflects vitamin B_6 activity in the body. A simple regimen of 100 mg of B_6 taken twice daily for 90 days raises EGOT to normal levels.

Reducing the repetitive movement during that time will speed healing. Because B_6 is a diuretic it reduces the edema usually associated with CTS. Individuals taking high doses of B_6 should be careful to increase water intake and perhaps may need to add magnesium and potassium supplements to replace these lost nutrients.[15]

Dr. Ellis has helped hundreds of CTS patients avoid surgery and prescription painkillers. However, where nerve tissue has been seriously damaged, he admits that surgery might be required. He suggests working closely with a trained nutritionist to develop a tailored personal profile. Since all vitamins in the B-complex typically work together, a B_6 deficiency probably points to other diet deficiencies. Although B_6 is present in a wide variety of foods, it is not available in large quantities. Since B_6 is lost through cooking and through the processing of refined foods, it is easy to develop a deficiency.

Vitamin B_6 is essential for the body's production of all but two of the twenty most important amino acids and for 118 known enzymes. A B_6 deficiency weakens the body's ability to synthesize collagen and elastin fibrils that bind tissues together. This condition makes tissues more vulnerable to injury and/or infection. Decreased collagen production takes its toll on cartilage throughout the body, but especially in the stressed CTS area where arthritis may develop. A severe vitamin deficiency weakens the immune system.

To call RA—and perhaps many other chronic diseases listed in Table 1—an "autoimmune disorder" is not precisely true. The immune system is indeed attacking the body's own cells, but they have been infiltrated by insidious pathogens which use the healthy cells to cloak themselves.

Systemic lupus erythematosus ("lupus") belongs to the RA category and is characterized as an autoimmune disease by the medical community. Lupus affects primarily women ages 18-45 but can occur in older people. It involves chronic inflammation that can affect many parts of the body including heart, lungs, skin, joints, muscles, kidneys, and the nervous system. As with many chronic illnesses, lupus is difficult to diagnose because there is no uniform pattern of symptoms.

Osteoarthritis (OA)

This condition is often called the "wear and tear" disease because it involves cartilage degeneration. OA occurs more frequently than RA. According to the Arthritis Foundation, OA affects about 21 million Americans, mostly women. It is cited as the main reason for nearly 400,000 knee and hip replacement surgeries every year.

Dr. Gabriel Cousens[16] has treated hundreds of patients over the past three years at his Arizona clinic. His therapy is a combination of exercise, massage, diet, and meditation. Dr. Cousens is both a medical doctor and a homeopathic physician. He has concluded that OA is caused by faulty nutrition, overindulgence in junk foods, and lack of exercise. The toxins trapped in the joints are a result of poor circulation, improper digestion, and sluggish organs unable to clear those toxins. His detoxification program has a 95% improvement record for OA patients.[17]

Tests for mycoplasma infection reveal that about 50% of human OA cases also display some degree of the RA form. Individuals with *both* types of arthritis pose a significant challenge to medical practitioners because therapeutic probing using gold or Plaquenil can be dangerous. Until bone scanning techniques were invented, it was common and convenient for doctors to assert that the patient had either OA or RA, but never both.

CARTILAGE DEGENERATION

Cartilage is an essential structural substance found throughout the body and is of four types:

1. Fibrocartilage, notable for tensile strength (the ability to resist breakage), found primarily between the vertebrae

but also in some interarticular areas of the joints. It contains numerous thick bundles of collagen fibers;

2. Articular, which is found in the joints, has the resilience to rebound from compression, and enables bones to slip over one another smoothly;
3. Morphological, such as that found in the nose and ears; and
4. Elastic, found at the front of the rib cage, allowing expansion with breathing action.

Connective tissue makes up one-third of our body weight, most of it in the form of collagen. Tightly interlaced collagen fibrils form better than half of human cartilage, giving it its compressible and elastic characteristics. These fibrils act as resilient "springs" to confine and compress the water-binding proteoglycan molecules in a cartilage matrix that can bind up to 1,000 times its weight in water. This matrix is constrained by the collagen network, creating an intrinsic pressure ranging from 2.5 to 5 atmospheres. Lubrication is maintained by compression and by the intact nature of the cartilage matrix.[18]

Destructive enzymes, proteoglycanase in particular, attack and break down the matrix. With this damage, the matrix's water-binding capability is decreased and absorption of nutrients is diminished. As cartilage erodes, its collagen fibers are exposed to wear, and cushioning effect is lost. The exposed fibril ends act as irritants within the joint capsule. As the immune system responds, the result is a release of chemicals and heat that promote reddening, swelling, and pain in the surrounding nerves and tissues. What follows is the destruction of collagen proteins that hold the cells together as functional connective tissues—synovia, blood vessel, and skin. Arthritics typically look older than their chronological age because their skin is deficient in collagen.

Scar tissue and bone gradually replace the eroded joint regions, causing irregularly shaped articulating surfaces. Age, weight-bearing stresses, and other external forces on joints over time contribute to the ultimate degeneration of cartilage, especially in the hips and knees.

Cartilage is highly susceptible to stress but the underlying subchondral bone bears much of the brunt of compressive forces. Exposed to repeated mechanical stress, this bone can become unusually stiff by a series of healed and calcified microfractures over time. The stiffer this bone, the more the nearby softer cartilage degenerates. Thus care of one's bones is as important as cartilage health for arthritic individuals.[19]

Cartilage erosion can have an etiological cause through what is called "chronic tension," which results in sustained isometric muscle contraction of numerous joints of the body, for example, sustained compression of intervertebral cartilage in the cervical spine and disks.[20]

In the case of OA, cartilage continues to erode and then to grow back. Irregular regrowth masses can eventually cover the entire joint. This accounts for the swelling visible from the exterior side of the skin as well as contraction and alignment problems. In advanced cases, the load-bearing cartilage of the joint becomes rough and pitted, damaged to the point where bone rubs against bone, and more severe pain occurs. A life-threatening joint complication can occur when the cervical spine becomes unstable through cartilage and bone erosion.

Bone friction and destruction is the characteristic feature of osteoarthritis. The same joints may be affected as with RA, but OA is a localized problem while RA joint pain moves to various sites in the body. Typically, OA is directly related to unusual wear or damage to the joints, or to loss of lubricating fluid between the joints, typically associated with the aging process.

In both RA and OA, joints can wear abnormally for a variety of reasons:

- injury damages cartilage, causing the immune system to go into tear-down mode to remove the injured tissues and cells;
- circulation is impaired, so lubrication material is not transferred effectively to the joint or sheath area to rebuild injured cells;
- poor diet does not provide strong skeletal material during childhood development or after injury;
- muscles do not adequately support the joint;
- constant application of misdirected mechanical forces puts excessive stress on the cartilage in a particular joint; and/or
- improper physical therapy and/or exercise can literally wear out the joint(s).

As the body tries to repair itself, cartilage may grow abnormally, seen as knobs under the skin and protruding from the area around the joint. Since there are no pain nerves within cartilage, deterioration generally goes unnoticed until pain and swelling occur. When the surface of the cartilage becomes abraded, the body sends antibodies to attack the exudates of debris that should have been removed by the white blood cells of a robustly functioning immune system. The antibodies' interaction with these sloughed-off bits results in pain and inflammation. Cartilage is shown as shaded areas in the skeletal drawing in Figure 3.

OA can affect both load-bearing joints of the knees, hips, and ankles as well as non-load-bearing joints of the fingers, elbows, and hands. OA is also characterized by calcium deposits, which can accumulate like bony spurs on pressure points and impinge on nerves. The pain and inflammation symptoms are similar to RA, but OA is considered to be a noninflammatory form of arthritis that is hereditary and incurable.

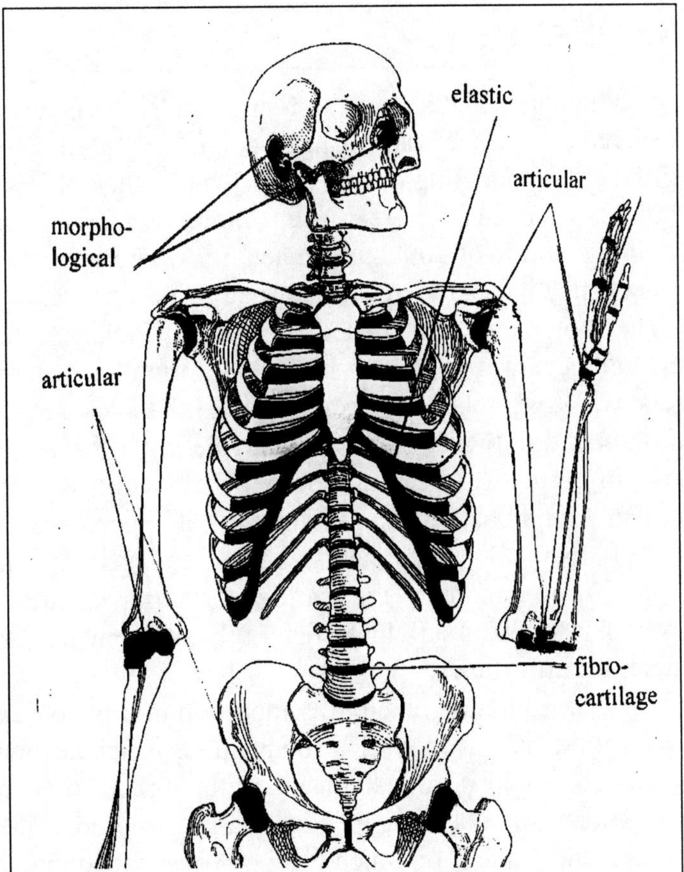

Figure 3. Human Body Cartilage (shaded)

Pets afflicted with OA respond well to an improved diet and glycosaminaglycan supplements, which fortify cartilage in diseased joints and help to reduce pain. Acupuncture, chiropractic adjustments and certain popular herbs such as boswellia and curcumin also help animals. Antioxidant vitamins assist in reducing pathologic inflammation.[21]

BONE HEALTH

The human skeleton is a surprisingly active structure of active metabolic tissue that changes continually throughout one's life. Bone modeling occurs in our youth when 100% of the bone surface is active. Adult bones undergo bone remodeling at a rate of 20% surface activity where older bone tissue is cyclically destroyed and replaced by new tissue.

The bone loss associated with OA indicates that destruction occurs at a faster rate than formation. Study[22] subjects with age-related osteoporosis who took omega-3 polyunsaturated fatty acids as fish oil supplements showed an increase in serum calcium, osteocalcin, and collagen. The study also found that evening primrose oil potentiates the effects of fish oil supplements. Since collagen is also important in maintaining the cartilage matrix, additional research has confirmed that fish oil supplements are beneficial for arthritics.[23]

The best source of calcium is food rich in this nutrient, such as yogurt and salmon. The body more efficiently and easily absorbs small portions consumed throughout the day. Calcium intake of 1,000 mg per day can restore some lost bone mass at any age. Too much calcium (over 2,500 mg per day) may cause absorption problems.[24] Read labels on commercial supplements. Elemental calcium is the ideal type. Formulations containing calcium carbonate, zinc, or aluminum arc harmful. Dolomite and bone meal products, sold as calcium supplements, contain lead and should be avoided.

Bone disease often signals an imbalance of the body's required essential minerals. High doses of cortisone-like drugs or thyroid medication can increase the risk of bone loss. A dysfunctional or overworked immune system may be linked to a calcium deficiency and bone loss. When a pathogenic organism invades the body, the immune system's response includes building a calcium nodule around the invader to protect the healthy cells from harm. Failing to find adequate calcium in the bloodstream, the immune system will take calcium from bones. A bone density scan is a useful test to determine whether the body is under attack by infection and unable to defend itself adequately.

COMMON CONVENTIONAL TREATMENTS

There are hundreds of remedies and formulations for arthritis relief, ranging from ancient herbs to highly sophisticated pharmaceuticals based on the premise that the disease is a metabolic disorder of unknown origin. Some of our present-day drugs are derived from proven herbal remedies or mineral salts such as gold and copper, but they are concentrated to near-toxic strength.

Conventional RA treatment often consists of simply prescribing drugs that relieve pain in the short term but does not systematically address the root cause of the problem. Naturopathic practitioners suggest herbs, diets, and purges that are not effective in the long term. Both groups are endeavoring to solve a highly complex problem with extremely limited knowledge and primitive tools, considering the incredible diversity of the microbial zoo and a human immune system that has evolved assorted mechanisms to combat the assaults of many shape-changing and adaptive invaders.

The way in which these two groups approach the problem of disease is philosophically the same. Both try to restore the body to balance. However, the body is not a static entity—pathogenic microbes continue to evolve and adapt to their changing *in vivo* environment—so there is no single prescription drug or herbal substance that will provide a lasting solution.

The body's dynamic collective and interacting mechanisms typify the ultimate control theory problem. There is much to be learned through cooperation and sharing, rather than the adversarial relationship that exists, sometimes overtly, between conventional medical doctors and practitioners of alternative or complementary medicine.[25]

Several celebrities, notably Dr. Deepak Chopra, Dr. Andrew Weil, and Dr. Gabe Mirkin have shown that medical doctors can and should seek out information from any source that will help heal their patients. By practicing what they call "integrative" or "functional" medicine, they are taking a holistic view of their patients, rejecting the us-versus-them relationship that has stifled progress in the treatment of chronic disease.

Prescription Drugs

A patient reporting arthritis symptoms of pain and swelling in the joints to a physician will usually be given a prescription for medication. The drugs most commonly prescribed to reduce inflammation are the nonsteroidal anti-inflammatory drugs (NSAIDs) in the ibuprofen family such as Indocin, Feldene, Relafen, Naproxen, and others. NSAIDs are designed to block prostaglandins. These drugs relieve symptoms but do not change the overall progression of the disease.

RA treatment may specifically include disease-modifying antirheumatic drugs (DMARDs) such as Methotrexate, Plaquenil, and Ridaura (auranofin or gold salts). DMARDs are intended to inhibit DNA, RNA, and protein synthesis, so they seem to affect the disease itself. This implies some form of cellular activity either by an infecting microorganism or in a body cell that is acting incorrectly.

A doctor will usually prescribe NSAIDs first, then progress to DMARDs. However, since severe joint damage can occur in the early stages of RA, it would seem that treatment with DMARDs should be given earlier in order to prevent further damage.

In severe or persistent cases, the doctor may prescribe powerful drugs such as Prednisone or penicillamine to slow the course of the disease and prevent cartilage and/or bone damage. About half of RA patients receive prescribed low doses of Prednisone, an artificial version of a hormone synthesized by the body's adrenal glands to relieve inflammation. However, these medications suppress some of the actions of the immune system. Our new high-tech drugs are not without possible serious long-term side effects, as shown in the examples in Table 2.[26]

One potential side effect of Prednisone is peptic ulcers. In 1994 the National Institutes of Health (NIH) reviewed numerous medical studies and concluded that a bacterium called *Helicobacter pylori* was the root cause of most peptic ulcers. The sloughing off of necrotic inflammatory tissue creates the ulcers in the stomach and duodenum. This conclusion had been announced over a decade earlier in 1982 when two Australian scientists, Doctors J. Robin Warren and Barry Marshall, conducted meticulous experiments and proved this fact. Their research showed that *H. pylori* is a common bacterial agent colonizing an estimated 30-50% of the world's population.

Table 2. Prescription Drug Side Effects

Drug name	Type	Some potential side effects
Indocin (indomethacin)	NSAID	hypertension, edema, blurred vision, corneal and retinal damage, tinnitus, hearing loss, rash, nausea, diarrhea, anemia, anorexia, renal dysfunction, gastrointestinal bleeding
Feldene (piroxicam)	NSAID	headache, anemia, drowsiness, rash, malaise, vertigo, dizziness, blurred vision, tinnitus, photosensitivity, liver toxicity, gastrointestinal bleeding
Relafen (nabumetone)	NSAID	dizziness, fatigue, insomnia, nausea, headache, nervousness, rash, edema, abdominal pain, diarrhea, gastritis, tinnitus
Naprosyn (naproxen sodium)	NSAID	headache, occult blood loss, nausea, pulmonary infiltrates, dizziness, heart palpitations, drowsiness, dyspepsia, liver dysfunction, constipation, visual disturbances, rash
Plaquenil*	DMARD	irritability, vertigo, tinnitus, fatigue, emotional changes, weight loss, blurred vision, retinal changes, abdominal cramps, diarrhea, nausea
Methotrexate (anti-metabolite)	DMARD	photosensitivity, diarrhea, ulcers, gingivitis, tubular necrosis, rash, liver dysfunction, nausea
Ridaura (gold salts)	DMARD	abdominal pain, stomatitis, diarrhea, nausea, kidney damage, anemia, jaundice, interstitial pneumonitis

Table 2. Prescription Drug Side Effects, cont'd

Prednisone ** (adrenocortoid)	DMARD	hypertension, acne, peptic ulcer, cataracts, glaucoma, increased susceptibility to infection, edema
Penicillamine (chelating agent)	DMARD	rash, anemia, oral ulcerations, nausea, dyspepsia, pancreatitis

* Plaquenil (hydroxychloroquine sulfate) is considered one of the safest drugs for treating RA and lupus. One of the antimalarials, it is derived from Peruvian cinchona tree bark. It was used extensively in the 1800s to treat these diseases.

** Prednisone is synthetic cortisone.[27]

At the time, they were ridiculed and their findings ignored by a medical establishment in the United States that has strong economic motives for keeping standard treatment of ulcers as a chronic disease in place. Today the antacid market is nearly $25 billion, and recurring ulcers mean regular visits to gastroenterologists.[28]

Natural herbal antibiotics can be effective for ulcers: the berberine compound found in both goldenseal (Hydrastis canadensis) and Oregon grape (Berberis aquifolium). Berberine kills a variety of harmful bacteria, including *H. pylori*.

Herbalists recommend taking licorice root extract (*Glycyrrhiza glabra*) with berberines. Licorice is an anti-bacterial, and also increases production of protective mucus in the stomach. Degycyrrhizinated (DGL) licorice is preferred to avoid water retention and high blood pressure.[29] One should discuss specific dosage with a qualified health care advisor.

Prescription antibiotics are often given to eradicate the *H. pylori* bacteria, but this treatment does not affect the recurring ulcers that are shown to be one of the side effects of NSAIDs and DMARDs. About 30% of stomach ulcers are caused by the corrosive effects of aspirin-type drugs, not by *H. pylori*. Because the two types of ulcer causes are unrelated, treatment for one type won't help the other.[30] The *Helicobacter pylori* Foundation provides details on the wide variety of *H. pylori* symptoms, tests, related diseases, and suggested treatments.[31]

In the 1930s, when some doctors began to suspect that RA might be an infectious disease, sulfasalazine (an antibiotic compound composed of sulfa and aspirin) was administered. In the 1950s the infection theory fell out of favor with the medical community, who adopted the autoimmune theory as the standard teaching that prevails to this day. Perhaps the infection theory was abandoned because mycoplasmal forms of bacteria were hard to detect with methods available at that time.

Sulfasalazine is now used successfully for ulcerative colitis, an inflammatory bowel disease (or Irritable Bowel Syndrome (IBS)). The successful use of sulfasalazine in treatment of RA for more than four weeks was reported in the mid-1980s.[32] Recent studies in the 1990s have shown sulfasalazine to be as effective as gold or penicillamine.[33] The positive action of the antibacterical component of sulfasalazine may indicate the role of bacterial infections of the intestine in the etiopathogenesis of rheumatoid diseases. However, the antibacterial component also enters the bloodstream where it is free to move to any site of infection and to suppress bacterial activity.

Although sulfasalazine has some immunosuppressive effects, it is hoped that the results of these studies will prompt a revisiting of the infection hypothesis among medical researchers.

Gold Salts

Sometimes injections of gold salts are prescribed to help control the inflammation of RA and to halt progression of the disease. It is still not fully understood how gold slows the progression of RA but studies have shown that gold reduces vascular permeability, lowering the number of white blood cells, slowing these cells' response to antigens, and thus diminishing the inflammatory response.[34] However, improvement may last only two to three years. If the RA returns, the physician usually prescribes another medication such as Methotrexate. Gold is used less frequently now than it was a decade ago.

Cartilage Transplants

Transplants have been under experimentation since 1915 using cartilage from a recently deceased young person. The success rate is 75-80% but surgeons are pressuring researchers to achieve a 90% rate. A relatively new procedure attempts to replace worn or damaged cartilage with healthy cells grown in a test tube, and then placed in the area in need of repair. The procedure has been tested in people with a type of early OA called "isolated cartilage defect", which occurs in young people and is usually the result of trauma, typically sports-related.[35]

The same problem occurs with any transplant—the body tends to reject the transplant as an "intruder." Immuno-suppressing drugs can reduce this reaction, but they are also toxic. Orthopedic surgeon Dr. Juan Rodrigo has performed more than 20 cartilage transplants on laboratory animals using a type of detergent, which partially digests the bone cells while leaving the cartilage cells undamaged. A break-through in this area remains elusive.[36]

Meniscal tears (torn knee cartilage) are the most common orthopedic surgical procedure. Although every year some 750,000 patients have a torn meniscus removed, only about three thousand transplants have been performed in the United States since 1990. Not every patient needs a transplant, and not all are fit for the surgery. The pre-surgery requirement is for stable, normally aligned, arthritis-free knees, and an upper age limit of 50-55. This is a "Catch 22": those most in need of the surgery do not meet the success criteria. Fortunately, there are other less risky options besides transplants to relieve arthritis pain and to restore mobility.[37] Supplements that help rebuild cartilage, Glucosamine and Chondroitin, are discussed in Chapter 7.

Pain is a symptom of some condition in the body that requires attention. Athletes often seek painkillers that permit them to continue playing sports despite the risk of further damage to an injured area. Drugs that suppress pain may allow continued movement when rest and temporary immobilization are required for the body to heal.

Arthroscopic Surgery

A new procedure that uses arthroscopic probes and lasers cauterizes nerve endings in the spine so that arthritics suffering from low back pain are afforded some relief. Either an orthopedic surgeon or a rheumatologist trained in arthroscopy can perform the examination. An MRI test is usually given prior to the surgery. The arthroscopic probe, when used along with other tests and a complete medical history, can be a valuable diagnostic tool. A dime-sized incision allows the thin tube of the arthroscope, tipped with a small, lighted lens, to magnify and illuminate areas within the joint. The examining physician is able to view and diagnose problems such as synovitis, cartilage damage, tendon and ligament tears, and loose fragments of bone or cartilage that may be present in the joint and causing irritation.

Arthroscopic surgery using a laser can repair torn cartilage or ligaments, remove loose pieces of bone or cartilage, or remove inflamed joint linings. Unfortunately, this treatment does not remove the cause of the disease, and deterioration continues. Incisions are much smaller than those incurred in conventional surgery, joint trauma is minimal, and recovery time is usually shorter. However, complications for any surgery may include infections, blood clots, and damage to blood vessels or nerves.[38]

An operation called arthrodesis, or joint fusion, freezes bones together, essentially removing the joint. Synovectomy is a surgical procedure to remove the synovial membrane. These procedures do not necessarily remove the pain. Joint replacement substitutes artificial joints for those worn away, and is usually done on the hips, wrists, elbows, shoulders, knees, and fingers.

Non-prescription Drugs

Over-the-counter (OTC) drugs such as aspirin, acetaminophen, and ibuprofen are usually suggested by doctors for mild cases of arthritis to alleviate joint pain, but even these less powerful chemicals have their own assorted side effects, depending on the individual and the duration of use: stomach pain, nausea, vomiting, heartburn, low-level bleeding in the bowel, fluid retention, anxiety, depression, dizziness, drowsiness, ulcers, skin rash, prolonged clotting time, and tinnitus (ringing in the ears).

Until very recently, quinine sulfate was available inexpensively OTC. This drug has been shown to be active against a variety of parasites (see Chapter 3). It has a marked positive effect against arthritis pain and inflammation but now quinine is available only by prescription.

COMMON NATUROPATHIC TREATMENTS

Because there are many herbs that strengthen the immune system, many others that improve circulation, and still others that relieve symptoms of inflammation, pain, and swelling, a comprehensive list is beyond the scope of this book. Appendix I lists those referenced consistently in texts dealing with naturopathic treatment for arthritis and related rheumatic ailments. While aspirin and ibuprofen may relieve pain, they can also lead to other health problems.[39]

The most powerful and safest anti-inflammatory agent is superoxide dismutase, an enzyme produced naturally by red blood cells. This enzyme is contained in many vegetables, as are vitamins A (betacarotene), C (ascorbic acid) and E (alphatocopherol). The potency of these vitamins is increased when combined with copper, zinc, and selenium. While a vitamin or dietary deficiency has not been shown as a cause of arthritis, allergies to certain foods or substances can affect the development and severity of a wide range of chronic diseases, including arthritis.[40]

The vitamins and supplements described in this book as immune system enhancers are given as examples of substances a doctor or nutritionist may deem important to include in a specific profile based on a particular individual's needs. In some cases, a commonly available, widely used, and otherwise benign vitamin or supplement might be contra-indicated because a pre-existing health problem or conflict with prescription medications could make it harmful.

Herbal medications may actually interfere with and complicate surgical procedures before the operation. Eight herbal substances pose some degree of risk during the perioperative period.[41] These are echinacea, ephedra, garlic, ginkgo, ginseng, kava, St. John's wort, and valerian. These eight herbs account for more than half of all single herb preparations sold in the United States. Negative reactions include: bleeding from garlic, ginkgo, and ginseng; cardiovascular instability from ephedra; and hypoglycemia from ginseng. Use of St. John's wort leads to increased metabolism of perioperative drugs, but some nonherbal dietary supplements such as glucosamine and chondroitin appear to be safe for perioperative patients.[42] There is a risk for adverse herb/drug interactions between anesthetics and kava and valerian. These herbs seem to increase the sedative effect of the drugs.

At present, information on adverse reactions is required at varying levels of detail at health care facilities across the United States. There is no mandate to capture data on the exact nature or extent of problems unless the patient reports evidence proactively.

Three factors contributing to under-reporting of adverse events are (1) physicians' failing to obtain a detailed history of non-prescribed medications from their patients; (2) patients' unwillingness to admit the use of herbal remedies to their doctors; and (3) patients' reluctance to report and seek treatment for adverse reactions. One study[43] found that the lack of disclosure and reporting is the patient's belief that either the doctor is not knowledgeable about herbal substances or that s/he may be prejudiced against non-conventional therapies.

Even if the data were to be reported, there are no mechanisms in place to logging, processing, interpretation, evaluation, or dissemination. Perhaps some day technology will allow biochip readouts or instant sample analysis without waiting for lab results, and will further be capable of transmitting patients' data directly to a central database. Until then, the quality of reported data is questionable, since herb-drug reactions experienced will be somewhat subjective and will vary among individuals.

Physicians should carefully interview patients who are candidates for surgery regarding their history of herbal medication usage and then take steps to prevent, recognize, and treat potentially serious interaction problems before surgery is performed. Both doctor and patient should be aware of pharmacodynamic or pharmacokinetic risks.

Although in most cases, patients may be advised to avoid herbal medications for 2-3 weeks before surgery, in others, abrupt withdrawal from herbal substances may be detrimental.[44] Doctor and patient must work together to determine the optimal course of action before surgery.

Homeopathic Remedies

Homeopathic philosophy is consistent with ideas about vaccination and immunization, namely, that "like heals like," according to the Law of Similars, the basic principle of homeopathy. This fundamental tenet states that a substance that causes a set of symptoms in a healthy person acts as a curative medicine when given to sick people who have similar symptoms. Thus a minute amount of the toxin is given to the individual to acquaint the body with the invader so as to train it to ward off future assaults.

The medicine is designed to make the patients feel worse before they feel better. It forces the immune system to react vigorously to the invading organism, thus training it thoroughly in resistance, unlike antihistamines, antibiotics, and cold medicines, which suppress the immune reaction and do not challenge the system to learn to repel the invaders. Homeopathic approaches that involve a cyclic alteration of repeated immune stimulation and gentle immune suppression facilitate transport of natural antibiotics to hidden sites of pathogenic organisms. This action is consistent with the Jarisch-Herxheimer effect described in Chapter 3.

Specific homeopathic remedies have been found to be consistently useful in relieving arthritis symptoms under the following conditions:[45]

- worse in warm weather, inflamed joints, intolerant of touch, and ill humored: *Colchicum* 6c.
- worse during stormy/changeable weather: *Rhododendron* 6c.
- when symptoms include pain and stiffness, made worse after rest, and in cold, damp weather, symptoms improve with continued motion: *Rhus toxicondendron* 6c.
- stitching pain, made worse by any motion, eased by rest: *Bryonia* 6c.

The amounts in homeopathic compounds are very carefully measured and diluted. Medicines diluted one part to 99 parts are called *centesimal* potencies and are labeled 6c, 30c, and so on. Sometimes the dilution factor is one part medicine to nine parts liquid and these *decimal* potencies are labeled 6x, 30x, and so on. Medicines diluted 15 times or less (15c, 15x, or lower) are referred to as low potencies, while those diluted 30c, 30x or higher are considered high potencies. The ingredients in an OTC homeopathic remedy for yeast infection that includes *Candida albicans* 30x illustrate the immunization principle of the Law of Similars.

An individual taking a homeopathic remedy should avoid all products containing mint (including jelly, candy, flavored toothpaste, mouthwash, and gum) during treatment. Other substances that affect homeopathic regimens adversely are camphor and caffeine. A physician trained in both homeopathic and conventional medicine should be able to advise the patient on these kinds of interactions.

Chinese Medicine

Chinese medicine suggests natural substances such as bupleuri root, pubescent angelica root, ledebouriellua root, timospora stem, licorice, cinnamon twigs, and Chinese skullcap for their anti-inflammatory effects.

Acupuncture may also be helpful. It is believed that acupuncture stimulates endorphins in the brain regions related to injury sites. The brain has a complex overlap of functions, so it may be that external stimulation sites map to those brain regions responsible for other parts of the body. Acupuncturists use detailed charts to map stimulus points to brain areas of responsibility for a variety of regions/organs.

This ancient Chinese method of healing has been scientifically analyzed using an electronic probe to test the instant effects of acupuncture on calcium (Ca) and sodium (Na) ions of normal and injured muscles *in vitro*. It was found that in normal muscles after acupuncture, Ca content of the plasma membrane obviously increased, while Na content tended to decrease. At ten minutes after acupuncture, Ca content resumed to normal but Na content increased three-fold. The results indicated that acupuncture could increase the penetrability of *normal* muscle membrane to Ca and the penetrability of *injured* muscle membrane to Na. This might be the vital mechanism of changing Na-Ca exchange of cell membrane and adjusting plasma Ca content.[46]

DMSO

DMSO (dimethyl sulfoxide), a solvent used in the wood pulp and paper manufacturing process, was hailed in the early 1960s as a "miracle drug" to relieve inflammation but the FDA quickly suppressed its use. It was not until 1978 that the FDA approved DMSO for use in the treatment of interstitial cystitis, a bladder inflammation, but has not yet recognized serious laboratory research for its use in the treatment of scleroderma, spinal paralysis, arthritis, bursitis, and, in some cases, cancer.[47]

The chemical formulation of DMSO consists of two methyls bound to sulfur plus oxygen. When oxidized, DMSO becomes di-methylsulfoxone, a sulfur-based antibacterial known as MSM (methylsulfonylmethane). DMSO also may bind to pain source nerve sites in the area of injury, reducing the stimulation capacity. DMSO facilitates the transfer of dissolved substances into the body. Through hydroscopic action, DMSO also facilitates fluid transport from the trauma site, reducing swelling and speeding elimination of waste tissue remnants. DMSO's reputation for relieving symptoms of swelling comes from this desiccating capability. A joint filled with excess fluid will respond quickly to DMSO as the fluid is drawn out from the affected area and the pressure is relieved. DMSO is widely used by veterinarians and ranchers to treat horses with sprains.

Since DMSO usage is still discouraged for human use by the FDA, it would be very difficult to formulate and sell a patch that transports some other useful substance "X" into the body through the many layers of skin and tissue. However, a combination of DMSO + X could be useful. X could be copper or gold salts, but this poses some danger if too high a concentration is used. X could be tetracycline or erythromycin or minocycline, but these antibiotics are not yet on the market for human consumption in the United States except by prescription.[48] MSM is available in health food stores as a dietary supplement. DMSO should only be used topically.

Care should be taken in the application of DMSO. Since it is a powerful conductor, anything that touches the solvent should be extremely clean—the area to be touched as well as the hands or device applying the solvent—lest harmful bacteria be introduced through the skin. Washing the hands immediately after applying DMSO is strongly recommended. Twenty grams of DMSO per kilogram of body weight is considered a lethal dose, so DMSO is relatively nontoxic. A 150-pound person would have to absorb three pounds of DMSO to reach a lethal level. However, DMSO and oxygen therapy should not be combined since chemical interactions with released oxygen are dangerous.

THE WD-40 MYTH

A popular myth has grown around the use of WD-40 as a joint lubricant and pain reliever for arthritis. The liquid is sprayed on the painful joint much as one would fix a squeaky mechanical hinge. To be used by the body, the substance must be absorbed through the skin. The thinner the skin, the more is absorbed.

To date, no credible scientific studies have shown any benefit from the use of WD-40 for arthritis. In fact, there may be cumulative harmful effects. The manufacturer's warning indicates that contact with skin and vapors should be avoided. WD-40 contains petroleum distillates, as do gasoline and oil. Problems ranging from mild skin rash to severe allergic reactions have been reported. Prolonged exposure can cause cancer and other serious health problems.

WD-40 has a documented dangerous synergism with insecticides, notably pyrethrin, the active ingredient in head lice medication.[49] Pyrethrin is made from dried, concentrated powder of flowers from the chrysanthemum family. Both the natural pyrethrin and synthetic pyrethroid insecticides mimic the hormone estrogen, which causes cell proliferation. Misuse of these insecticides can result in proliferation of breast cancer cells as well as endocrine disruption, kidney problems, and nerve damage.[50]

Proponents of WD-40 may be experiencing a placebo effect or may realize some benefit from increased blood circulation in the affected area as the substance is massaged into the skin. Breathing the vapor may have a temporary pain-killing effect, but delicate linings in the nose, throat, mouth, and lungs may be damaged.

OXYGEN THERAPIES [51]

Oxygen treatments have been shown to be beneficial in cases of viral or bacterial infections that suppress the immune system. Most bacteria associated with RA are anaerobic or borderline anaerobic. Thus they would be expected to respond to oxygen therapy. Furthermore, there is a synergy between oxygen and antibiotics. However, the FDA is currently discouraging oxygen treatments for valid reasons: the therapy has a very narrow safe dosage range and requires precision in the amount administered. There are several types of oxygen therapies:

- Hyperbaric treatment with pure oxygen (O_2) at two atmospheres has been used to treat AIDS, arthritis, Chronic Fatigue Syndrome (CFS), mononucleosis, MS, and infections with anaerobic bacteria. Hyperbaric oxygen therapy (HBOT) is believed to enhance the antimicrobial effects of antibiotics. It is commonly used to treat deep-sea divers who have "the bends." This treatment is commonly used in Europe, lasting 1-2 hours in a hyperbaric chamber two or three times per week for several months.

HBOT has been documented to be beneficial in MS treatment.[52] The Institute for Molecular Medicine has recently established a new treatment protocol for MS patients based on detection of chronic bacterial and viral infections. HBOT can only suppress chronic infections because the microorganisms are borderline anaerobes; it cannot completely destroy them. The suppressing action is enhanced

The chamber works by forcing oxygen into compromised cells and tissue, thus allowing the normal infection-fighting function of white blood cells to proceed. This oxygen treatment has been used in cases of "flesh eating bacteria." [53] The *Streptococcus A* bacterium is a mutated strain of the microbe that causes strep throat, a common childhood disease. The bacterium isn't precisely "flesh eating" but its action has the same effect; it produces toxins that deprive the cells of oxygen until they die;

- Ozone (O_3) inhalation or ingestion, which must be done very carefully as ozone inhaled directly is poisonous. Ozone generators sold commercially as home appliances to clean the air pose a potential hazard since improper use can burn the lungs. Ozone is dissolved in water to form hydrogen peroxide (H_2O_2). This treatment is not advised for arthritics since H_2O_2 stimulates destructive inflam-mation in tissues;
- H_2O_2 is an effective and non-toxic topical antiseptic. The molecule is unstable and when warmed, degrades into water and oxygen. H_2O_2 at 10% is actively virucidal and sporicidal. A 3% solution is often used to cleanse and disinfect wounds, since anaerobic bacteria are particularly sensitive to oxygen. Dilute H_2O_2 injections or infusions seem to facilitate the immune response and

disable some pathogenic organisms. Some cells of the immune system generate H_2O_2 while other *in vitro* enzymes act to suppress H_2O_2. This treatment is considerably less expensive than hyperbaric treatment, but involves some degree of risk if administered intravenously.

Hydrogen peroxide is produced naturally in the body as part of the histamine reaction and subsequent inflammation. An element of the cell called peroxisome has the job to produce H_2O_2 to destroy invading viruses, bacteria, and other contaminating substances that try to attack the cell. The presence of additional H_2O_2 facilitates the histamine reaction, which in turn increases the severity of the inflammation. Some invaders also can generate H_2O_2 that in some unknown way must benefit the invader.

Peroxides must be administered with extreme caution since misuse can produce anaphylactic reactions in some hypersensitive individuals. Treatments can be effective if a diluted, low dose is tried first, then very gradually building up to a stronger solution. Similarly, ozone should be dissolved in a saline solution and slowly infused, gradually building up to the optimal level over time.

---

[1] Clark (1997) pp. 14-15.

[2] See www.drmirkin.com/joints/J159.htm for supportive references.

[3] Excerpted from the *Illustrated Health Encyclopedia*, online at www.pittsburgh.com/shared/health/adam/ency/article/000431.html.

[4] Centers for Disease Control. MMWR 50(17):334-336, 2001.

[5] Clark (1997) p. 4.

[6] Clark (1997) p. 8.

---

[7] Seachrist, Lisa. "RA'S Gender Differences." *Arthritis Today*. July/August 1996.

[8] Barnes and Galton (1976), p. 203.

[9] Clark (1997) p.26.

[10] Dr. Samuels (1991, p. 26) claims, along with the majority of conventional physicians in the medical establishment, that RA is recognized as an autoimmune disease, i.e., a condition in which the body becomes allergic to its own tissue. He also states that "a tremendous amount of research has been done on RA but its cause remains unknown."

[11] More detail regarding each of these illnesses can be found at the Autoimmune Related Diseases Association's website, www.aarda.org.

[12] The author's personal experience led to this observation. Soon after a severe "flu" swept through the company ranks one winter, employees who typically spent hours each day at computer terminals suddenly complained of wrist pain. Dozens of requests for wrist support braces were made. Many of these workers were career secretaries who had never before experienced carpal tunnel problems before having the "flu." My belief is that latent mycoplasmal infection was reinvigorated by exposure to *Streptococcus*.

[13] Rosenfeld, Dr. Isadore. "When You Can't Get a Grip." *Parade Magazine*, September 17, 2000.

[14] Thomson, Bill. "Pioneer of Carpal Tunnel Surgery Predicts B6 Therapy." *Natural Health*, July/August 1993.

[15] Challem, Jack. "Cure Carpal Tunnel Without Surgery." *Natural Health*, July/August 1993.

[16] Cousens (1999).

[17] Vitetta-Miller, Robin. "Recipes for Relief." *Natural Health*, October 1999.

[18] Cailliet, Rene. "Disuse Syndrome: Fibrositic and Degenerative Changes," in Brena and Chapman (1983) pp. 67-68.

[19] Colbin, Annemarie and Hunt, Paula. "Build Strong Bones." *Natural Health*, May/June 2000.

[20] Op. cit., Cailliet, p. 70.

---

[21] Wynn, Dr. Susan G., a veterinarian discussing the problem of arthritis in pets at www.altvetmed.com.

[22] Broadhurst, C.L. and Sinther, M. "Evening Primrose Oil: Pharmacological and Clinical Applications," in Mazza and Ooma (2000) pp. 213-264.

[23] Volker, et al. (2000).

[24] Ott, Christopher. "The Surprising Benefits of Calcium." *Natural Health*, January/February 2002.

[25] A *Natural Health* Debate with Dr. Wallace Sampson and Dr. Lewis Mehl-Madrona. "Alternative Medicine: Under the Microscope." *Natural Health*, September/October 1998.

[26] Source: *Physician's Drug Handbook*. The 2001 edition (9th) has just been published. See http://store.springnet.com. Side effects for tetracycline, in low doses, are mild cramps, nausea, diarrhea, and lightheadedness until the body adjusts to the medicine. For an online guide covering more than 250 over-the-counter drugs and their side effects, see www.arthritis.org/answers/DrugGuide/default.asp

[27] Unattributed feature, "Cortisone: Still Useful After 50 Years." *Arthritis Today*, November/December 1998.

[28] Brian O'Reilly. "Why Doctors Aren't Curing Ulcers." *Fortune*, June 9, 1997.

[29] Vukovic, L. "Home Remedies." *Natural Health*, July/August 2000.

[30] Dunkin, Mary Anne. "Those Other Ulcers." *Arthritis Today*, July/August 1996.

[31] See www.helico.com.

[32] Bax, D.E. and Amos, R.S. "Sulphasalazine: a Safe, Effective Agent for Prolonged Control of Rheumatoid Arthritis. A Comparison With Sodium Aurothiomalate." *Ann Rheum Dis* 1985; 44: 194.

[33] Samuels (1991), p. 134. See also Feltelius, et al. (1986).

[34] Samuels (1991), p. 132.

[35] Rick Boling. "New Cartilage for Old." *Modern Maturity*, September/October 1995.

[36] UC Davis Health System. "Cartilage Transplants Remain a Focus of Research." *Matrix*, Volume 4, No. 5, August 1997.

---

[37] Roback, Missy. "Knee Cartilage Transplant Offers Hope to Some." *CBS Health Watch*, July 2000. Via Medscape.

[38] Dunkin, Mary Anne. "Arthroscopy." *Arthritis Today*, September/ October 1998.

[39] Ott, Christopher. "Stop the Pain." *Natural Health*, May/June 2000.

[40] Clark (1997) p. 46.

[41] Ang-Lee, Michael K.; Moss, Jonathan; and Yuan, Chun-Su. "Herbal Medicines and Perioperative Care." *JAMA*, July 11, 2001. Vol 286, No. 2, pp. 208-216.

[42] Op. cit.

[43] Blendon, R.J.; DesRoches, C.M.; Benson, J.M.; Brodie, M. and Altman, D.E. "American's Views on the Use the Regulation of Dietary Supplements." *Arch Intern Med.* 2001; 161:805-810.

[44] Op cit., Ang-Lee, M.K., et al. Also see Waltman, Alicia. "Talking Alternative Medicine with Your Doc." *Natural Health*, May/June 2001.

[45] Smyth (1994) p. 346.

[46] Qu Zhuqing, et al. (1993). Via Medline website.

[47] DMSO has been shown to suppress inflammation, kill leukemic cells, and to protect cells and organisms *in vivo* against the damaging and lethal effects of cold and of radiation. Collected laboratory results were published as individual research papers in *Annals of the New York Academy of Sciences*, Vol 141, Art. 1. "Biological Actions of Dimethyl Sulfoxide." March 1966.

[48] Minocycline is available from www.lifestylepharmacy.com, a New Zealand supplier, and from other foreign sources.

[49] See www.safe2use.com/pests/lice/poisons.htm.

[50] NCAP's *Journal of Pesticide Reform*. Spring 1999, Vol. 19. No. 1. Also see www.fhradio.org/fm/archives/1998/2142(FM).html.

[51] This section contains general information from several websites, primarily www.io.org and www.ncf.carleton.ca.

[52] Naubauer, R.A. "Protocol for the Treatment of Multiple Sclerosis with Hyperbaric Oxygen." *J. Hyperbar Med.* 1990;5:53-54.

[53] Grant, Amy. "*Streptococcus A*—Necrotizing Fasciitis." EmergencyNet NEWS Service (ENN), June 15, 1994.

2. HOW THE IMMUNE SYSTEM WORKS

Observing pathogenic microorganisms, one is tempted to assign an almost human intelligence to their actions. They seem to strategize, cunningly evade detection, and skillfully organize to wage war to overcome opposing elements of the immune system. This is a fallacy, of course, but for ease of explaining the infection connection to a lay audience, this book will characterize interactions between pathogens and the immune system's defenses in familiar military combat terms.

Microorganisms have no capability to think. They are simply able to adapt at higher rates of selection, to mutate rapidly, and to react to specific stimuli. During their short life cycles, most die early, but the survivors select out and replicate with new imprinting.

Similarly, coordination among elements of the immune system appears to be intelligently orchestrated by the participating cells and organs, but it is really an example of nature's evolved design of the human body.

In-depth research into the function of the immune system has only been performed since the 1970s. Before that time, immune system status was used only as an indicator of one's general health. For instance, white blood cell counts were tested; a high count indicated that the body was trying to fight an infection. Antibiotics were then prescribed as heavy artillery to destroy the infection, unfortunately suppressing the immune system in the process. Corticosteroids (cortisone compounds) were then given to combat inflammation. These drugs, too, suppress the immune system.

In the 1940s and 1950s, tonsils were removed routinely in cases of throat infections. We now know that the tonsils are an important element of the immune system, part of the body's first line of defense against disease. Tonsillectomies were a contributing factor in the poliomyelitis epidemic of the 1950s because the operation removed lymph nodes essential to a fully functional immune system. The medical community thus unwittingly brought about this iatrogenic epidemic.

The appendix is another supposedly useless organ that is routinely removed. However, it is an important part of the immune system. Appendicitis is a warning of a much bigger problem. Removing a healthy appendix or noninflamed tonsils is akin to disabling the trouble light on your car's dashboard because you don't like the color red. Appendix removal should only be performed when appendicitis is a consideration and if there is danger of rupture and peritonitis. Scans are now available to diagnose appendicitis.

Immunologists now insist that the tonsils should not be removed only under highly serious circumstances. Yet every year more than a million tonsillectomies are performed, and some states still have laws that the appendix must be removed if the lower abdomen is opened for other surgery.

Sensing a vital loss to the immune system, 20% of the time the body will gradually regrow tonsils and an appendix. The greatest risk of death following any surgery is a nosocomial (secondary) infection contracted during recovery at the hospital. This is because nearly all surgeries depress the immune system to some extent, leaving the body vulnerable to infection.

Not all aspects of the immune system are fully known. What we do know is that the medical community tends to view afflictions such as cancer as a local, specific disease. However, it may be that cancer is merely a symptom of a larger problem—a malfunctioning immune system. Conventional medicine seems focused on treating the symptoms rather than looking deeper to the root cause of illness.

Statistics show that during the period 1987-1997 the number of Americans treated for depression rose from 1.7 million to 6.3 million.[1] The percentage of patients who used immunosuppressing drugs such as Prozac increased from 37% to nearly 75%. Those receiving psychotherapy declined from 71% to 60%. As antidepressants are aggressively marketed, we can expect this trend to continue. We can also expect an increase in chronic illnesses that are associated with damaged immune systems.

The medical community has perhaps ignored the immune system for so long because its components and interrelationships are not readily observed. Medical specialists in other systems—digestive, circulatory, nervous, respiratory, and so forth—see these systems as easily described and can observe their physical connections. By contrast, immune system connectivity is on the molecular level. Moreover, it almost seems to have a primitive intelligence, acting on the principle of action/reaction, i.e., stimulus/response.

To illustrate: if a microscopic piece of an organ enters the bloodstream through disease or injury, the immune system will muster defenses to fight the foreign invader. Having done so, the immune system will have been trained to attack the original organ. This is the start of an autoimmune response, unless the suppressor T-cells stop the body's attack on itself.

In the following sections, a brief overview of the inner workings of the immune system is presented in layman's terms in order to set the stage for the chapters to follow.[2]

THE LYMPHATIC SYSTEM

The most discernible physical part of the immune system is the lymphatic system. On a molecular level, the entire immune system pervades the body, since even the smallest cell can create chemicals to aid in the defense of the entire system. The two major parts of the lymphatic system are the primary and secondary organs.

Primary Organs

These are the thymus gland and, collectively, the bone marrow. The thymus is located just beneath the breastbone. It functions at its peak during adolescence. The thymus is the most powerful organ of the immune system, and resides at its center.

Bone marrow is the soft tissue located in bone cavities. Bone marrow produces specialized lymphocytes (T-cells and B-cells) to travel through lymph vessels to the secondary organs and into the blood stream. Bone marrow is the source of stem cells, which become leukocytes and lymphocytes. Leukocytes travel through the blood stream on sentry duty, on the alert for invaders.

Within the cortex of the thymus gland, the thymosin hormone is secreted which helps bone marrow lymphocytes mature into T-cells.

Secondary organs

The main organs in this class are the lymph nodes, spleen, tonsils, liver, Peyer's patches in the small intestines, and appendix. These are locations where the molecular elements of the immune system assemble to combat germs, viruses, and allergens. The spleen is an important immunologic filter of the blood.

A healthy, uncompromised, functioning lymphatic system is effective in protecting the bloodstream from malignant cells, bacterial cells, or particulate matter in the form of spores. The lymphatic system acts as a unit, with filtration taking place not only in the lymph nodes themselves but also along the lymphatic capillaries and trunks.

Lymph nodes are small, ovoid structures located in various places in the body along the route of the lymphatic vessels. These nodes trap antigens and filter them out of the lymph fluid, which is composed of tissue fluids routed from all over the body to the lymph nodes for cleaning and subsequent return to the blood stream.

In almost all kinds of injury there is an increase in lymph flow from the injured tissue that helps to reduce pressure by removing fluid. The lymph flow also carries away cell debris and other chemical exudates that might lead to further inflammation if they remained at the site.

Of the total volume of fluid that moves from the blood into and around the tissues, approximately 90% reenters the cardiovascular system. The remaining 10% enters the blind-ended lymphatic capillaries by osmosis and diffusion. From these capillaries, the tissue lymph fluid flows through a series of progressively larger vessels to two large lymphatic vessels that resemble veins.

CELLULAR COMPONENTS

At the cellular level, the variety and amounts of chemical substances capable of being produced by immune system cells to kill invaders are immense. The immune system must be ready to combat a vast array of predators capable of attacking the body. Rather than stockpile an arsenal of coded chemical weapons in advance, the immune system manufactures its killer chemicals only when the chemical marker on its surface identifies an invader. This is done on the spot, when the invader is confronted. If the invader is new to the body and multiplies quickly, it may take several days for the immune system to produce and mobilize enough defensive components to counter the colony.

Infections are the most common causes of human disease. They are produced by bacteria, viruses, parasites, and fungi. Before reaching the infection stage, the invader must run a gauntlet of immune system defenses. Antibodies are present at all the body's main gateways of entry and exit. However, if the invader finds an unprotected opening, e.g., through the skin, it must now contend with patrolling killer cells and other sentries that will sound the alarm.

The two major white cell (leukocyte) types of the immune system are lymphocytes and phagocytes.

Lymphocytes

T-cells. These are the more common of the two chief kinds of lymphocytes (the other being B-cells), beginning development in the bone marrow before maturing in the thymus and accounting for approximately 70% of all lymphocytes. T-cells are the main regulators of the immune system. T-cells are of four major types:

1. *Helper T-cells*, which initiate the immune response to foreign antigens immediately. They also activate a second, more long-range defense called the humoral, or antibody, response performed by the B-cells. Their quantity is measured as a CD4 count;
2. *Inducer T-cells*, which oversee the development of T-cells in the thymus;

3. *Suppressor T-cells*, which limit the immune response after helper T-cells have successfully fought off the invaders. Their quantity is measured as a CD8 count. Normally there are about twice as many helper T-cells as suppressor T-cells. In immune deficiency diseases like AIDS, the CD4 to CD8 ratio is seriously out of balance, and the body is vulnerable to opportunistic infection; and
4. *Effector or cytotoxic T-cells*, which kill infected cells by binding highly specific receptors on their surface to antigens, breaking them apart. They learn to recognize invaders by previous exposure to macrophages. A subset of these T-cells is naturally cytotoxic without prior imprinting in the lymphoid organs. They are called natural killer or NK cells.

Natural Killer (NK) Cell Action

This T-cell activity merits special attention, because it is the primary indicator of a strong, healthy immune system. White cells (leukocytes) are measured to indicate the presence of infection. Unlike other white cells, the number of NK cells stays constant. NK cells are the first line of defense to an assault on the body. An NK cell will attach itself to an invading cell, such as *Candida albicans* or a cancer cell, and inject it with small granules it carries. These small granules act like explosive charges, destroying the foreign cell's membrane within a few minutes. After injection, the NK cell moves on to the next invader cell.

Healthy NK cells are able to attack two or more invaders simultaneously. Individuals with low NK activity cannot effectively fight off such conditions as Chronic Fatigue Syndrome, cancerous tumors, viral infections, and various autoimmune diseases such as lupus. The four-hour

51Chromium-release assay test can determine NK cell activity. See Chapter 7 for ways to increase NK cell activity naturally.

B-cells. B-lymphocytes also begin in the bone marrow and mature there. B-cells have a shorter life span than T-cells. As they mature, B-cells become specialized plasma cells that reside in the lymph nodes and in the spleen. When stimulated by an antigen, these B-lymphocytes become antibody-producing factories.[3] Once they have created a specific antibody to combat a particular pathogen, these B-cells remember this information to be ready for a future attack. This process is called "building resistance." The immune system requires sulfur-containing amino acids for the formation of antibodies. These amino acids must be a part of regular nutritional intake for the immune system to function properly. Diet and supplements are discussed in Chapter 7.

Antibodies

There are two types of immune response: (1) cell-mediated and (2) humoral antibody response. The first is characterized by the production of cells that recognize and bind antigens on the surface of foreign cells. This binding action kills cells in the case of viral infections and induces other cells (macrophages) to participate in the immune system reaction. The cell-mediated response involves T-lymphocytes.

The humoral antibody response refers to antibodies that circulate in the bloodstream and bond to antigens. This bonding renders the antigens easier for phagocytes to ingest. The humoral antibody response involves B-lymphocytes, and activates a system of blood proteins called complement, which destroys the antigen.

Antibodies are Y-shaped protein molecules called immunoglobulins (Ig) produced by the B-cells. There are five classes of antibodies: IgA, IgD, IgE, IgG, and IgM. All are functionally distinct from one another, but all are designed to defend against invading bacteria, viruses and microbes.

IgA and IgE are found in our bodily secretions, i.e., in saliva and in the mucous membranes of the lungs, genitals, and intestinal tract. IgA antibody production increases during exercise, lovemaking, and laughter. The latter is the source of the phrase "laughter is the best medicine." While IgA is on the alert for invading bacteria and viruses, IgE work with sentry-like mast cells to combat allergens and parasites. IgE is the antibody responsible for allergic (anaphylactic) reactions.

An antibody does not destroy an invader by itself, but seizes the enemy with one of the branches of its "Y," holding it for destruction by complements C1 through C9. These complex blood proteins attack in a linear formation, piercing the cell wall of the invader cell so that its insides spill out. Macrophages and neutrophils are then signaled to dispose of the mess. The complements contain carbon, hydrogen, oxygen, and nitrogen, and they bind to B-cells and some of the immunoglobulins. IgG is the major serum antibody activating complement and binding to phagocytes. Antioxidant vitamins enhance the health of complements.

The first immunoglobulin synthesized in response to a foreign antigen is usually IgM, and the effect occurs during the first week after exposure. Over the following weeks, production of immunoglobulin switches to IgG. Subsequent exposure to the antigen stimulates IgG production directly.

Phagocytes

We have examined the first type of immune system cells (lymphocytes). The second type (phagocytes) move through the blood stream to an injury site where they either destroy the invader or produce antibodies to do so. A few types of phagocytes can ingest other cells, microbes, and foreign particles. Vitamin C enhances the motility of phagocytes, that is, their ability to be attracted to a target and travel to it. Excessive levels of zinc suppress this ability.

Phagocytes destroy their target by releasing strong free radicals such as hydrogen peroxide and superoxide anion. Phagocytes store antioxidants vitamin C and the amino acid glutathione, regulating the balance between free radicals and antioxidants to ensure their survival during the attack.

There are two main groups of phagocytes: myeloid cells (granulocytes) and monocytes. Myeloid cells contain toxic granules of nitric oxide used to engulf and digest invaders. Examples of granulocytes are basophils, mast cells, neutrophils, and eosinophils. Monocytes are short-lived, their task being to dispose of waste produced after immune system battles. They also destroy pathogens like bacteria, viruses, and cancer cells by creating nitric oxide from the amino acid L-arginine.

These specialized phagocytes become macrophages (from the Latin "big eaters"), which eat their fill of these post-battle wastes, die, and are expelled from the body as the pus and mucus seen at the site of the infection. The phlegm we expel during a cold is the collection of macrophages—dead immune cells. Tumors protect themselves by producing the enzyme arginase that breaks down L-arginine. A study in England suggests that a diet supplemented with L-arginine may be beneficial in treating cancer. [4]

Mast cells

These large cells act as lookouts, triggering a quick response to an invasion of allergens or parasites. IgE in turn triggers the release of histamines to increase immune response and blood flow. When we take antihistamines at the first sign of an allergic reaction, we are reducing the symptoms but at the same time suppressing the immune system and allowing the attack to get out of hand. The symptoms of allergic reaction are really a manifestation of natural histamine production. One of the best ways to relieve the symptoms (whether in the lungs during an asthma attack or in the sinuses) is to increase consumption of pure water.

Mast cells are large cells found just under the skin, in the gut, in the nasal passages, lungs, and urinary tract. They are found in unusually high numbers in the bowels of those suffering from Crohn's Disease and Irritable Bowel Syndrome (IBS).[5]

The use of antiallergy and asthma drugs that suppress mast cell action should be reassessed. Future research may reveal that there is an association between these drugs and vulnerability to respiratory illnesses and infectious diseases. Effective therapeutic use of antihistamines may require more or less use in specific circumstances or in a certain timed sequence with other drugs.

Recent studies support the hypothesis that mast cell activity can lead to resistance to certain infections.[6] A Duke University team found a molecule called CD48 on the surface of mast cells. The CD48 molecule recognizes a protein called FimH formed on the hair-like tips of many infectious bacteria. Sensing this FimH protein, the mast cell alerts the immune system by releasing a substance called Tumor Necrosis Factor-alpha (TNF). Being able to stimulate

CD48 activity, as needed, could mean progress in the treatment of people with dysfunctional immune systems.

Hormones

Investigators were for a time in the 1950s convinced that hormonal deficiency was the cause of arthritis. Hormone therapy may provide some relief for RA sufferers; however, the benefit derives from the regulation of the immune system. Since every cell in the body participates in the immune system, a brief discussion of the endocrine system and hormones is in order.

The endocrine system's ductless glands and the hormones they secrete on demand enable changes in the metabolic actions of the body's tissues. Hormones enable the body to cope with stress, infection, trauma, and changes in temperature. They control reproduction, growth, and the development of essential bodily fluids. The endocrine glands include the hypothalamus, thymus, pituitary, thyroid, parathyroid, adrenal medulla and cortex, pancreas, testicles, ovaries, and, during pregnancy, placenta. The gut makes several hormones that regulate digestion. The kidneys generate a hormone that stimulates red cell production. The brain contains at least 45 different kinds of neurotransmitters, many of which act as hormones elsewhere in the body.

The thymus has two functions: an important gland of the immune system and an endocrine organ assisting in the defense of the body against infection. The thymus produces hormones that stimulate T- and B-cells to develop some measure of immunity against microbes and tumors by prompting interferon production.

A cell under fatal attack by a virus creates a type of protein called *interferon* to warn other cells of the serious impending infection. The warned cells create antiviral substances to stop the virus from replicating in uninfected cells. Synthetic interferon created in the laboratory is sold at high cost as a cure for cancer and for Hepatitis C. The drug has serious side effects and does not always work as advertised.

Interleukins are hormones that coordinate the battle conducted by immune system cells. One type of interleukin points T-cells to their targets and tells them when to create interferon, to escalate the immune system response by calling upon NK cells, and to stimulate B-cells to produce antibodies. The body creates interleukins naturally when one is excited, happy, exercising, indulging in a satisfying project, pursuing one's bliss, and generally enjoying life. Both interferon and interleukin are lymphokines, the type of hormone that both infected cells and T-cells create to mobilize the other cells in the immune system.

The adrenals produce steroid hormones, including cortisone, which reduce inflammation by strengthening the membrane of lysosomes, the cell structures that release inflammatory substances. Inflammation of local tissues is designed to stop the spread of infection to other parts of the body. When too much cortisone is present, the lymph glands wither, and this in turn depresses immunity.

The natural hormones usually have no harmful side effects, unlike their synthetic counterparts. When the body produces too little of a particular hormone or enzyme, physicians can usually treat the condition successfully by augmenting or replacing the substance. In cases of hormone excess, operation or radiation is the usual treatment.

Proteins and Enzymes

Collagen as a structural protein is a component of almost every tissue in the body. In most of the rheumatic diseases, the collagen of the blood vessels is destroyed as well as the connective joint tissues. The enzyme collagenase is stored primarily in white cell granules called lysosomes. When an irritant attaches to tissue cells, white cells rush to the site to release lysosomes of collagenase and other digestive enzymes whose purpose is to destroy the foreign invader causing the irritation. If excessive collagenase is released because there are too many localized white blood cells, the result is the destruction of surrounding tissues as well as the invader.

A palliative solution is either to remove the surplus white blood cells or to chemically inhibit the enzymes they produce. While this technique will stop the spread of inflammation, it may leave the irritant in place and does not stop the disease. Most NSAIDs work to limit lysosomal enzyme action.[7]

---

[1] Olfson, Mark, MD, MPH; Marcus, Steven C., PhD; Druss, Benjamin, MD; Elinson, Lynn, PhD; Tanielian, Terri and Pincus, Harold A., MD. "National Trends in the Outpatient Treatment of Depression." JAMA. 2002; 287:203-209.

[2] An excellent well-illustrated overview can be found in "Life, Death and the Immune System." Special Issue of *Scientific American*, September 1993. See also Dixon (1986) and Roitt, et al. (1989).

[3] Rosenberg (1992) pp. 79-80.

[4] *Alternatives*. November 1994; 5:17.

[5] Galli, Dr. Stephen J., et al. "Mast Cells Stimulate Immune Response Against Bacteria." *Proceedings of the National Academy of Science*, July 1999; 96:1-6.

[6] Op. cit.

[7] Clark (1997), p. 110.

3. HOW INFECTION WORKS

Inflammation is the way the body generally responds to infection or other form of trauma, such as impact or muscle damage. We are all familiar with the signs of pain, swelling, warmth, and redness associated with this kind of trauma. These symptoms are beneficial because cells of the immune system are attracted to the injured area where they fight the infection, then clear away the debris in preparation for tissue regrowth and repair.

CAUSES OF INFLAMMATION

Chemicals known as cytokines and prostaglandins control the infection process, and are released in an orderly and self-limiting manner. When the immune system is functioning properly, inflammation is beneficial. It is the body's way of ridding itself of potentially harmful agents such as bacteria and viruses.

A significant problem arises when the process does not end at the appropriate time. That is, a trauma or infection may trigger inflammation, but the immune system continues to fight in an unabated active state. This is the essence of the autoimmune theory that the medical community ascribes to RA. During this complex process, the body responds by moving calcium to the site, forming nodules—dry, gritty, calcium hydroxyapatite crystals—that clump around the invading microbes. These nodules can be seen as "hot spots" on a radioisotope scan picture or MRI.[1]

Many of the natural chemicals generated by the immune system are those that cause the pain of RA and, over time, can damage cartilage. The drugs prescribed to relieve RA pain are in fact trying to inhibit this natural chemical overproduction but they do not remove the root cause of the inflammation.

In RA, inflammation is directed toward the synovium, or joint lining. Nearby blood vessels enlarge, new blood vessels form, and joint fluid increases, creating tenderness and pain in and around the joint, usually with stiffness, visible swelling, and redness. A low-grade fever, along with swollen lymph nodes—glands of the immune system that produce lymphocytes—may indicate systemic or regional inflammation. Fatigue is one symptom of inflammation. Calcium nodules of accumulated inflammatory tissue may appear in the lungs and on the skin. The more prominent and painful these nodules, the more serious the RA condition. Many patients with known infections exhibit RA signs and symptoms although they are not formally diagnosed with RA.

All forms of RA have an inflammatory component, show evidence of connective/synovial tissue damage, and are under the aegis of a process *resembling* the autoimmune reaction. This is perhaps because the invaders bind to normal cells and can still occasionally be detected as foreign. In a genuine autoimmune reaction, the body attacks its own cells, but in RA the reaction is actually the body's natural defense against an infection in the connective tissues. This struggle is the cause of the inflammation, pain, and disfiguring effects of RA since the disease agent is connected to the cell. When the disease agent is removed, the fight ceases. However, the autoimmune theory has become so entrenched in American medical school teaching that other options have not been considered until very recently.[2]

One example of a misnamed "autoimmune disorder" where the linkage to mycobacterial infestation is usually undetected is the development of acute rheumatic fever following a streptococcal infection. Individuals who show evidence of nodules at the joints—a classic and disfiguring symptom of arthritis—are frequently those who have a history of streptococcal infections, usually going back to childhood.[3]

Dr. Brown found that diagnostic tests could detect streptococcal antibodies still present, along with the residual strep bacterial L-forms. He recommended that antistreptococcal treatment using penicillin (or one of its derivatives) first be used to lower the streptococcal level before attempting to eradicate these L-forms. Mycobacteria and other bacteria have the ability to lose part or all of their cell walls when attacked by antibiotics. This transformation to an L-form allows these microbes to elude antibiotic attack and regrow cell walls later.

The problem with using penicillin derivatives is that drug allergies may occur over time, and this limits their usefulness. Furthermore, penicillin induces the bacteria-to-L-form transformation without being effective in combating the L-forms.

Now, however, with Polymerase Chain Reaction (PCR) analysis of synovial fluid it is possible to detect the genetic material of the mycoplasmal microorganisms, L-forms and other agents of rheumatoid arthritis and reactive arthritis. Much of the research is originating outside the United States, but American scientists are gradually beginning to explore the possibility of bacterial infection in RA, confirming the findings of Dr. Brown.[4] Patients with other diagnoses such as Lyme Disease or Fibromyalgia and who test positive for mycoplasma or Chlamydia also exhibit RA signs and symptoms. A detailed discussion of PCR testing appears in Chapter 6.

Studies have isolated antigens to several gastro-intestinal pathogens from the synovial fluid in patients with reactive arthritis. The most common pathogens found were *Salmonella, Shigella, Yersinia, Borrelia, and Campylobacter.*[5]

THE ROLE OF MYCOPLASMAS

Mycoplasmas were discovered in 1898 and given different names starting in 1910. In 1941 the first classification and nomenclature system was established, but did not catch on because of the ambiguity between mycoplasmas with bacterial L-forms. In 1956, the current classification system was adopted consisting of a single order, *Mycoplasmatales*, containing a single family, *Mycoplasmataceae*, with a single genus, *Mycoplasma*, and fifteen species. Today there are over 100 documented species,[6] although more recent PCR analysis indicates that some previously named species may be identical. Not all mycoplasmas are harmful. Some are benign (in the tissues, blood, and gut) and others can be pathogenic (in the joints and synovial tissue.)

Mycoplasmas are but one class of hundreds of types of organisms residing in our bodies, part of the indigenous microbial flora primarily of the pharynx and genitourinary tract.[7] Most of the time these bacteria are benign, but when they increase in abnormal numbers or a new strain is detected, the body's immune system reacts to suppress the condition, just as it does when an externally caused infection occurs. Dr. Brown found that the mycobacteria and mycoplasmas could be two causes of arthritis as well as lupus and Scleroderma, since they seem to bind to host cell membranes and make those cells a target for a defensive immune system response.

Mycoplasmas seem to have an affinity for certain parts of the body and attach themselves there, waiting for the right time to emerge. Experimental animal research has shown that some strains of mycoplasmas, once isolated, migrate without exception to the joints.[8] Drs Joel Baseman and Joseph Tully point out that, "It has been suggested that [*M. arthritidis*]-related superantigen-like molecules may exist in mycoplasmas of human origin triggering auto-immune and other inflammatory pathologies."[9] When this assertion is credibly tested it will show that mycoplasmal infections are the *trigger* for autoimmune disorders and will perhaps lead researchers to look beyond the traditionally held belief that such disorders occur because the immune system is malfunctioning.

Microorganisms stimulate an autoimmune reaction in the following ways:

- Incorporating host antigen structures into their cell membranes. I.e., when mycoplasmas are released from cells they bud from the cell membrane like viruses but in contrast to viruses, they do not exclude all host glycoproteins (antigens) from their membranes when they are released. These host antigens can stimulate a concomitant immune response when the host responds against the microorganism;
- Certain microorganisms, such as mycoplasmas and some bacteria, use molecular mimicry to "hide" from the host's immune system. This can set off an autoimmune response to the normal antigen being mimicked;
- Some bacteria carry "super antigens" that strongly stimulate the host's immune response; and

- Some bacteria and viruses kill normal host cells, releasing large quantities of normal antigens that may trigger an autoimmune response.

The current medical theory regarding autoimmune disorders is based on the notion of the immune system attacking a single invading/infecting organism in the *in vitro* form, as observed in a test culture, not *in vivo*, i.e., within the body. Infections such as malaria, protozoas, and streptococcus have been studied *in vitro* at prestigious medical centers such as the Lister Institute in France. However, mycoplasmas and L-forms are resident, *in vivo* parasitic "invaders" that become active from time to time to obtain nutrients, expel wastes, breed, and migrate out of the body to form new colonies. These actions precipitate an allergic reaction that appears to be an autoimmune disorder since no external cause for the reaction is detected by current testing methods.

In April 1994, National Institutes of Health (NIH) researcher Dr. Polly Matzinger, head of the T-cell Tolerance and Memory section at the NIH's National Institute of Allergy and Infectious Diseases (NIAID) proposed that what spurs the immune system is a distress call from dying cells. Matzinger argues that T-cells require a signal from critical white blood cells (dendritic cells, which inhabit every tissue of the body) to initiate action. The dendritic cells lie dormant until cells nearby call out in shock. This provides a specific example of the general description by Dr. Brown for the reaction of microbes to antibiotics and resultant Jarisch-Herxheimer reaction.

Dr. Matzinger's nontraditional point of view about the immune response is under investigation at the NIH and elsewhere.[10] Her observation that T-cells don't attack *all* "foreign-looking" substances, e.g., milk proteins from newly lactating breasts in pubescent females, led her to question the central "self/nonself" metaphor of immunology held since the early 1900s. She claims that immunosuppressive drugs such as cyclosporine are often ineffective because they block signals between T-cells and transplants but don't block the alarm that cells in shock send to dendritic cells.

Shape-Changing Organisms

We know from the study of many forms of life that metamorphic changes during the lifespan of an organism run from initial seed through several shape and structure changes, with interim stable forms that adapt to the particular life phase and to the environment, and then change back to seed form again. This ability to alter shape and structure is called pleomorphism. It is probably the combined result of evolution and the many climatic and environmental changes the evolving organism has faced and to which it has had to adapt over hundreds of millions of years and perhaps trillions of trillions of generations.

Thus, the vulnerability of one shape or form to an attack or environment change can be circumvented by a shape change so that the organism will evolve specific R-factors to ensure resistance to an attack.

In the laboratory, L-forms so closely resemble mycoplasmas because both lack cell walls that at one time all mycoplasmas were referred to as L-form bacteria. We know now that mycoplasmas have no enzymes, a feature required to transition to an L-form.

According to Dr. Brown, mycoplasmas and bacterial L-forms are vulnerable to various attacks by tetracycline antibiotics in a different way than penicillins, which attack the normal streptococcus cell/cell chain forms, causing mycoplasmas to transition to the L-form (with reduced or absent cell wall) as an act of survival. Erythromycin and the tetracyclines have broad-spectrum effects on mycoplasmas and other forms of infection when used in a low-dose, long-term manner. Sometimes to kill both forms of an organism it is necessary to use both a penicillin and a tetracycline. Current medical doctrine may still suggest that these antibiotics should not be used together.

Penicillin antibiotics temporarily decrease the phagoctyic, or germ-eating, capacity of leukocytes. The tetracycline family of antibiotics is different from other antibiotics in that it affects the interior of the cell and not the membrane. Specifically, tetracycline inhibits 30-40% of the normal folic acid synthesis, which eventually kills the invading microorganism. It is well to note that aspirin-type medications, such as NSAIDs used conventionally in high doses to treat RA, also deplete folic acid.[11] The question is: Should folic acid supplements be used to offset the loss caused by tetracycline or NSAIDs, or will restoring folic acid to the normal level help the infectious microorganism survive? Further scientific research is needed to determine this balance.

Chronic pneumonia is a good prototype for what happens when a mycoplasma infection becomes fixed around a certain area.[12] Nodules of granulation material—inflamed tissues that surround the infectious organism for months—produce the characteristic cough of the disease. A similar phenomenon happens around the RA sufferer's joints.[13] The body must be trained to defend itself with minimal help from external agents such as antibiotics. This is the reason for very low tetracycline dosage over a period of weeks or months. However, there are certainly circumstances where the only means to cure a chronic cough or other persistent infection is with antibiotics of a specific type, prescribed for short duration.

Souvenirs of Childhood Illnesses

We carry mycoplasmas and L-forms with us as remnants of childhood infections such as pneumonia, strep throat, bronchitis, rheumatic fever, or other early illnesses. Mycoplasmas are not viruses, since they do not require living cells in which to grow. Mycoplasmas are included within a separate class (Mollicutes) of bacteria because they have lost the ability to develop a cell wall. This makes them harder to see and much harder to culture *in vitro*.[14] They are specifically adapted to certain cellular environments by their genetic nature, which is quite robust in its complexity, having adapted and evolved over millions of years. Micro-organisms such as mycoplasmas often lie dormant, waiting for conditions to be favorable for propagation. This would explain conditions such as rheumatoid arthritis, Chronic Fatigue Syndrome (CFS), or Gulf War Illness, which seem to strike suddenly.

It is not necessary for the whole mycoplasma micro-organism to be present for a reaction in a joint or tissue to be provoked. Mere fragments are sufficient to create a powerful antigenic reaction that causes the body to produce antibodies to counter it. These antigens are constructed by the host's cells from bits of pathogenic protein and cellular proteins called major histocompatibility complex (MHC) molecules. The processing and assembly of antigens are the keys to understanding the flexibility, specificity, and thoroughness of all immune responses.[15] The antibody reaction may be mainly against a "host antigen" carried on the mycoplasmal membrane.

Affinity of mycoplasmas or L-forms of cellular bacteria for the tissue and fluid of the joints has been recognized since the 1890s. Experiments by Dr. Brown and Jack Nunemaker in the 1930s demonstrated that the L-form they studied was a variant of the *Streptobacillus* organism.

The cellular bacteria was able to lose its capsule and cell wall and enter a state in which it could become invisible, pass through a filter, and return to the parent form, re-growing its cell walls. *Chlamydia* is another example of a bacterial organism capable of both walled and wall-less states.[16] L-forms can reproduce but the rates are slower than that of the cellular form.

This cloaking capability explains how L-forms are able to "go underground," transmutate, and reemerge after the immune system attack on the bacterial form has subsided, returning to assault injured cells aggressively. An immune system weakened by addictive drugs, anti-depressants, or improper diet is unable to produce the quantity and quality of natural antibodies to stave off this new attack.[17]

Studies in 1994-1996 on ear infections in children concluded that L-forms as atypical forms of bacteria may play an important role in the bacteriologic aspect of secretory *Otitis media*. Both Turkish[18] and New Zealand[19] research groups point out the failure of conventional culture methods to identify the responsible pathogen(s). Further, the researchers admit that some agents are capable of changing bacterial behavior and consequently the clinical course of action. A Russian study[20] identified persistent forms of bacteria that performed antigenic mimicry or otherwise protected themselves against the host's immune system response.

These studies indicate that a comprehensive reexamination of L-forms is long overdue. This could open up a whole new field of infectious-disease pathology where new methods are developed for the isolation and identification of causative agents in bacterial infections. New theories of etiology provide an understanding of bacterial vulnerability.

Mycoplasmas and Autoimmune Diseases

There are several reasons why mycoplasmal infection can play a role in autoimmune diseases:

- **Cell shape modification**. As mycoplasmas replicate within invaded body cells and are released from host cells, they seize antigens from the surface of the host cell and incorporate these within their outer surface membranes. The immune system detects the hybrids and learns to antagonize parts of familiar antigen shapes. Then it launches a response against these semi-familiar antigens, in turn triggering an autoimmune reaction. Mycoplasmas may also attach to familiar blood lipoprotein molecules so that the body's immune responses are confused, and cross-reactivity results.
- **Infiltrated T-cells**. Standard microbiology textbooks state that the host's cells carry MHC molecules on their surfaces. In infected cells, these MHC molecules bind to and display small peptides from the parasite. It is this combination of MHC molecules and peptides that forms antigens recognizable by T-cells and what makes them candidates for destruction. What the textbooks may overlook is that infiltrated and compromised T-cells will not attack infected cells that carry fellow parasitic organisms.
- **Mimicry of normal cells**. Mycoplasmal antigens seem to be able to mimic host antigens or to attach to familiar blood lipoprotein molecules. The body's immune responses are confused, and cross-reactivity results.
- **Apoptosis simulation**. Another possibility is that mycoplasmas can cause apoptosis or "programmed

death" of host cells, after which normal host antigens are released and the body reacts with an autoimmune response.[21] A defective apoptosis gene has been found to be a factor in prostate cancer.[22] Mycoplasmas are found in seminal fluid. Similarly, a defective apoptosis gene might contribute to the continued viability of mycoplasma-invaded prostate cells.

THE PUZZLE OF RA FLARE-UPS

One of the enduring puzzles of so-called autoimmune disorders is that they all go through cycles of exacerbation and remission. Researchers and physicians must integrate the insights from their specialized fields with the knowledge we have gained about nutrition.

Recognizing that bacteria and their L-forms trigger allergies, which can be suppressed, and that remissions can be maintained by low-dose, long-term anti-mycoplasma antibiotic therapy is an important beginning. Hundreds of experiments on animals have proved that mycoplasmas are important cofactors in arthritis and other chronic rheumatic disorders and that the tetracycline family of antibiotics suppresses mycoplasmal infections.

Mycoplasmas are capable of long-term intercellular *in vivo* survival and slow replication, so they may be resident and waiting for some trauma or barometric pressure changes to activate them when the host's immune system has moderated its operation. Thus the progression of the infection is cyclical, with waves of reemergence followed by withdrawal to less detectable forms.

Therefore, when mycoplasmas act as antigenic substances, triggering internal allergic responses, they release toxins intermittently to a sensitized area, subsiding and then reappearing. Antibodies move through the body via white blood cells and platelets, and it is through this means that RA migrates from shoulder to hand to knee as the antibodies launch counterattacks against local toxins. The antibodies move on to new battlefields whenever migrating antigens like mycoplasmas flare up. Dr. Brown compares the antibodies' movement and fight against antigens to smoke jumpers carried by airplane from one brush fire to the next. Wherever some "fires" are temporarily quenched, the body enjoys some brief respite.[23]

There are several bacterial components capable of inducing arthritis. For example, experiments using animals with *Streptococcus* have shown that systemic injections of group A *Streptococcus pyogenes* lead to acute arthritis that peaks in a few days, then subsides, only to recur as inflamed joints a few weeks later, eventually causing joint destruction. There are several enigmas in the streptococcal arthritis model that parallel those of reactive arthritis, one of which is that arthritis (and other chronic disorders such as CFS and Fibromyalgia) can be precipitated by an assortment of completely different organisms. Researchers admitted that "the mechanism of recurrence of acute episodes in humans has yet to be defined."[24]

This type of ebb and flow explains the types of flare-ups that RA sufferers describe. It also explains the apparent causal relationship between changes in the weather and RA pain. Clinical evidence shows that two environmental factors can cause flare-ups: (1) a sudden drop in barometric pressure and (2) the presence of high humidity in conjunction with this drop. In the 1930s, Dr. Joseph Hollander, head of rheumatology at the University of Pennsylvania performed studies of the effects of barometric pressure on rheumatoid disease along with such other factors as temperature, humidity, and oxygen. Volunteers were confined to sealed, climatically controlled rooms, recording their impressions of how they felt each hour while subtle changes in their environment were made. The barometric effects were approximately those of atmospheric conditions prior to a storm. The aches and pains reported by volunteers corresponded to a sudden release of antigens to a sensitized area, confirming Dr. Brown's theory that shape-changing or migrating mycoplasmas could be acting as antigenic triggers.

The mechanism of migration of the infectious forms from host to host has not been determined. It might be related to this barometric pressure change. Prior to storms and wet weather periods, there are increases in colds. As the microorganisms migrate out of the body they stimulate respiratory distress, thus broadcasting their seeds via effluvia (e.g., sneezing) to other mammalian hosts.

RA patients also experience a higher incidence of flare-ups in the late spring and early fall. Some physicians[25] see an allergy connection, but attribute these reactions to specific environmental substances that are assimilated into the body and reach reactive sites throughout the body via the bloodstream. However, such externally caused allergic reactions do not explain sensitivity to barometric pressure.

The closer one gets to sea level, the higher the concentration of oxygen. Arthritics do not fare as well at higher altitudes as they do nearer sea level, because in the thinner air their cells are starved for oxygen. This explains the pain and swelling in the joints arthritis sufferers experience after a long airplane journey.

Trauma to joints and tendons may cause structural changes, further reducing oxygen transport and limiting removal of fluids and wastes in the region of the injury. The lack of oxygen in the traumatized area increases pressure and swelling. Several of the herbal remedies described in Appendix I improve blood oxygenation.

SUPPRESSING MYCOPLASMAS

Dr. Brown and his associates accumulated significant evidence that mycoplasmas and their L-forms were at the root of RA, as seen in the impressive list of published laboratory results included in *The Road Back*. They discovered that tetracyclines were a group of antibiotics that could kill or radically suppress mycoplasma and L-form growth in the laboratory. They also found that tetracyclines could help RA conditions to improve when administered in a low, controlled dose over a long period (months to years), depending on the severity of the condition and whether there were other bacterial complications adding to the sensitizing process. In these cases other antibiotics could treat the other bacteria. Specific and detailed antibiotic treatment protocols can be found on the Internet.[26]

Dr. Brown's research findings explain why arthritis remedies such as quinine, bee venom, gold salts, and copper have been used over many centuries: it is because these substances have also been found to be effective in suppressing the growth of mycoplasmas *in vitro*.

Quinine

The colonial British stationed in Africa learned of the benefits of quinine in the 1800s as a cure for malaria, a mosquito-borne *Plasmodium* parasite. Quinine is derived from the bark of several species of *Cinchona* and during the 17th century was brought to Europe from South America, where it was used to allay fever and pain, dilate the larger blood vessels, and generally relax muscle tissue. Quinine contains alkaloids, which are active organic compounds containing at least one nitrogen atom. Traditional usage is a very small dose, which is more toxic to the parasite than to the host. Alkaloids are potentially toxic in large amounts (e.g., morphine).

Quinine sulfate is both inexpensive and effective in reducing bursitis, tendonitis, and synovitis pain. Sadly, it has been removed from the commercial market in the United States, Europe, and South America since malaria is not considered to be the global scourge it once was. Other antimalarial drugs are effective against arthritis, but they are more expensive and also require a prescription.

Bee Venom

Analysis of bee venom shows that it contains the proteins mellitin and apamine, which cause the pituitary and adrenal glands to produce cortisone. This natural hormone is an effective and dramatic anti-inflammatory that does not produce the devastating side effects of artificial cortisone. A succession of bee venom immunization treatments has been reputed to be a cure for arthritis. However, this approach runs the risk of death in some individuals by fatal anaphylactic shock. The treatment is therefore avoided by the medical profession for insurance reasons.[27]

Copper and Gold

Copper jewelry is often advertised as an arthritis pain reducer. The way copper works is similar to gold. Skin acid dissolves the copper into Cu++ ions in sulfate and chloride forms. The green color visible on the skin after contact with copper or gold indicates the presence of sulfate. A very small amount of the cupric ions are absorbed through the skin and pass into the blood and tissue near the point of contact. Copper in concentrations of more than 10 mg[28], like gold salts, can be poisonous, but a more diluted amount works to suppress mycoplasmas and L-form metamorphosed *Streptococcus pneumonia*. Copper (2mg) as an amino acid chelate is sold in health food stores as a mineral supplement. Oysters are rich in copper.

Tetracyclines

For thirty years, Dr. Brown's persistence in claiming that RA should be viewed as a bacterial allergy, treatable with anti-mycoplasmic tetracyclines, has run counter to the prevailing view of how antibiotics should be administered. Antibiotics such as penicillin have always been seen as a short-term, high-dosage response used to treat pneumonia, strep throat, bronchitis, and other bacterial disorders. They are not usually prescribed over an extended period because physicians believe, rightly, that germs will become more resistant to the antibiotic.

This reasoning applies to the typical course for a prescribed antibiotic treatment, which is 10-14 days. If the patient shows no signs of significant improvement, another class of antibiotic is usually given. Also, if the antibiotic *is* effective so that the mycoplasmas die and the patient experiences an uncomfortable Jarisch-Herxheimer reaction, s/he may opt to discontinue the antibiotic treatment and not resume.

The form and dosage are very important, but pills are more convenient than injections or painful intravenous drip infusions. However, that latter are the best ways to administer antibiotics, since the concentration is higher and more controlled. Also, infusion or injection avoids the GI tract and thus minimally changes the environment of any of the hundreds of natural and useful organisms that reside in the digestive system.

Dr. Brown emphasized that a low dose of tetracycline over a long period of time will not have the usual effect of a sudden influx of antibiotics, which can interfere with the ability of the immune system to limit fungal infections such as *Candida albicans*. Since the mid-1980s, streptomycin-resistant forms of bacteria have developed because of the use of pills, which were not 100% effective, and short-term assaults that left behind a cadre of evolved, resilient organisms.

There are four different tetracyclines presently available: simple tetracycline, oxytetracycline, doxycycline, and minocycline (trade name Minocin).

Tetracycline antibiotics kill bacteria by disabling the ribosome part of their cell structure and inhibiting the cell's metabolism. Ribosomes are one of the required components necessary for protein synthesis from amino acids. Bacteria develop resistance by shielding themselves with one type of protein and creating another to eject the antibiotic from the cell.[29] Drug companies are working on ways to target these defensive proteins.[30]

Dr. Brown's research showed that when tetracycline is used to suppress the defensive envelope the organism builds around itself, the body's own disease-fighting capability can combat it effectively and the RA is eventually driven into remission. Tetracycline antibiotics are among the few that are effective against virtually all species of mycoplasmas, with relatively low toxicity and few side effects.[31] Physicians have used oxytetracycline for decades to treat adolescent acne with minimal adverse effects.

Drs Baseman and Tully further vindicate Dr. Brown and his antibiotic approach, saying, "The occurrence of various *Mycoplasma* and *Ureaplasma* species in joint tissues of patients with rheumatoid arthritis, sexually transmitted reactive arthritis, and other human arthritides can no longer be ignored. A clinical trial of long-term (6 to 12 months) antibiotic (doxycycline) therapy before cartilage destruction might prove beneficial in managing such frequent and often debilitating infections."

Dr. Brown also found that those individuals who use oxytetracycline over a period of months or years tend to avoid colds, pneumonia, and other respiratory diseases. Other benefits include elimination of chronic cough and reduction of Irritable Bowel Syndrome. Tetracycline antibiotics are effective against a wide range of bacteria and L-forms.[32] The following are the plus and minus factors of using tetracycline[33]:

- side effect reduction/prevention: none known;
- depletion of, or interference with, potassium, folic acid, Vitamins B_2, B_6, B_{12}, C, and K;
- sensitivity to sunburn;
- supportive interaction with Vitamin C, probiotics, Vitamin B_3 (niacinamide only, for *bullous pemphigoid dermatitis herpetiformis*);
- adverse herbal interaction to goldenseal, Oregon grape, barberry; and
- reduced drug absorption/bioavailability of minerals (aluminum, calcium, magnesium, iron, zinc)

Minocycline

According to Dr. Mercola, who prescribes Dr. Brown's protocol with proven success, Minocin has a distinct and clear advantage over simple tetracycline and doxycycline in three important areas:

1. Extended spectrum of activity
2. Greater tissue penetrability
3. Higher and more sustained serum levels

Dr. Mercola advises taking Lederle brand Minocin since nearly all generic minocycline is clearly not as effective in penetrating tissues. He also stresses that Minocin not be given with iron, else over 85% of the dose will bind to the iron and pass through the colon unabsorbed. Dr. Nicolson further advises that *all* metals and mineral supplements be avoided while taking Minocin. Full details of Dr. Brown's antibiotic protocol, modified and improved by Dr. Mercola and written for physicians, are shown in Appendix II.

Test results from individuals suffering from arthritis who participate in double-blind tests with tetracyclines are not typically interpreted correctly because these tests are designed to look for a rapid linear response within a six-month period. Some chronic disease conditions do not react to a long-term, low-dose antibiotic treatment in such a short amount of time. Some conditions may require years. When the treatment is discontinued, a relapse occurs. These antibiotics are so effective in suppressing mycoplasmas that a reaction called the Jarisch-Herxheimer effect develops. This phenomenon is described later in this chapter.

One 1995 study[34] showed that RA may be caused by, exacerbated by, or have relapses triggered by a persistent infection of *Mycoplasma* or *Chlamydia*. Treatments with minocycline have shown positive results. This study is significant because it was conducted over the course of nearly a year. Some of the 219 participants were as young as 18 years of age. The improvement associated with the minocycline treatment suggests that a longer, protracted infection such as that caused by mycoplasmas contributes to RA. Another minocycline study showed as much as 50% improvement for 65% of the test subjects.[35]

Dr. Gabe Mirkin notes that five significant controlled studies show that minocycline drops the rheumatoid factor towards zero and helps both to alleviate pain and to retard cartilage destruction in rheumatoid arthritis patients.[36] In his August 1999 newsletter[37], Dr. Mirkin cites a study[38] showing that more than half of RA sufferers are infected with mycoplasma. He has treated his patients successfully with minocycline.

Dr. A. Robert Franco, head of the Arthritis Center of Riverside, CA, has treated over a thousand RA patients successfully with Dr. Brown's antibiotic regimen since 1988.[39]

The featured presentation at the American Academy of Rheumatology in 1997 demonstrated that minocycline is the safest and least costly drug for RA, and is also the most effective when given before extensive cartilage damage has occurred.[40] Dr. Mirkin deplores the fact that despite hundreds of papers showing that hundreds of different infections cause arthritis, most rheumatologists continue to treat RA with immunosuppressing drugs because they consider RA to be an autoimmune disease. According to Dr. Mirkin, these dangerously toxic drugs shorten the patient's life by an estimated ten years and increase cancer risk six fold.[41] The drugs are highly expensive, and merely dull pain rather than target the infection.[42]

Correcting Intestinal Flora Imbalance

Despite its success in fighting infection, long-term use of antibiotics runs the risk of upsetting the balance of intestinal microflora. This condition is called dysbiosis. Rotating the antibiotic every 4-5 years, even within the same antibiotic family, decreases the possibility of developing tolerance or damaging the ecology of the gastrointestinal (GI) tract.[43] The goal is to prevent chronic intestinal Candidiasis, but *Clostridium* toxins could perhaps present an even bigger problem.

Clostridium difficile is a major pathogen that causes a spectrum of antibiotic-associated intestinal disease from uncomplicated diarrhea to severe, life-threatening entero-colitis. It is nosocomial, i.e., usually contracted in hospitals and nursing homes. *C. difficile* disease is caused by the over-growth of the organism in the intestinal tract, primarily in the colon. The pathogen appears unable to compete successfully in the normal intestinal ecosystem, but can compete when normal flora are disturbed by antibiotics, allowing overgrowth of *C. difficile.* This organism then replicates and secretes two toxins: an enterotoxin that causes fluid accumulation in the bowel, and a potent cytotoxin.[44] These toxins are similar to the Borrelia-produced Lyme Disease toxin as well as other fat-soluble toxins resulting from exposure to substances like pesticides and molds. Lyme Disease and toxins are discussed in Chapter 5.

Supplementing the diet with *Lactobacillus acido-philus* and *L. bifidus* in refrigerated, powdered form helps maintain the ecological balance of normal intestinal flora that may be killed during antibiotic therapy. These probiotics are usually made from concentrated globulin whey protein. Those allergic to milk or dairy products should not use these substances. Timing is important. Dr. Nicolson recommends taking probiotics 2-3 hours after ingesting antibiotics for maximum benefit.

According to Dr. Mercola, recent studies[45] show that up to one third of beneficial bacteria products labeled "probiotics" do not contain the bacteria listed on the bottle. Moreover, they may actually contain some harmful strains. Ask for specifics on product content from the health food store or get specific recommendations on a trustworthy brand from Dr. Mercola's website, www.mercola.com.

Limiting the presence of antibiotics in the GI tract is important for another important reason. When antibiotics cause bacteria to change to their L-forms they are then more able to share and exchange plasmids—a virus-like form that enables genetic exchanges between micro-organisms. Plasmid exchange can result in a mutated bacterium that has learned how to combat antibiotics.

THE JARISCH-HERXHEIMER EFFECT

When the antibiotic is working effectively against the microorganism, a phenomenon called the Jarisch-Herxheimer effect sometimes occurs. The symptoms are those of an allergic reaction.[46] This effect may occur when a physician treats, for instance, a streptococcal infection with a penicillin-group antibiotic. One explanation is that the *Streptococcus* is not found at the site of the irritation, nor is it protected by inflamed or scarred tissue, as a mycoplasma would be.

The Jarisch-Herxheimer effect may at first appear to be an allergic reaction to the drug itself, and the physician (or the patient) may discontinue antibiotic treatment for that reason. However, the two responses can be distinguished. Allergic reactions to drugs are typically immediate and rapid, involving different actions of cytokines, and may be manifested as stomach upset, rash, or headache. The Jarisch-Herxheimer reactionon the other hand, manifests itself as an exacerbation of existing symptoms. It is caused by the rapid death of a colony of parasitic microorganisms releasing their internal toxic contents *in situ*.

According to Dr. Brown, with a bacterial allergy the mycoplasma creates a toxin barrier around itself that keeps the immune system's natural disease-fighting antibodies at bay. Tetracycline simply suppresses the toxin, the mycoplasma's means of defense. The fact that tetracycline causes the Jarisch-Herxheimer reaction demonstrates the presence of infection.[47] There may be more to it than that. With precise testing for mycoplasmal microorganisms and L-forms, perhaps by PCR or biochip methods, it may be possible to trace the origin of the infection and to see the relationship, for instance, between folic acid and fat-molecule destruction.

Dr. Mercola has found that those of his patients who follow strictly prescribed nutritional guidelines in his food program (Appendix V) in parallel with the improved Dr. Brown protocol (Appendix II) rarely experience a Jarisch-Herxheimer reaction.[48]

Natural antibiotic or antibacterial substances such as immune system-enhancing herbs and tonics may also produce a Jarisch-Herxheimer effect. As soon as this "allergic reaction" is noted, the individual should stop intake of the substance because the body's immune system needs time to train itself to deal with the infection and become stronger. Supplements of vitamins C and B_6 are helpful in countering the body's excessive histamine production during the course of the reaction.

This treatment method may seem counterintuitive, but it follows standard allergen immunization principles. The Jarisch-Herxheimer effect to some extent indicates success, but it cannot be endured for long without considerable discomfort, so treatment should be temporarily suspended or dosage reduced. Periodic resumption should be tried until the person gradually becomes immunized to the allergy trigger. The allergic reaction diminishes as the population of the invading organism is driven to zero. Cortisone or other corticosteroids or antihistamines may be used in conjunction with tetracyclines to permit higher doses of the antibiotic with acceptable levels of allergic reaction.

TOXIN BUILDUP

When antigens and antibodies clash, the result is destruction of cells and a sudden release of toxins, which are composed of a variety of diverse components—proteolytic enzymes, kinins, kallikreins, histamines, and other irritants.[49] The result of the struggle is pain and inflammation. As the mycoplasma antigen migrates to a new area, the antibodies follow it to this new combat zone, leaving the former battlefield to rest and heal, but toxins are left behind.

This pattern illustrates the migratory nature of RA. Arthritics complain of shoulder pain for a week or so, then pain in the hands or feet. The toxins released by the antigen-antibody conflict are often trapped in pockets of the bursa and are not promptly expelled through the various elimination organs of the body. These trapped toxins can create a mass of fluid or scar tissue that can bring pressure to bear upon the joints when blood vessels expand. Gravity assists in trapping toxins in the lower-extremity joints of the knees and feet. Excess weight and ill-fitting shoes, especially high heels, will exacerbate the pressure and pain on these swollen, irritated tissues.

Ways to expel these accumulated toxins are localized massage, herbs that stimulate circulation and eliminate toxins, increased water intake, and daily low-impact aerobic exercise followed by elevation of the lower legs to above-heart level several times per day using a slant board. The toxins will be loosened and drain into the bloodstream to be eliminated by the kidneys, skin, and lymphatic system. Topical application of DMSO may also be helpful in reducing pain and swelling, in combination with topical oil of wintergreen.

Clearance of bacteria from soft tissues appears to be of low priority importance as a host-defense mechanism during soft-tissue infection.[50] It may be that this is the reason mycoplasmas are able to establish a foothold early and have time to adapt to later assault by antibiotics.

Cloaking organisms like *Mycobacterium tuberculosis, M. pneumoniae,* and *Chlamydia pneumonia* seek out and bind to specific types of molecules, including fats found in the blood (lipoproteins). Fats are diverse in sizes and shapes. Not all fat cells provide ideal camouflage for the organism and others are only marginally useful, so the cloaking mechanism is rendered defective.

The relative concentration of useful versus harmful fats is little understood and most of that knowledge is in the form of epidemiological statistics. Shape-related matching mechanisms and cell surface modification techniques should be studied further and modeled by computer simulation to explore not only RA accretions but also cardiovascular syndromes such as plaque and tachycardia. The effect of Coenzyme Q_{10} and folic acid need to be studied in relation to the activities of cloaking, shape-changing microorganisms.

Neutralizing Harmful Toxins and Enzymes

Dr. Brown realistically asserted that harmful microbes cannot be completely eliminated. The aim of the antibiotic regimen is to keep the pathogenic mycoplasmas within manageable bounds so that the body's own immune system can keep them from becoming uncontrollably virulent and invasive.

In those cases where the particular pathogen is unknown or in doubt, it is more effective to target and neutralize the irritants as a first step, without identifying the organism producing them. Clues might be found in the toxin or enzyme made by the microbe, e.g., the correlations listed in the IBM Bio-Dictionary Annotation between *Mycoplasma pneumonia* and the COX-2 enzyme.[51]

Certain enzymes generated in turn may reveal the particular strain of pathogen responsible. The Arthritis Trust's findings[52] confirm Dr. Brown's suspicion that *M. pneumoniae* was a prime candidate as a causal factor of arthritis. However, today's commonly available tests are not definitive or comprehensive enough to identify all strains of a given pathogenic organism.

Strain-specific antibiotic susceptibilities may be needed to permit selection of the most effective antibiotic/*M. pneumoniae* vaccine combination. *M. pneumoniae* vaccine is used to treat pigs but is not available for humans.[53]

While the *S. pneumonia* vaccine protects against multi-strains of that bacteria, this exposure can lead to colonization with mutated *S. pneumonia* L-forms that may act in similar ways to mycoplasmas.

Anti-Toxins

Certain anti-toxins have been developed for specific life-threatening conditions such as tetanus, botulism, spider bites, snakebites, and box jellyfish stings.[54]

Gamma globulin, also known as Immunoglobulin (IG, a blood extract similar to an anti-toxin) was used in the past as a non-specific anti-infection passive immune booster.[55] The purity of such blood extracts is subject to question today due to the levels of infection in the blood supply.

One aspect of RA allergic flare-up appears to be related to certain toxins, for example, salmonella toxin, where studies have found arthritis-causing HLA-B27.[56]

ALLERGIC REACTIONS

If, as Dr. Brown asserts, RA is due to a kind of infectious allergy where mycoplasmal microorganisms and L-forms reside in joints and emit irritants to which the body reacts, this would explain why the person afflicted with RA has periods during which s/he feels reasonably well. During these lulls, it could be that bacteria or their L-forms release just a small bit of the toxin. Another explanation may be that the L-forms revert to cellular forms temporarily, or the organisms may develop a cholesterol "coat," or perform a sort of cloaking that is somewhat imperfect.

Mycoplasmas are cyclic in nature. They often persist in metabolically inactive states where a few are released from cells, followed by more active states where many are released. Whatever the trigger, over a period of months or years the body creates fixed-tissue antibodies that are poised and ready to react to the released toxins whenever and wherever they appear. The body thus learns to react to mycoplasmas in the same way it learns to react to a substance like poison ivy. The first contact causes the body to produce a specific type of antibody tailored to the allergen. The periodic reaction between antibody and antigen causes irritation. Antibody reactions alone cannot suppress mycoplasmal infections. This may be why efforts to develop vaccines against mycoplasmas have not been successful.

Keeping the body's systems in balance requires acceptance of the fact that our bodies are constantly changing. Living organic systems are always in a dynamic state. The best comparison we can make is to control theory, where "balance" means oscillating within an acceptable range. For an allergic reaction, the oscillation looks something like the cycle shown in Figure 4.

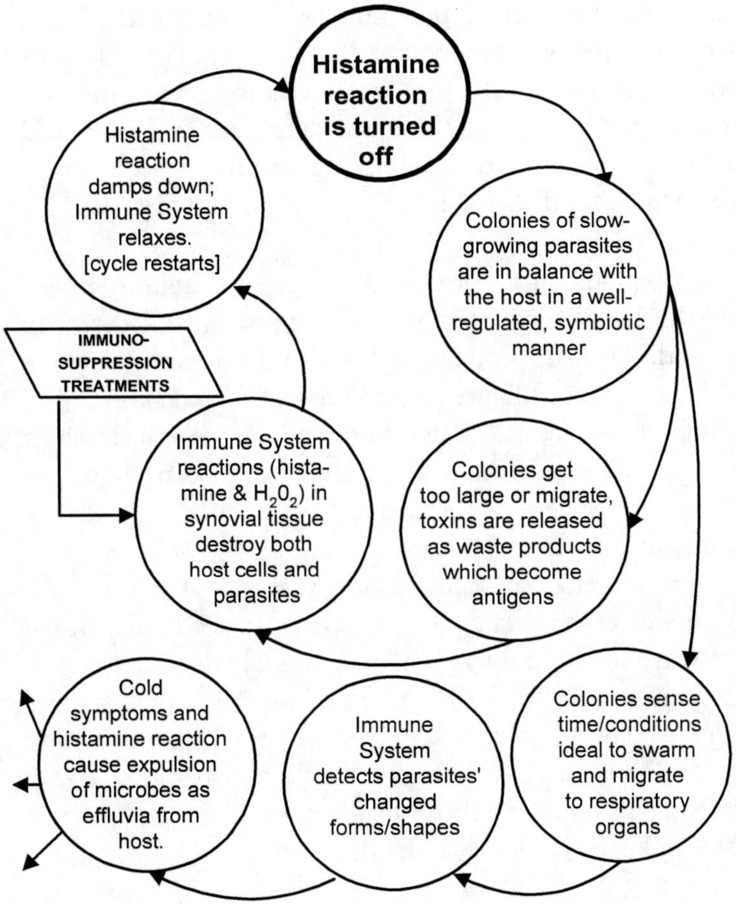

Figure 4. Histamine Reaction Cycle

Antihistamines block the action of histamine, a chemical produced by the immune system. Histamine is usually bound up in granules found inside mast cells—specialized immune cells found in the skin, nasal passages, and the gastrointestinal and respiratory tracts. An allergic response, whether to an internal or external substance, is really a stimulation of the immune system to develop a specific antibody, immunoglobulin E (IgE). The IgE antibodies attach themselves to mast cells to prepare to ward off the invaders. As the offending substance (e.g., ragweed pollen) enters the body, it bumps against these primed mast cells and sets off their histamine chemicals.[57] H_2O_2 is also released.

Commercially produced chemical antihistamines work by blocking the action of histamine once it has been released. Over-the-counter (OTC) antihistamines have a long track record of success and are considered safe if used in moderation and according to directions.[58] Antihistamines such as chlorophineramine maleate have been shown to reduce the severity of rheumatoid arthritis attacks by mitigating joint pain.

However, one should not rush to swallow antihistamines at the first sign of sneezing. Instead, one should find ways to avoid allergens from animals, molds, grasses, detergents, and foods by identifying the circumstances under which allergies strike, then removing the offending agent. The process may be as simple as cleaning furnace filters or installing electrostatic air cleaners in the home or office to keep dust levels to a minimum.[59]

Naturopathic remedies

If external remedies are called for, one might try a gentler approach than OTC chemicals. No matter what the allergy, German researchers have discovered that eating onions reduces the amount of histamine produced by mast cells.[60] Vitamin C (with bioflavonoids) and pantothenic acid have been shown to be natural antihistamines. Vitamin E and selenium stabilize cell walls, while vitamin A decreases the permeability of cells in skin and in the mucous membranes. This is important because undesirable pathogens can enter weakened cells during an allergy attack.

Vitamin B-complex, especially vitamin B_6, has been shown to decrease allergic reactions, especially when taken together with vitamin C in large amounts.[61] This is because the B vitamins enhance the immune system. Those individuals with chronic illness have a low absorption rate so liquid B vitamin supplements in sublingual form (drops administered under the tongue) are most effective.[62]

Homeopathic Remedies

Homeopathic relief for allergy and sinusitis usually consists of:

- *Belladona* 3X;
- *Sanguinaria canadensis* 3X; and/or
- *Spigelia* 3X.

When a homeopathic medicine is labeled "X" it means the dilution is 1:9. When described as "3X" it means the dilution is vigorously shaken, then diluted again 1:9 and shaken; the procedure is repeated a total of three times.[63]

---

[1] Samuels (1991) p. 31.

[2] Brown and Scammell (1988) pp. 7-8. The autoimmune theory is underscored repeatedly in immunology textbooks such as Rose, et al. (1986) and also in various articles in *Arthritis Today*, the publication of the Arthritis Foundation. E.g., Purpura, Mary. "One Person's Stress is Another Person's Challenge." *Arthritis Today*, March/April 1997, and also Dinsmoor, Robert and Kahn, Cynthia, "Smart Drugs." *Arthritis Today*, January/February 1996.

[3] Brown and Scammell (1988) pp. 78-79.

---

[4] See www.rheumatic.org for paper citations, case studies, laboratory results, abstracts, and so forth. An impressive paper by Dr. Joseph M. Mercola, "Protocol for Using Antibiotics in the Treatment of Rheumatic Diseases," can be found at www.mercola.com. The paper was presented at the 31st Annual Meeting of the American Academy of Environmental Medicine in Boston, MA in October 1996. Dr. Mercola lauds Dr. Brown's pioneering work in mycoplasma research and tetracycline treatment. The paper essentially expands on Dr. Brown's and Henry Scammell's fundamental work, *The Road Back*. Dr. Mercola offers an improved version of the original protocol using minocycline in Appendix II of this book. This text is written by a physician for physicians and may be difficult for the layperson to understand.

[5] Blumberg, Dr. Darren R. and Sloan, Dr. Victor S. of the Robert Wood Johnson Medical School, New Brunswick, New Jersey in a letter "Classification of Reactive Arthritides." Also see Veys E.M. and Mielants, H. "Enteropathic Arthropathies." In: Klippel, J.H. and Dieppe, P.A., editors. *Rheumatology*. St. Louis: 1994.

[6] Personal communication with Dr. Garth Nicolson, January 2002.

[7] "Mycoplasmal Infections," a well-documented, detailed overview, is provided without charge to Institute for Molecular Medicine visitors.

[8] Research conducted primarily by Dr. Albert Sabin, who worked with Dr. Brown at the Rockefeller Institute during the 1930s. Also see Simecka, J. W., et al. "Mycoplasma Diseases of Animals." in Maniloff (1992) section V, chapter 24.

[9] All quotes attributed to Drs Baseman and Tully in this chapter may be found at www.medscape.com/other/EID/1997.

[10] Matzinger, P. "Tolerance, Danger and the Extended Family." *Annual Reviews in Immunology*, 1994. 12:991-1045. Dr. Matzinger's now famous "Danger Model" is described clearly in layman's terms at http://cmmg.biosci.wayne.edu/asg/polly.html. For further details see http://www2.mni.uwo.ca/3m/previous/matzinger.html.

[11] Toppo (1986), p. 52.

[12] Cassel, G.H and Mekalanos J. "Development of Antimicrobial Agents in the Era of New and Reemerging Infectious Diseases and Increasing Antibiotic Resistance." *JAMA* Feb 7 2001; 285(5), 601-605.

[13] Brown and Scammell (1988) p. 39.

---

[14] Drs Baseman and Tully (1997): .”..pathogenic mycoplasmas are among the most difficult microorganisms to grow from clinical specimens and remain frequent contaminants of primary and continuous eucaryotic cell lines and tissue cultures. In some instances, mycoplasma contamination is obvious since infected eucaryotic cells exhibit aberrant growth, metabolism, and morphology. However, mycoplasmas often establish covert and chronic infections of target cells that lead to either invalid and misleading data or introduction of mycoplasmas or their products into reagents dedicated to therapeutic or research purposes.”

[15] Engelhard, Victor H. “How Cells Process Antigens.” *Scientific American*, August 1994.

[16] Personal communication with Dr. Garth Nicolson, January 2002.

[17] Viruses are also able to manufacture proteins that switch off or dampen cellular immune responses. A virus’s DNA is capable of infecting or destroying a cell, eluding the immune system by mutating and gene-swapping. Garrett (1995) pp. 572-5.

[18] Ataoglu, H.; Goksu, N.; Kemaloglu, Y.K.; Bengisun, S.; and Ozbilen, S. “Preliminary Report on L-forms: Possible Role in the Infectious Origin of Secretory Otitis Media.” *Annals of Otology, Rhinology and Laryngology*. June 1994; 103:6, 434-8.

[19] Watson, P.; Voss, L.; Barber, C., et al. “The Microbiology of Chronic *Otitis media* with Effusion in a Group of Auckland Children.” *New Zealand Medical Journal*. May 1996; 109:1022, 182-4.

[20] Bukharin, O.V. “[The Biomedical Aspects of the Persistence of Bacteria], (Biomeditsinskie Aspecty Persistentsii Bakterii.).” *Zhurnal Mikrobiologii, Epidemiologii I Immunobiologii*, Supplement. August/ September 1994; 1: 4-13.

[21] Nicolson, Garth L.; Nasralla, Marwan Y.; and Nicolson, Nancy L. “The Pathogenesis and Treatment of Mycoplasmal Infections.” *Antimicrobics and Infectious Disease Newsletter*. 1999; 17(11): 81-88.

[22] See http://www.psa-rising.com/medsci/p53.htm.

[23] Brown and Scammell (1988) p. 149.

[24] Toivanen (1988) pp. 160-162.

[25] Mandell (1983) chapter 5.

[26] See www.rheumatic.org and www.mercola.com.

---

[27] Horstman, Judith. "Bee Venom." *Arthritis Today*. November/December 1998.

[28] Sittig (1985).

[29] Ongoing microbiology research by Dr. Stuart Levy, Tufts University.

[30] Notably Paratek and GlaxoSmithKline.

[31] Roberts, Marilyn C. "Antibiotic Resistance." in Maniloff (1992), section V, chapter 31.

[32] Appendix: "Antibiotics: Efficacy Against Susceptible Pathogens." *Physician's Drug Handbook* (1993) pp. 1139-1145.

[33] For details and scientific references see www.puritan.com, www.healthwell.com, and www.medical.healthnotes.com.

[34] Tilly (1995) via Medline.

[35] O'Dell, J.R.; Paulsen, G.; Haire, C.E.; et al. "Treatment of Early Seropositive Rheumatoid Arthritis with Minocycline: Four-year Followup of a Double-blind, Placebo-controlled Trial." *Arthritis and Rheumatology* 1999;42:1691-1695.

[36] See www.drmirkin.com/joints/J106.htm.

[37] Mirkin, Dr. Gabe. "Mirkin Report for Healthier Living." August 1999.

[38] *Rheumatology* 1999;38(6): 504-509

[39] See www.thearthritiscenter.com/arthritis_info.htm#Anchor-Infections-11481. This is an excellent and comprehensive website. The Arthritis Center is located at 4000 14th Street, Suite 511, Riverside, CA 92501. Phone: (909) 788-0850.

[40] O'Dell, et al. "Minocycline Therapy for Early Rheumatoid Arthritis Continued Efficacy at Three Years." Annual meeting of the American College of Rheumatology. November 9, 1997.

[41] Mirkin, Dr. Gabe. "Mirkin Report for Healthier Living." August 1999.

[42] Mirkin, Dr. Gabe. "Reactive Arthritis." June 3, 1999. From the Internet at www.drmirkin.com/joints/J159.htm.

[43] *Protocol for Antibiotic Therapy*, from The Road Back Foundation at www.roadback.com.

---

[44] Wells, Carol L. and Wilkins, Tracy D. "Clostridia: Sporeforming Anaerobic Bacilli." See http://gsbs.utmb.edu/microbook/ch018.htm. Botulism and tetanus are other forms of Clostridia.

[45] See www.mercola.com/2001/jul/11/probiotics.htm.

[46] Brown and Scammell (1988) chapter 15.

[47] Brown and Scammell (1988) chapter 23.

[48] See www.mercola.com/forms/wellness_condensed.htm for Dr. Mercola's comprehensive "Eating Plan for Optimal Health." He has helped thousands of his patients who make a commitment to this admittedly difficult but ultimately rewarding dietary plan. A brief outline of this plan appears in Appendix V.

[49] Brown and Scammell (1988) chapter 7.

[50] Olszewski (1987) pp. 123-127. See also *Arthritis Today*, March/April 1997, and Dinsmoor, Robert and Kahn, Cynthia. "Smart Drugs." *Arthritis Today*, January/February 1996.

[51] See http://cbcsrv.watson.ibm.com/Annotations/MP/chunk_083/MPcox2 and http://cbcsrv.watson.ibm.com/Annotations/MG/chunk_017/MG_gi_1045749.txtFT.html.

[52] See www.arthritistrust.com/topics/mycoplasmaL.html.

[53] See www.pfizer.com/ah/stelresp/techaward.html

[54] See www.merck.com/pubs/mm_geriatrics/sec16/ch132.htm.

[55] See www.mckinley.uiuc.edu/health-info/dis-cond/vacimmun/immunglo.html.

[56] See www.m.u-tokyo.ac.jp/english/organization/InternalMedicine/DepartmentofHematologyandOncology.html. Also see Maksymowych, W.P.; Ikawa, T.; Yamaguchi, A.; Ikeda, M., et al. "Invasion by *Salmonella typhimurium* Induces Increased Expression of the LMP, MECL, and PA28 Proteasome Genes and Changes in the Peptide Repertoire of HLA-B27." *Infection & Immunity*. 66: 4624-32, 1998 and Ikawa, T.; Ikeda, M.; Yamaguchi, A.; Tsai, W.C., et al. "Expression of Arthritis-causing HLA-B27 on Hela Cells Promotes Induction of C-Fos in Response to *in vitro* Invasion by *Salmonella typhimurium*." *Journal of Clinical Investigation*. 101: 263-72, 1998.

[57] Michaud (1989) chapter 9.

---

[58] One of the most benign is the generic antihistamine chlorpheniramine maleate, a world standard, which appears as the active ingredient in many commercial OTC anti-allergy products.

[59] Culhane, Kari W. "Allergy Antidotes for Kids." *Natural Health*, March/April 2000.

[60] Michaud (1989) pp. 64-5.

[61] Mandell (1983) pp. 232-3. Megadoses of any vitamin are not recommended over time. The large amounts suggested here are for a specific and intense allergic reaction, not for daily intake, even as a preventive measure.

[62] Personal communication with Dr. Garth Nicolson, January 2002.

[63] Ullman (1991) presents an excellent and comprehensive treatment of the topic.

4. LINKS BETWEEN INFECTION AND ARTHRITIS

Antibiotic-resistant bacteria were practically unknown 50 years ago. Today they are a worldwide health problem. Such illnesses as strep throat, pneumonia, meningitis and tuberculosis are becoming increasingly harder to treat. By some estimates, more than 60,000 Americans die each year from drug-resistant infections.[1] Hospital-borne infections alone help kill between 80,000-100,000 people in the United States each year. In 1992, 42% of all staph infections in large U.S. hospitals were caused by strains that had grown resistant to methicillin[2], one of the only drugs available to treat staph. That is a 10% increase in staph infections over a decade.[3]

Drug-resistant *Streptococcus pneumoniae* (DRSP) presents a growing public health challenge as worldwide studies increasingly report pneumococcal strains resistant to penicillin and other drugs. In the mid-1990s, *S. pneumoniae* was determined to be a leading cause of illness and death in the United States, accounting for an estimated 3,000 cases of meningitis, 50,000 cases of bacteremia, 500,000 cases of pneumonia, and more than seven million cases of *Otitis media* each year. The prevalence of DRSP infection has not been a reportable condition but the CDC has been actively working to solve this problem. An important first step in 1994 was to build a laboratory-based, electronic surveillance system to capture DRSP data.[4] Using these statistical data, researchers can study the epidemiology of DRSP and eventually be able to minimize DRSP complications through control and prevention.

More than 20% of all enterococcus infections in U.S. hospitals' intensive care units and in nursing homes are now resistant to vancomycin, until recently considered the antibiotic of last resort.[5] Researchers are hunting for new antimicrobial agents, and pharmaceutical companies are developing synthetics like Zyvox and Cidecin to combat microorganisms that have become resistant to traditional drugs thought to be "magic bullets" since the discovery of penicillin in 1944. Bacteria and parasites sometimes undergo random mutations, making them more resistant to an antibiotic. The process of exchanging DNA with other resistant microbes via plasmids *in vivo* confers that resistance upon the receptor organism.

When powerful antibiotics are used, the intent is to kill *all* enemy microbes, but those that survive multiply and remember the combat and learn from it. By the 1950s, most staph infections had become highly resistant to penicillin. Part of the problem was that doctors prescribed penicillin indiscriminately for all sorts of complaints, often in response to patients' demands for antibiotics. We know now that ear infections and some sinus infections are not only caused by bacteria, but also by fungal infections.[6]

By including antimicrobial agents in household cleansers, cosmetics, and lotions industry is exacerbating the problem and making it easier for pathogenic microbes to develop resistance.

Antibiotics are included in feed for livestock. However, the FDA's Center for Veterinary Medicine plans to disallow fluoroquinolones in poultry feed after campylobacter was found in 88% of samples of poultry for sale in Minnesota's supermarkets. Campylobacter is a known cause of diarrheal disease; 20% of the poultry samples were fluoroquinolone resistant.[7] Part of the problem is improperly prepared food, e.g., unsanitary conditions or undercooking.

Drug-resistant tuberculosis and malaria are re-emerging as serious health problems in developing countries. In 1992, New York City hospitals reported 3,800 new cases of TB. One-third of these victims showed drug resistance to rifampin, an anti-TB drug viewed as effective, and streptomycin, also considered reliable. Most of the TB cases were AIDS sufferers, hospital residents, prison inmates and the homeless. There is no quarantine requirement now in place for individuals with TB, since it is considered a "conquered" disease.

According to the CDC, sudden and unexplained illness may be the result of newly emerging infectious organisms. Of 45 mystery diseases reported between 1995-1997, only 13 could be traced to a known organism. Some illnesses may be a mystery because no test has been developed to diagnose them.[8] The CDC, in its capacity as a gatherer and interpreter of statistical data, should establish databases similar to the DRSP project to capture infection symptoms, test results, and treatment outcomes.

The Human Genome Project holds great hope for discovering causes and cures for a wide variety of diseases, as do projects to gene-map pathogenic microorganisms. However, microbes will not stop evolving and developing resistance to new generations of drugs. The microbial arms race will never end.

THE WIDESPREAD USE OF CHEMOTHERAPEUTIC DRUGS

The routine use of antibiotics and other immunosuppressive drugs worldwide has trained bacteria to adapt and evolve in order to survive. The result is a variety of extremely hardy and often virulent microbes that defy conventional treatment, which is usually prescribed bombardment with the traditional drug of choice.[9] These drugs are sometimes simply a retooling of existing drugs, repackaged and marketed under a new name. Since it is difficult and time consuming to test and pinpoint the cause of a medical problem (e.g., an ear infection), an appealing shortcut is to prescribe a broad-spectrum antibiotic.

The typical pattern is to prescribe stronger or different antibiotics with each successive infection. A sick child with the sniffles is quickly given antibiotics intended to assault and vanquish the enemy "bug." By their first birthday, about half of all children have had at least one ear infection. The prescribed treatment is usually amoxicillin or trimetho-primsulfamethoxazole.[10] Unfortunately, the middle ear's beneficial bacteria are also killed off in this wholesale slaughter.

The process is akin to spraying one's entire backyard with potent insecticide to kill off a few specific unwanted pests. The result is that the poison also kills benevolent garden visitors such as bees, some birds, and predator wasps that feed on aphids. Overuse of chemotherapeutic drugs, like the overuse of insecticides, is a Pyrrhic victory. In time, as a drug is used more and more frequently, the susceptible germs die off but the resistant, pernicious ones reproduce. The more people use antibiotics, the more pressure is put on bacterial populations to develop immunity until the pathogenic germs become resistant to multiple drugs. Physicians may eventually be forced to return to less effective treatments abandoned many years ago, before antibiotics were introduced, as the number and type of omni-resistant germs continues to grow.

Much of the fault of this untargeted and widespread drug use in the United States lies with the American patients, who have come to expect a prescription for a quick fix for their discomfort. Some physicians contribute to the problem because they want to practice state-of-the-art medicine and have little or no interest in exploring any unconventional remedies that do not bear the American Medical Association's (AMA) endorsement.[11]

Pharmaceutical companies play a role as they aggressively promote new medications in order to recoup research and development costs and start making a profit. Managed-care companies compound the problem by hesitating to pay for expensive tests to determine which particular chemotherapeutic drugs are the proper treatment, so the low-cost approach is to routinely treat with penicillin to start, and then to move on to other formulations depending on patient response.[12]

Antibiotics

The typical Health Maintenance Organization (HMO) allocates 10-12% of its budget for medications.[13] An estimated 30% of the budgets of hospital pharmacies are directed toward the purchase of antibiotics.[14] Too frequent use of antibiotics and/or partial treatment (not following the 10-14 day regimen) has allowed surviving bacteria to gain strength and mutate into more resistant and robust forms.

Today, doctors are more discerning about routinely prescribing antibiotics. However, patients are often at fault for failing to follow the doctor's orders. Some take just enough of the medication to make the symptoms subside, and then save the rest of the pills for another time to avoid making another appointment. The body's system is not fully rid of the original infection, so the remaining microbes are left to develop into a pernicious, drug-resistant form. Some patients are not disciplined enough to follow the medication instructions through the full course and quit when they feel better. Some use past-date medications belonging to friends or family members because they are unwilling or unable to pay for a doctor visit and tailored prescription.

The same effects of misuse will result if the prescribing doctor does not first test to determine the cause of the problem and how sensitive it is to various drugs. However, most RA-associated microorganisms rarely grow in cultures, so molecular tests such as PCR must be employed. Antibiotics work in one of four ways:

- blocking the formation of the cell wall in the next generation of germs;
- preventing bacteria from making essential proteins;
- attacking or dissolving bacterial cell membranes; or
- blocking production of bacterial DNA, thus stopping replication.

Bacteria can generate overt enzyme counterattacks to break down antibiotics. They also can adapt to the new chemical environment by building a tougher membrane wall or changing slightly whatever biochemical process the antibiotic was supposed to affect. They accomplish this in places on the DNA chain or with new enzymes that are not blocked by the antibiotic. Ideally, all sites on the DNA chain would have to be blocked to prevent the propagation of bacteria.

Agricultural antibiotics

Animal arthritis traced to *Bovis pleuropneumonia* was first documented at the Pasteur Institute in 1898. These viral-like microbes are a particular strain of a pleuropneumonia-like organism (PPLO), which we now know as *Mycoplasma mycoides*, is highly transmissible. PPLOs can cause a variety of arthritic, respiratory, reproductive, and neurologic disorders in different animal species.[15] Dr. Clark speculates that the potential for economic impact on the agriculture industry led to concerted efforts to find and eliminate the cause of these diseases in livestock.

Since the early 1950s, farm animals have been routinely dosed with antibiotics to keep them healthy so they will in turn grow faster and be ready for market. Production of medicated feed additives is big business. The Animal Health Institute estimated that in 1984 farm animals consumed a total of $292.4 million in antibacterial additives. In 1986, an estimated 50% of the antibiotics manufactured in the United States were fed to, injected into, or applied to livestock.[16] Overuse is worse overseas. In 2001, the estimate is 70%. This translates to 16 million pounds annually in the mid-1980s to nearly 25 million pounds today.[17] Overuse is worse overseas.[18]

Genes for drug resistance are carried not only on the chromosomes but also on extrachromosomal elements called plasmids, which control their own replication. The plasmids of bacteria found in the small intestine are called "R-factors." These plasmids may carry several resistance genes —to penicillin, streptomycin, erythromycin, sulfonamides, and tetracycline. As a result of plasmid transfer, resistant R-factors were found in pathogenic *Staphylococcus aureus* soon after penicillin was introduced in the 1950s. The plasmids from livestock make their way into our food chain. Allowing farm animals to live and breed among drug-resistant microorganisms results in a national food supply of meats or meat products contaminated with antibiotic-resistant bacteria.[19]

Regrettably, one cannot tell whether the meat and animal products, including eggs and dairy products, carry drug-resistant mycoplasmal microorganisms. The consumer must either resolve to eat fewer animal products, seek out organically grown farm products, or accept the risk of absorbing strains of resistant bacteria. In any case, meat, especially chicken, sausage, and hamburger, should be thoroughly cooked before consumption.

To halt this transfer of antibiotic-resistant, disease-causing bacteria to humans, only those antibiotics not used for clinical applications should be given to livestock. Furthermore, hospitals should rotate the use of antibiotics they routinely administer. For example, alternate macrolides, tetracyclines, and sulfonamides with chloramphenicol, penicillin and streptomycin in three- to four-year cycles. Antibiotics like colistin, vancomycin, ristocetin, neomycin, and polymyxin should be reserved for special cases.[20]

Irradiation of food products

Our government needs to require meat sterilization as a global solution to the contamination problem. However, studies have shown that sterilization by irradiation is not completely safe despite USDA claims to the contrary. While irradiation effectively kills meat-borne infections, it introduces new and equally harmful effects. For years it has been known that laboratory animals develop Vitamin K deficiencies leading to blood clotting disorders, internal bleeding, carcinomas, and other serious symptoms after consuming irradiated beef.[21]

Shortly after the tragic cases of Thalidomide-caused birth effects were documented in the 1960s, the World Health Organization stated that "Irradiating can bring about chemical transformations in food and food components resulting in the formation of potential mutagens, particularly hydrogen peroxide and various organic peroxides.[22]

Two decades later, the mutagenicity and cytotoxicity of irradiated foods and food components remained a problem. Embryonic deaths and severe mutations in laboratory animals were still being reported.[23] A recent article in *Nutrition* cautioned that increased concentrations of a mutagen in irradiated food increases the risk of cancer.[24]

The irradiation is done by three methods: gamma rays, X-rays, or high voltage electron beams. The low dose treatment can significantly reduce levels of pathogens such as:[25]

- *Salmonella*, *Campylobacter jejuni*, and *Escherichia coli* (in fresh meat and poultry)
- *Trichinella spiralis* (in fresh pork)
- *Cysticercus cellulosae* (pork tapeworms)
- *Taenia saginata* (beef tapeworms)
- *Staphylococcus aureus*
- *Lisiteria monocytogenes*
- *Aeromonas hydrophila*
- *Toxoplasma gondii*
- *Cyclospora*
- *Clostridium botulinum*
- *Bacillus cereus*

Only the enteric viruses and the endospores of the genera *Clostridium* and *Bacillus* are highly resistant to low ionizing radiation.[26]

Radiated products must bear special labels carrying the international symbol of irradiation (a "radura") and a statement indicating that they were treated. This symbol is shown in Figure 5.

Figure 5. Radura Symbol of Irradiation

The nutritive molecule-degradation of irradiated food is not well understood to determine whether it provides a significant health hazard. However, the vitamin and mineral depletion of preserved foods is well known, and is the basis of the health/vitamin/nutraceutical industry. There is some concern over free radical production by irradiation, increased fat rancidity, and enzyme inactivation.

Irradiation of meat products is analogous to the pasteurization of milk. While pasteurization kills harmful bacteria, it also destroys beneficial enzymes as well as altering the proteins albumin and casein to produce damaging effects.

Even some strong proponents admit that irradiation of beef and poultry for the consumer market is a way for the industry to get around USDA regulations prohibiting unsanitary slaughterhouse practices.[27] More on this controversial issue can be found on the Internet.[28]

Dr. Mercola advises purchasing only non-irradiated meat. There is a very slim chance one might acquire a mild food borne infection. Should this happen, he suggests one teaspoon of healthy gut bacteria such as acidophilus or bifidus taken every hour for 4-8 hours until balance in restored and the individual feels better.[29]

Health food stores sell non-irradiated beef, but although it is labeled "organic" it is not "real beef" because the animals are fed grain, not grass. Cattle do not eat grains naturally—they eat grass. Omega-6 fats are potentially harmful; omega-3 fats are desirable. Grain-fed beef can have an omega 6:3 ratio higher than 20:1.[30] This means that it has a 35-75% fat content, and over half of this is saturated fat. By contrast, grass-fed beef has an omega 6:3 ratio of 3:1, which is comparable to fish. Less than 10% of grass-fed beef is saturated fat. Health problems correlate with omega 6:3 fat ratios higher than 4:1.

Benefits of eating grass-fed beef[31] are:

- a natural source of omega-3 fats
- high in CLA (Conjugated Linoleic Acid), a fat that reduces the risk of cancer, obesity, diabetes, and a number of immune disorders
- high in beta carotene
- contains over 400% more Vitamins A and E
- virtually devoid of risk of Mad Cow Disease and *E. coli*

CLA is found in fats of animals raised naturally on pastures rather than those fattened on grains in a feedlot. Beef with a high CLA content will enable weight loss without other diet measures and exercise.

Beef is not the only meat product generating health concerns. Free-range chickens eat vegetables high in omega-3 fats, along with insects, fresh green grass, fruit, and small amounts of corn. The eggs of these chickens have an omega 6:3 ratio of 1.5:1 whereas the egg from a grain/corn-fed chicken has a ratio of 20:1.

Fish, while generally a leaner food choice than beef, is heavily promoted as a good source of the omega-3 fats. Sadly, a growing percentage of fish harvested for market are found to be contaminated with mercury. The larger the fish, the higher the measure of contamination, but catch location is an important factor. There is less danger from eating deep-water than bay-caught fish. The United States government presently warns pregnant women to avoid eating fish.

Omega-3 fatty acids are essential for normal growth and may play an important role in the prevention and treatment of coronary artery disease, hypertension, arthritis, cancer, and other inflammatory and autoimmune disorders. Omega-3 deficiencies have also been tied to dyslexia, cancer, violence, depression, memory problems, weight gain, arthritis, heart disease, eczema, allergies, inflammatory diseases, diabetes, and many other conditions.

Most experts believe that Mad Cow Disease is related to stockyard animals' living conditions, type and quality of their food, and pesticides in their environment. Because testing for Mad Cow Disease is extremely difficult and bacteria may take several decades to incubate, it seems prudent to avoid grain-fed beef. Choosing grass-fed beef also lowers the danger of *E.coli* infection because stockyard cattle are fed the flesh of other animals (dogs, cats, pigs, horses, old dairy cattle) that might be carriers of the bacteria.

Few supermarkets, even specialty markets, carry grass-fed beef. The best way to purchase grass-fed beef is to purchase from a local rancher who is raising free-range cattle.[32]

SURVIVAL STRATEGIES OF MICROBES

Antibiotics were first discovered in the 1940s. By 1965, there were over 25,000 antibiotic formulations on the market.[33] Laboratory tests find that many of these products are only marginally effective, and some allow bacteria to thrive. Bacteria are organisms that are determined to survive. This may mean changing shape, modifying cell walls, transforming into L-forms, mutating, encysting, conjugating, adopting camouflage, going dormant until a suitable opportunity to emerge again presents itself, hitchhiking on another organism, migrating to another host, or developing a protective (cholesterol) coating to deflect attack. Not all microorganisms use all of these techniques, but such actions and capabilities are encoded in the DNA of many organisms, to be used when the need arises.

During the mid-1980s, physicians noting an alarming increase in pediatric ear (*Otitis media*) infections routinely prescribed antibiotics, only to find that by 1990 about one-third of all ear infections were due to *Pneumococcus* strains that were resistant to penicillins.[34] Author Mark Lappe's book *Germs That Won't Die*, published in 1981, decried the improper use of antibiotics and predicted wholesale production of pathogenic new organisms. His critics charged that he grossly exaggerated the scope of the problem. Ten years later, he was vindicated.

By 1992 a number of organisms, including strains of cholera *Escherichia coli*, *Cryptosporidium*, and the Legionnaires' Disease bacteria, had developed a tolerance to chlorine. Microbes were able to survive in doses of chlorine that in the past had killed their species. To ensure safe drinking water, higher and higher doses of chlorine are being used. Evidence of chlorine failure can be seen in the surge of Legionnaires' Disease, *Giardia* infections, and cryptosporidiosis infections among people who use chlorinated hot tubs, swimming pools, and public spas.[35]

By 1993, nearly every common pathogenic bacterial species had developed some degree of clinically significant drug resistance, and over two dozen of these strains posed life-threatening crises to humanity by having learned to tolerate the most commonly available antibiotic treatments.

Resident bacteria that we all carry in our bodies at any given time can outwit antibiotics as they evolve chemical weapons to best competitors for survival. Killing all but a few percent of a colony of bacteria still leaves the equivalent of "weed seeds" to spawn the next resistant generation. *Streptococcus pyogenes* (rheumatic fever) bacteria colonize human connective tissue, causing arthritis-like pain in the joints and potentially lethal infections of the heart. This bacterium was thought to have been wiped out by the 1970s in industrialized nations, yet a rheumatic fever outbreak in 1985 occurred in Salt Lake City, Utah and new cases were still being found in the 1990s.[36]

A 1995 federal survey found that 25% of the individuals sampled had pneumococcal infections resistant to penicillin and at least three other commonly prescribed antibiotics. Representing the group with the highest proportion of drug-resistant infections (41%) were white children aged 6 and under.[37]

The CDC reports that as of 1996 *Streptococcus pneumoniae* is responsible for at least one third of the 24 million outpatient visits for *Otitis media* and for half a million cases of pneumonia and meningitis in the United States each year. The CDC attributes 40,000 U.S. deaths each year to pneumococcal infections. *Pneumococcus* has shown increasing resistance to penicillin, the preferred drug for treating this type of infection.[38]

Of course, general respiratory infections caused by *Streptococcus* have not decreased much at all in the poor countries of the world. The World Health Organization estimated in 1992 that about 800,000 of the deaths among children each year were due to *Streptococcus pneumoniae* and overall, about 80% of those deaths were traced to bacterial infection of the lungs. In developing nations where antibiotics are available, village paramedics, lacking training and laboratory support to correctly distinguish viral from bacterial and mild from acute disease, may overuse antibiotics. The result is a set of antibiotic-resistant pneumococcal strains thriving globally, some able to defeat the action of several antibiotics administered simultaneously.

A cluster of seven deaths attributed to Group A *Streptococcus*, dubbed "flesh eating bacteria," attracted attention to this virulent strain in 1994, although it is by no means new. About ten cases of necrotising fasciitis are reported in any given year throughout England and Wales.[39]

T-Cell Infiltration

Shortly after retroviruses were discovered in the early 1970s, research scientists theorized that if a retrovirus inserted itself near certain host genes, those cellular segments of DNA where transposons rarely go would be activated and cause wild cell growth. Animal experiments demonstrated that cancer could be caused by retroviruses by virtue of their ability to invade and disrupt cellular DNA.[40] In 1979, researchers found evidence of a virus *inside* the immune system's T-cells (disease-fighting white blood cells) in human patients.[41] Despite this (and other) evidence of microbes infiltrating T-cells, the body's front line of defense, a study done in 1995 at the Mayo Clinic admitted surprise at finding that sets of T-cells are "different" among patients with RA and those who do not have RA.[42]

The disease process initiated by mycoplasmal microorganisms is usually very slow, characterized by periods of dormancy. Because many are able to hide themselves in various ways inside animal or human tissue and even, as viruses sometimes do, within the T-cells, they are difficult to detect. Different types of T-cells have various proteins protruding from their surfaces that serve to identify their function and form to other parts of the body. These sugar/protein markers allow cells to recognize each other in "friend or foe" fashion. It was only in the 1980s that scientists achieved the ability to distinguish one population of T-cells from another.

HOW MICROBES SPREAD

The greater the number of people infected, the greater the chance of mutation by microorganisms. As populations increase and people become more mobile, greater opportunities exist for bacterial and viral spread and mutation. In a climate of constant change, it is inevitable that microbes will discover a particular mutation that will give them a high probability of success in defeating the human immune system, promoting their survival and allowing them to pass more efficiently from person to person.[43] This observation is usually made regarding viruses, but if RA is indeed a bacterial infection, then it must be capable of spreading like other bacteria.

Person-to-person sharing of strep throat, pneumonia, and other respiratory diseases lead to development of organisms that later show up as elements of RA. Transmission of pathogens by insects is discussed in Chapter 5.

So-called "opportunistic infections" such as pneumocystis, meningitis, and candidiasis attack immunodeficient humans. The immune system overloads if exposed to too many microbes. A type of pneumonia organism resident in nearly every human being's system is kept in check by the immune system until that system fails to perform efficiently for a variety of reasons such as: improper diet, negative environmental factors, exposure to cold weather, drug use, fatigue, and so forth. The time is ripe for the opportunistic *Pneumocystis carinii*, which is associated with AIDS, to assert itself, grow, and spread to another human host. Similar etiology operates for *Mycoplasma pneumonia* and *Streptococcus pneumonia.*

Human antibodies (leukocytes) seek out antigens—proteins coating the virus—and surround them snugly to devour and incapacitate them. If these antigens are genetically changed, even slightly, so that they are not in the expected form, natural antibodies may not be able to lock on to these mutated forms with as snug a fit. The immune system must then reformulate its leukocytes to the new shapes. This takes time for a new generation of customized antibodies to be developed.

Recent research in cellular biology and virology has identified shape-shifting organisms, but much more remains to be done. Plasmids and transposons[44] move among microbes trying to gain entry to cells. L-forms, viruses, and mycoplasmas can readily interact with plasmids. Plasmids play a role in the evolution not only of bacteria but also possibly of all species on earth. Many contain genes called "integrons" that facilitate the integration of their DNA into any of the host organism's genomes. DNA thus moves not only between assorted bacterial species but also between entire families of organisms, e.g., between:

- bacteria and yeasts;
- plants and bacteria; and
- complex parasites and host cells, including T-cells and macrophages.[45]

Streptococcus pneumonia bacteria are not very efficient at absorbing plasmids, as are other bacteria, but they compensate for that failing by being voracious DNA scavengers.[46] *S. pneumonia* L-forms minus the cell wall can easily interact with foreign plasmids.

Staphylococcus also uses plasmids, genes, mobile DNA, mutations, and conjugative sharing of resistance factors to overcome whatever drugs are set against it. *Staphylococcus* is everywhere—in human bodies as well as in mammalian pets, on object surfaces and in garden soil. Many varieties of *Staphylococcus* are not pathogenic. We interchange *Staphylococci* on a daily basis, through handshakes and by handling common objects, but most of the time our immune systems render it harmless. If the bacterium enters a cut or wound, it finds an environment favorable to growth and stimulates an immune system response. While the cut or wound takes the full attention of the immune system, the bacteria find a home.

In 1992, some 23 million Americans received preoperative antibiotics before surgery. Over 900,000 (about 4%) of these patients developed postsurgical bacterial infections, most of which were traced to *Staphylococcus*.[47]

Spanish Flu

During the Spanish Flu pandemic of 1918-19, the human immune system could make antibodies against only two of the over seven hundred proteins that were observed to protrude from the outer envelope of the virus. Those who were able to generate these antibodies survived. The Flu sickened one billion people worldwide, and killed over twenty million.[48] Over the years, as more sophisticated research methods were developed, virus specialists concluded that influenza was a sort of microbial chameleon that had learned to adapt or die through the millennia of its existence.[49]

When the complex organization of the influenza virus was examined, RNA spirals were found to be entwined around themselves, and were coated with protective proteins. These coated spirals form genetic structures similar to chromosomes found in human and animal cells. When the virus reproduces itself, the spirals unwind to make duplicate sets of proteins and RNA. In the process, parts of the spirals could overlap and be copied, so that once reassembled, the offspring were a somewhat different version of the parent. This random genetic change could either be fatal or survival-oriented for the virus, and the new form could be lethal to the human host because the new shape no longer matches the immune cells trained to fight the old shape.

Pneumonia Epidemics

Virologists in the mid-1970s discovered that as flu viruses invade a cell and multiply in great quantities, their packaged chromosomes migrate to the outer wall of that cell and push through the cell membrane just hard enough to pull a glob of the membrane around themselves to create an outer protective coating. This process is called "budding." The newly created virus buds protrude from the host cell, attached by a strand of cell membrane until the time is right to detach and migrate to the lungs, nasal passages, or tear ducts of their human host. The new shape causes additional immune system responses that promote the expulsion of the virus from the body of the host. This process explains high transmissibility and virulence, such as that evidenced by the 1968 Hong Kong flu pandemic.[50]

Pneumonia Mutations

In the early 1960s *M. pneumoniae* was recognized as a primary cause of chronic pneumonia. According to Drs Baseman and Tully, "Today *M. pneumoniae* remains an important cause of pneumonia and other airway disorders, such as tracheobronchitis and pharyngitis, and is associated with extrapulmonary manifestations such as hematopoietic, exanthematic, joint, central nervous system, liver, pancreas, and cardiovascular syndromes."[51]

It should be noted that the appearance of mycoplasma infections occurs most often in persons whose immune systems are compromised, but may be found in those who are ostensibly healthy. Anyone with an immune deficiency is susceptible to a wide variety of microbial infections in which mycoplasmas may be prominently involved. In fact, immunosuppressive chemotherapy increases the risk of mycoplasmal infections.

Erythromycin, tetracycline, and minocycline are seen to be effective chemotherapeutic agents for L-form and mycoplasmal infections.[52] Most other broad-spectrum agents have limited ability to suppress mycoplasmas. Penicillin antibiotics force cellular forms into L-forms. The L-forms grow slowly, and appear to tunnel, coat, and cloak, going to a dormant phase untouched by antibiotics. Recovery depends on an effective host immune system.[53]

Laboratory tests finding *M. pneumoniae* in the human urogenital tract lead to the hypothesis that these micro-organisms are behaving like parasites, masking their genetic and chemical characteristics to travel unopposed to other favorable sites in the body. This action permits alternative modes of host-to-host transmission, such as sexual activity.[54]

According to Drs Baseman and Tully, "Many mycoplasmal pathogens exhibit filamentous or flask-shaped appearances and display prominent and specialized polar tip organelles that mediate attachment to host target cells. These tip structures are complex, composed of a network of interactive proteins, designated adhesions, and adherence-accessory proteins. These proteins cooperate structurally and functionally to mobilize and concentrate adhesions at the tip and permit mycoplasmal colonization of mucous membranes and eucaryotic cell surfaces."

Further confirming the parasitic nature of myco-plasmas, they go on to say, "…mycoplasmas exhibit limited biosynthetic capabilities; are highly fastidious and dependent upon the host microenvironment and complex culture medium for growth; have been observed in intimate contact with mammalian cell surfaces and within target cells; may be capable of initiating fusion with host cells through their cholesterol-containing unit membranes; and survive long-term recommended antimicrobial treatment in humans and tissue cultures."

Since multiple pathways of interaction with target cells is the way the *Mycoplasma* species operates, associations of mycoplasmas to human diseases remains controversial because of the desire to find a simple theory of the disease's etiology. What is needed is a set of careful, convincing laboratory studies with sophisticated equipment and techniques. Application of PCR techniques to samples from a wide range of arthritic and other potential infection sites has shown multiple strains of cooperating organisms including both cellular, L-forms and mycoplasmas.[55] This leads to the conclusion that multiple antibiotics, carefully combined and precisely directed to specific organisms, will be needed in the future.

Escherichia coli Mutations

The generally held belief that mutations were random was challenged in 1988 by British biologist John Cairns of the Harvard School of Public Health. Using recombinant DNA techniques, Cairns made a set of *Escherichia coli* mutations that had specific and unusual nutritional needs. He then altered the bacteria's environment in the laboratory, depriving the mutated bacteria of chemicals they could not manufacture on their own. Results of this experiment showed that the *E. coli* would specifically change two separate sets of genes to adapt to its new situation and survive, in far less time than a random mutation would allow.

Further experiments proved that *E. coli* mutants were able to withstand attacks from either viruses or antibiotics *before* those substances were introduced to the bacteria's environment. This finding demonstrates that *E. coli* DNA has native genetic memory of previous encounters with organisms that encoded the suppressing antibiotic molecules.

According to Cairns, transposons and plasmids act within the "great biological soup" of shifting genes to give one organism the capabilities normally carried by another. This shows the mechanisms behind evolution and that evolution can occur at a rapid rate if recipe swapping is facilitated by the use of cell wall-dissolving antibiotics. Human beings thus could be viewed as the result of four billion years of gene swapping. In 1994, researchers at Rockefeller University and the University of Alberta, Canada confirmed Cairns' findings.[56]

Ongoing research in microbial pathogenesis is providing evidence of the generality of these principles. That is, the microbes' reproduction rate decreases to provide better survival odds against the next antibiotic attack. When antibiotics dissolve the cell walls, plasmids from one organism's L-forms can more readily be traded with those of another, possibly different, organism.

Studies of various pathogenic *E. coli* strains showed that there was a tradeoff between genes for virulence and those for antibiotic resistance. Discoveries of new *Mycoplasma* strains that demonstrate stronger resistance to tetracycline and erythromycin antibiotics sustain the disturbing assertion that mycoplasmas may become undefeated in the long term.

POSSIBLE LINKS WITH OTHER DISEASES

Disruptive influences over the course of history have enabled microbes to adapt to a much wider range of ecological changes. Examples are the opening of new trade routes, increasing urbanization, the Industrial Revolution, the development of irrigation farming, and the systematic use of antibiotics in the treatment of a wide variety of ailments. It is little wonder that infection, spread so easily and suddenly, can account for a wide variety of chronic health problems. Pathogenic microbes seek stability in their relationship with their human hosts. Virulence decreases as parasite and host mutually adapt to one another.

The immune system requires hundreds of distinctly different types of cells—from tiny, free-floating lymphocytes to huge, slow-moving macrophages—to recognize a harmful incoming organism and then do the appropriate signaling to the immune system to muster its defenses and destroy it. However, if the incoming microbes are small enough to disguise themselves as friendly cells, even to the point of hiding within T-cells, they can take root in the body and modify genes in normal cells. Here they can switch off the cellular detection genes, thus living like reproducing bacteria clumps to form cysts, benign tumors, and/or cancerous masses.

The question is: if there is a link to cancer, what other diseases could trace their root cause to shape-shifting, evasive microbes? For example, syphilis is caused by the bacterium *Treponema pallidum*, the same spirochete that causes the childhood skin disease known as yaws, which has been known since ancient times. Advanced urbanization brought these diseases into the cities where the organism adjusted to its new environment and spread easily in more densely populated quarters.

Recently, various mycoplasmas have been linked as cofactors to AIDS, Gulf War Illness, Tuberculosis, Chronic Fatigue Syndrome, Multiple Sclerosis, Amyotrophic Lateral Sclerosis (ALS or Lou Gehrig's Disease), Fifth Disease, Lyme Disease, Salpingitis, Crohn's disease, and various arthritides.[57] Rheumatoid factors (or R-factors) have been observed in a number of diseases other than arthritis:

chronic infectious diseases like leprosy, various parasitic diseases, tuberculosis, and subacute bacterial endocarditis; liver disease (in the form of chronic active hepatitis); lympho-proliferative syndromes, and sarcoidosis.[58, 59]

Dr. Joseph Tully, in an article[60] for the International Organization for Mycoplasmology, lauds Dr. Brown and his colleagues for their basic research, clinical expertise, and persistence in advocating antibiotic treatments for a variety of chronic illnesses traceable to mycoplasmal infection.

The Arthritis Center has tabulated an impressive list of arthritis-causing microorganisms.[61] Ongoing research is documenting the causal relationship between a wide range of diseases and mycobacteria, mycoplasmas, bacterial L-forms and the R-factor. A few of these disorders are described more fully below as examples. AIDS and Lyme Disease are discussed in the next chapter.

Fifth Disease ("Slapped Cheek Disease")

This condition is so-called because it is the fifth major childhood skin rash doctors regularly treat. It is spread by airborne effluvia from the nose and mouth of an affected individual. Initial symptoms of Fifth Disease (*Erythema infectiosum*) are similar to those of a mild cold. By the third week, a red rash generally appears on the cheeks giving a "slapped cheek" appearance. A pink, blotchy, itchy rash covers the upper arms and legs lasting 5-10 days. Arthritic symptoms of aching joints and fatigue are characteristic. The disease can also affect adults.

The B19 parvovirus is one specific infectious agent identified in Fifth Disease. Genetic influences, co-factors associated with other microbial infections, parasites, and/or environmental factors appear to be at work, because many people contract Fifth Disease and later fully recover without experiencing joint pain or other arthritis symptoms. An estimated 20% never completely recover.[62]

A measurable overlap exists between susceptibility and infection, offering a pointer to essential research on other chronic conditions. DNA residues in fluid drawn from a painfully swollen joint have shown evidence of past infections.[63]

An infection during pregnancy may increase the risk of miscarriage or spontaneous abortion. In people with chronic red blood cell disorders, such as sickle-cell disease, infection may result in severe anemia. Infection has also been associated with arthritis in adults.[64] Blood tests to check for immunity or infection are available.

Salpingitis

Studies of the etiopathogenesis of salpingitis indicate it seems to develop as an ascending infection from the lower genital tract. Salpingitis is an inflammation of the fallopian tubes leading to fibrosis. According to Cornell University researchers, the most important microbiological agents include anaerobic *Streptococci, Chlamydia trachomatis, Mycoplasma hominis, E. coli,* and *Ureaplasma hominis*.[65] Julkunen first suggested a relationship between salpingitis and rheumatoid spondylitis in 1962.[66] Further research has found an association between HLA-B27 and salpingitis, which suggests the existence of an independent inflammatory rheumatic agent.[67]

The notion of individual susceptibility has been studied only recently as a part of the research effort to investigate human genetics. It is logical to assume that chronic arthritis develops because genetically susceptible individuals handle infection differently depending on the robustness of their immune systems. If a dysfunctional immune system is faced with an invader skilled in molecular mimicry, the contest is over before it's begun. A powerful antigenic agent with cloaking capability is able to activate a massive T-cell response to a nonspecific target, leading to the development of chronic arthritis and the appearance of an autoimmune disorder.

Gulf War Illness/Gulf War Syndrome

A range of as-yet undiagnosed illnesses continues to be reported by Gulf War veterans ten years after that conflict. Over 100,000 U. S. veterans still suffer from various illnesses attributed to their service.[68] The sum of the conditions documented is called collectively Gulf War Illness (GWI), although as yet no one disease has been designated as the cause. Some of these conditions are not unique to Gulf War veterans and have been reported prior to the 1990s period of exposure.

A variety of infections are common in the Persian Gulf region—sandfly fever (also called Phlebotomus fever, pappataci fever, or three-day fever), Dengue fever, Sindbis, Rift Valley fever, typhus, brucellosis, spotted fever, schistosomiasis, and echinococcosis—but these have not been diagnosed among the veterans. Other infections that may possibly relate to GWI are Epstein-Barr, mycoplasma, and clostridium.[69] One must not dismiss chemical and biological warfare agents as possibly related factors. This topic is hotly debated and outside the scope of this book.

It is interesting to note that members of the French armed forces sent to the Gulf were uniformly treated with antibiotics. One is led to infer that incidences of mycoplasmal and bacterial infections were thus prophylactically suppressed, since returning French veterans reported only a few instances of GWI.

Dr. Nicolson's current hypothesis is that the combined effects of multiple toxic exposures (including multiple vaccines), chemical, radiological and biological exposures, may have produced GWI in predisposed, susceptible individuals. Gulf War veterans were exposed to a wide variety of chemicals, insecticides, fumes and smoke from burning oil wells, and inhalation of fine sand. They were also given several vaccinations against possible biological warfare agents. Dr. Nicolson proposes that these vaccines may have been given too close together. A CDC study asserted that no mycoplasmas were found in anthrax vaccine administered in stages over an 18-month period.[70]

This finding does not rule out Dr. Nicolson's multiple-vaccine theory, which is supported by studies noting that pre-schoolers today are routinely inoculated with as many as twenty-two assorted vaccines, compared to three given in the 1940s. Research may reveal a link between autism, a neurological disease typically striking children between 18-36 months of age, and impaired immune systems traced to a barrage of childhood vaccines. A 273% increase in reported cases of autism since 1987 may indicate an epidemic in progress.[71]

Undetectable microorganism contaminants in vaccines could result in illness, and may be more likely to do so in those persons with compromised immune systems. Since contamination with mycoplasmas has been found in commercial vaccines, the vaccines used in the Gulf War should be considered as a possible cause of veterans' chronic illnesses.[72]

Most of the signs and symptoms in a large subset of GWI patients can be explained by chronic pathogenic bacterial infections, such as mycoplasma and *Brucella* infections. Studies of over 1,500 U. S. and British veterans with GWI, reveal that approximately 40-50% of GWI patients have PCR evidence of such infections, compared to 6-9% in the non-deployed, healthy population.[73] According to one United States Senate study[74], GWI has spread to family members, and it is likely that it has also spread in the workplace.

Mycoplasma fermentans, most commonly detected in over 80% of those GWI patients testing positive for any type of mycoplasma, is found intracellularly. Since this sort of infection is unlikely to produce a strong antibody response, it may explain the lack of serologic evidence for these types of intracellular infections.[75]

Three types of symptoms were seen to be about three times more prevalent among Gulf War veterans than other test subjects: chronic fatigue, muscle and joint pain, and neurocognitive problems. The Institute of Molecular Medicine found in 1996 that joint pain and fatigue were the two chief complaints of a study of 18,075 GWI study participants.[76]

Another recent study[77] concluded that none of the *known* infectious diseases seemed likely to cause GWI, although an unknown variety cannot be ruled out. The study recommended further investigation into the role of mycoplasma infection to determine a causal relationship. Testing using nucleoprotein gene tracking may be able to detect the bacteria and can then be used to validate results obtained by PCR testing.

A federally funded study[78] found high rates of positive tests for mycoplasmal infection in ill Gulf War veterans. In this study, many of those who tested positive responded well to antibiotic treatment that resolved severe symptoms. Antibiotics used were doxycycline, minocycline, and others, administered over a 6-12 month period. It is important to note that the relapse is inversely proportional to the number of six-week trials used in the treatment. After only one six-week period, all patients relapsed. After three periods (18 weeks), 73% relapsed. The rate was down to 19% after 6 periods (36 weeks).[79]

Some in the scientific community have criticized the study results, asserting that comparing blood samples from a pre-deployment time period to the postwar testing period did not reveal increased rates of mycoplasma antibodies. This is understandable, since blood sample comparison is a poor way to find mycoplasmas; most patients with mycoplasma don't test positive for antibodies.[80]

Psychiatrists often decide in the absence of contrary laboratory findings that GWI is a manifestation of a somatoform condition such as Post-Traumatic Stress Disorder, rather than the result of organic or medical problems. However, most veterans have made it clear that while stress is a contributing factor, it is not a major factor. They insist that stress-related diagnoses do not accurately portray their illnesses. This view was supported by a 1997 General Accounting Office (GAO) Report.[81]

Critics also question the validity and reliability of the new nucleoprotein gene tracking test method developed by Dr. Nicolson and his associates.[82] The tests are highly specific and very sensitive—though not as sensitive as PCR—and analyze white blood cells for the presence of mycoplasma infection, so far identified in about 60% of Fibromyalgia Syndrome (FMS) patients, 60% of Chronic Fatigue Syndrome (CFS) subjects, and 45% of GWI patients. *Mycoplasma* species were identified in the synovial fluid of about 60% of patients with rheumatoid arthritis using PCR tests.[83] Dr. Franco's research has shown that 54% of his patients with FMS have mycoplasma infection, compared to 15% of healthy controls.

In Dr. Nicolson's words, "Once these [infections] are identified, then they can be treated with a regimen of antibiotics, vitamins and nutritional support.... At least three quarters of the people that start this treatment have recovered. Not everybody recovers and we attribute that to the fact that a lot of people have multiple reasons for their chronic conditions...In some cases people get temporary relief by going on hyperbaric oxygen."[84]

Mycoplasmas are microorganisms that prefer low oxygen tension. That is, when the body's tissues are starved for oxygen, the condition will stimulate the growth of these borderline anaerobes. This explains why symptoms of individuals with mycoplasma infections are worse after a long airline flight. GWI is particularly evident in helicopter pilots for this reason.

Illnesses such as asthma, genitourinary infections, CFS, HIV/AIDS, GWI, Fibromyalgia Syndrome (FMS), Irritable Bowel Syndrome (IBS)), and perhaps endocarditis are another manifestation of mycoplasmal infection.[85] Increasing and widespread instances of carpal tunnel syndrome (*tendonitis synovitis*) are possibly caused by *Mycoplasma synoviae*. PCR testing can prove or disprove this theory. A major study is underway to consider autism in children and depression in adults as chronic illnesses linked to mycoplasmal infection.[86]

Although there are approximately 50 different types of mycoplasma, 6 have been found to cause disease in humans. One species in particular, *M. fermentans (incognitus)*, has been detected in some tested Gulf War veterans and their families. It is known to grow in the body at a very slow rate. The infected individual will start to exhibit CFS or FMS symptoms at first: a low-grade fever and/or a sense of "flu" that settles in the lungs. The condition becomes chronic, and additional symptoms develop—joint pain, reduced mobility, chronic fatigue, vision problems, cognitive problems, muscle spasms, and a burning sensation—all coming on very slowly.[87] Details on FMS symptoms and treatment appear in Appendix II.

It is tragic that someone who may have a chronic illness like Fibromyalgia and who could be helped by the long-term antibiotic regimen described in this book is instead treated with a short course of antibiotics, often in several rounds spaced weeks or months apart. This approach is useless to combat a mycoplasmal infection at the root of chronic disease. A recent study detected *multiple* mycoplasmal infections in the blood of patients diagnosed with CFS and FMS.[88]

Multiple Sclerosis (MS)

MS is a neurological disease in which the blood/brain barrier is damaged. Edema and swelling cause the release of plasma proteins into the central nervous system, triggering an inflammatory response. The disease is intermittent, so initial diagnosis is difficult and is usually made only after several disabling attacks have damaged the nervous system.

MS has perplexed those who continue to search for a cause. One assertion is that the culprit is a spirochete, an organism in the same class as the one that causes Lyme disease. For MS, the microbe will define a new group of bacteria, which is very common and present in the majority of the population but generally present in higher numbers in persons who demonstrate MS symptoms. Elevated levels of these bacteria and a commonly resident yeast have been recovered from cerebrospinal fluid.[89] However, to date no solid double blind controlled research has been done to substantiate either claim. Since yeast may play a role in CFS, perhaps it might have some role in MS as well. PCR techniques and biochip testing hold promise to help sort out the conflicting theories.

Another research path[90] has examined the Human Herpes Virus Six (HHV-6) as a possible cause. HHV-6 is a disease contracted in infancy causing a high fever and rash. Although the children recover, the HHV-6 stays dormant in the nerves until an opportune time to emerge. At that time the virus damages the nerves' myelin sheath, producing the symptoms of MS.[91] HHV-6 DNA is detectable by PCR testing. Drugs developed for HIV may be able to cure MS. Patients with MS have a high incidence of mycoplasmal infections

Other research indicates that MS is either caused by or exacerbated by *Chlamydia pneumoniae* infection, which can be cured with doxycycline over several weeks.[92] Dr. Luther Lindner, a pathologist on the faculty of Texas A&M University, reports antibiotic therapy being used successfully to treat MS.[93] Treatment with hyperbaric oxygen has also enjoyed some success.[94]

Cerebrospinal fluid (CSF) is examined using PCR tests to detect the presence of immune system proteins known to be associated with MS. The CSF test can also detect the presence of oligoclonal bands. These bands are evidence of an autoimmune response and are found in 90 to 95% of MS patients. Since they are detected in other individuals with other diseases, the presence of bands is not a conclusive diagnosis for MS.[95]

Prescription drugs provide some temporary relief, but have not been able to stop the progression of or reverse the symptoms of the disease. These drugs also introduce adverse side effects. Persons with MS admit to using a variety of alternative methods and supplements: e.g., EPA fish oil, borage oil, and lecithin help to suppress autoimmune reactions and to rebuild the myelin sheath. Coenzyme Q_{10} and Vitamin B_{12} (sublingual preferred) are also beneficial for cell rejuvenation.[96]

Tuberculosis (TB)

In 1985 it was determined that fewer than 30,000 Americans had contracted tuberculosis each year since 1977. The majority of these were elderly European expatriates who had carried the *Mycobacterium tuberculosis* microbes in their bodies for decades, falling ill only when their aging immune systems failed to keep these microorganisms or their L-forms within an acceptable range. Because there were so few instances of TB, by the mid-1980s federal and state politicians had slashed TB control and surveillance budgets. They didn't realize that the emerging epidemic of HIV would cause associated outbreaks of tuberculosis. In the strictly Darwinian sense of "survival of the fittest," TB proliferation is beneficial to the human species in general since it kills off the HIV carriers and the rate of HIV propagation is reduced.

Changing social conditions of addictive drug use, poverty, and increased urban density also provided fertile ground for TB. Any condition that taxes the immune system—be it malnutrition, influenza, amoebas, tropical parasites, cancer, pneumonia, or other illness—gives *M. tuberculosis* an opportunity to exploit the vulnerability of its host. In 1991, direct costs for TB treatment topped $700 million and kept going up, but there were no funds budgeted to cover these costs.[97] The CDC reports that as of 1996, TB is a reemerging disease threat, causing an estimated 13 million deaths worldwide each year and accounting for 25% of preventable deaths among adults. Worldwide, more deaths are caused by tuberculosis than any other infectious disease. This situation has not changed since the 1980s.[98]

Barry Bloom, a TB expert for the World Health Organization and a researcher at the Albert Einstein School of Medicine in the Bronx deplores the U.S. government's attitude toward infectious diseases. He claims that there is a generation gap separating people who know something about TB and those who don't, since antibiotics were assumed to have eradicated the disease in the 1940s. Following this assumption—that all funding for TB research stopped as a budget decision—we find that the only experts remaining in America are some 40 scientists from that era who are now at retirement age. Russia is active in TB research and is the source of several important papers on the *M. tuberculosis* L-form and its often extreme virulence.

The same budget-driven view has been true of mycoplasma and L-form research in the United States. Despite mounting evidence of their pervasive and pathogenic potential, many in the U.S. medical community have assumed mycoplasmas away as obscure and benign organisms.

A willingness to overcome a legacy of indifference toward mycoplasmas and to clear away the many longstanding assumptions regarding their role will have high payoff in the understanding of rheumatoid arthritis and other chronic diseases. Sophisticated, high-tech testing methods increase the sensitivity of the tests for pathogenic factors, and will undoubtedly lead to widespread confirmation of many of Dr. Brown's conclusions.

Amyotrophic Lateral Sclerosis (ALS)

ALS, also called "Lou Gehrig's Disease," affects both the central and peripheral nervous systems. ALS patients exhibit progressive weakness and paralysis of muscles as the upper motor neurons in the motor cortex and the lower motor neurons in the brain stem and spinal cord are gradually destroyed. The etiology of ALS is still a mystery, but recent research suggests that one or more infectious agents, such as enterovirus, may play a causative role. Several hypotheses have been proposed[99] including:

- Glutamate toxicity
- Oxidative stress
- Mitochondrial dysfunction
- Autoimmune disease
- Infectious disease
- Toxic chemical exposure
- Heavy metals concentration such as lead, mercury, aluminum, and manganese
- Calcium and magnesium deficiency
- Carbohydrate metabolism
- Growth factor deficiency

Mycoplasmal infections, notably *M. fermentans*, have been found in over 85% of ALS patients. These pathogens, like enteroviruses, have the ability to penetrate the central nervous system and also to cause persistent neurological symptoms.[100] Both enteroviruses and myco-plasmas are able to cause slow, chronic infections that can eventually result in cellular dysfunction and cell death.[101]

VACCINES

Recent developments are multivalent (multi-strain) vaccines for such conditions as influenza, *Otitis Media* and *Pneumococcus*. These vaccines are now widely available in the United States and hold definite promise for preventive care, for children and older persons if administered with discretion.

The slowly progressing rheumatic infections—whether viral, mycoplasmal, or bacterial L-forms—are all prime candidates for suppression by vaccines which even if they do not target the exact microbe can also stimulate the immune system to re-energize its defenses.[102]

Where the primary reserve host is man, the use of vaccines has reduced the incidence and infection rate of a disease to insignificance, e.g., with smallpox and polio. In persistent disease cases, such as rabies, multi-dose vaccine treatments are necessary. In general, multi-doses (i.e., booster shots) of many vaccines are found useful if not essential to preserve levels of immunity. This may also apply to vaccines like the pneumococcal or mycoplasma vaccines that work against microbes known to express enzymes like COX-2, known to be associated with arthritis.

Vaccines, together with use of appropriate antibiotics, antienzymes, antitoxins, antiviral drugs, and/or apopotosis-inducing drugs in cases where the organism invades host cells would seem to provide a more effective multi-pronged attack on the microbe's vulnerabilities in several of its forms/stages.[103]

Some antiviral drugs act to defeat the cell attachment "ligand receptor" link mechanism. *Mycoplasma fermentans* (*incognitus*) is reported to have a very similar to HIV cell link structure on its surface. This implies that its ability to invade host cells may be inhibited by an anti-HIV compound working to disable the ligand receptor.

Leprosy vaccine tests in India are thought to have stimulated reactions similar to the Jarisch-Herxheimer effect, inducing the immune response against existing leprosy infections, similar to the TB skin test.[104]

In such cases, a prophylactic antibiotic regimen in addition to the vaccine might be a fruitful area for further research, leading toward infection identification and more rapid patient cures. However, there are more vaccine candidates than funds. Development and production is costly and dangerous to the developers who must culture the pathogen, work with its host and not become infected themselves. Such development and production facilities may also generate significant amounts of bio-hazardous wastes that require meticulous control and destruction. Progress in vaccine R&D is limited mainly by funding.

Status of work in this field can be disclosed using the Internet by using a search engine such as Google with keywords *vaccine* and either *disease name* or *organism name* or *condition*, e.g., *Scleroderma*.

Vaccines are being developed against epidemics that are again becoming global threats—malaria, tuberculosis, and leprosy.[105]

Many vaccines against various problem microbes have been developed for domesticated animals. Use of these vaccines can suppress the microbe in the animal population and reduce the chances of food-borne infections in humans. Human vaccines need to be developed against the same or similar colonizing pathogens such as Chlamydia, Gonorrhea, Shigella, Salmonella, Giardia and Clostridium.[106]

---

[1] Kearns, Brenda. "20 Tips for Beating Superbugs." *Your Health*, January 23, 1996.

[2] For full details on Methicillin-Resistant *Staphylococcus aureus* (MRSA), see www.cdc.gov.

[3] Benko, Laura B. "Cubist's New Class of Drugs to Treat Stubborn Infections," in *Investor's Business Daily*, April 3, 1997. The article describes Cubist Pharmaceuticals, Inc.'s plans to develop an entirely new type of antibiotics that will treat bacterial and fungal infections. The target is a $26 billion annual market. This is an estimated ten% of the global drug market.

[4] See www.cdc.gov/ncidod/EID/vol1no2/cetron.htm for details of the CDC's Action Plan for combating drug-resistant *Streptococcus pneumoniae.*

[5] Nash, J. Madeleine. "The Antibiotic Crisis." *TIME*, 1/15/2001.

[6] Mayo Clinic research, reported by Janice M. Horowitz, "It's Not Just Athlete's Foot." *TIME*, 1/15/2001.

---

[7] CNN (New York) press release. "Campylobacter: Poultry-borne Germ Causing Hundreds of Deaths." Web posted October 20, 1997 at www.nutriteam.com/poultry.htm.

[8] Krieger, Lisa (*San Francisco Examiner*) reporting on annual meeting of Infectious Disease Society of America held in San Francisco, 1997. "New Agents for Disease?" *South Bay Daily Breeze*, September 17, 1997, pg A5.

[9] Michaud and Feinstein (1989) chapter 8. See also Witkin (1985).

[10] "Ears, Infections, Antibiotics, and Our Kids." Unattributed *HealthNet News* feature, Fall 1996.

[11] This may be for insurance reasons, or because they consider the evidence anecdotal and unscientific for the natural healing properties of herbs/massage/meditation/etc., or they prefer to treat patients according to the traditional methods they were taught in medical school. The physicians' denigrating attitude toward naturopathic medicine is summed up by Dr. Paul G. Donohue, M.D. in "How You Can Control Arthritis." *To Your Good Health*, Summer 1992. "When a real cure is devised for a disease, the old 'grandma remedies' rapidly die. But until then, they flourish." In other words, ignore any consideration of alternative theories, no matter what evidence of success exists.

[12] A small representative sample of media reporting on this topic includes: Coleman, Brenda (Associated Press). "Study: Antibiotics Are Overprescribed." *South Bay Daily Breeze*, September 17, 1997, pg A5; "Antibiotic-Resistant Bugs on the Rise, Federal Study Finds." *Los Angeles Times*, August 24, 1995, pg 2; "Drug Resistance: the New Apocalypse." Special issue of *Trends in Microbiology*, Vol 2, No. 10, October 1, 1994; Cohen, M. L. "Epidemiology of Drug Resistance: Implications for a Post-anti Microbial Era." *Science*, vol. 257, 1992; Cohen, S.J., Halvorson, H.W., and Gosselink, C. A. "Changing Physician Behavior to Improve Disease Prevention." *Preventive Medicine* vol. 23, 1994; Levy, Stuart B. "The Challenge of Antibiotic Resistance." *Scientific American,* March, 1998; Salmon, D. K. "The Truth About Antibiotics." *Parent'sMagazine,* November, 1995; Spake, Amanda. "Losing the Battle of the Bugs." *U.S. News OnLine*, 10 May 1999; LaFee, Scott (Copley News Service). "Bacteria Wages War on Antibiotics." *South Bay Daily Breeze*, November 5, 2001, pg B3.

[13] Personal Communication with Dr. Tsuyoshi Okada, July 2001.

---

[14] Roberts, Marilyn C. "Antibiotic Resistance." In Maniloff (1992) section V, chapter 31, p. 513.

[15] Clark (1997) p. 34.

[16] Goodman-Malamuth, Leslie. "Animal Drugs." *Nutrition Action*, May 1986.

[17] Report of the Union of Concerned Scientists, as reported by Maggie Fox, Reuters Health and Science Correspondent. "Drug Use in Animals Seen Higher Than Thought." January 8, 2001.

[18] Thompson, Dick. "Drugged Chicks Hatch a Menace." *TIME*, May 31, 1999.

[19] "The Effects on Human Health of Subtherapeutic Use of Antibiotics in Animal Feeds." National Academy of Sciences, Washington, DC, 1980.

[20] Moore, James; Strachan, Acacia; Miller, Whelton; and Ricardo, Cristina. "Antibiotics Used in Animal Feed Create Long Term Health Hazards for Humans." Senior seminar project, Department of Chemistry and Biochemistry, University of Delaware, December 1, 2000.

[21] *Journal of Nutrition*, 69:18-21, 1959. Cosponsored by the Surgeon General of the US Army. See also *Federation Proceedings*, 19:1045-1048, 1960. Cosponsored by the Surgeon General of the US Army.

[22] *Bulletin of the World Health Organization*, 41:873-904, 1969. Cosponsored by the US Atomic Energy Commission and Food and Drug Administration.

[23] *Mutation Research*, 80:333-345, 1981 and *International Journal of Radiation Biology*, 18:201-216, 1970.

[24] "Food Irradiation." *Nutrition*, 16:698-701, 2000.

[25] Agriculture Research Service. "Background: Food Irradiation." December 10, 1997.

[26] See www.avma.org:80/onlnews/javma/aug96/s080196m.html.

[27] Osterholm, M.T. and Potter, M.E. "Irradiation Pasteurization of Solid Foods: Taking Food Safety to the Next Level." *Emerging Infectious Disease*, Vol. 3(4), 1997.

---

[28] Use the search engine at www.mercola.com or use Google with key words "irradiation" and "beef."

[29] Dr. Mercola's proven "Eating Plan for Optimal Health" can be found at www.mercola.com/forms/wellness_condensed.htm. Comprehensive dietary guidelines as well as lifestyle modifications are presented which, if diligently followed, will result in improved health and well-being. A recipe book is also available at this website.

[30] *J. Anim. Sci.* 2000. 78:2849-2855.

[31] See Dr. Mercola's scientific literature page at www.mercola.com.

[32] Find a Midwest source for beef purchase at www.mercola.com.

[33] Garrett (1995) p. 36.

[34] Ibid., pp. 414-415 and pp. 670-4.

[35] Ibid., pp. 428-30.

[36] Ibid., p. 416.

[37] Monmaney, Terrence. "Antibiotic-Resistant Bugs on the Rise, Federal Study Finds." *Los Angeles Times*. Vol. 115, No. 30, p. 2 August 24, 1995.

[38] Via the Internet at www.cdc.gov from the CDC Division of Bacterial and Mycotic Diseases. Newly identified bacterial pathogens with unusual patterns of drug resistance constitute the focus of this subagency of the CDC.

[39] "Horrible." Unattributed feature article. *The Economist*, May 28, 1994, p. 52.

[40] Garrett (1995) pp. 226-8.

[41] Ibid., pp. 232-3.

[42] Study results summarized by Lori Oliwenstein. "Understanding T-Cells," *Arthritis Today*, January/February 1996. The scientists, whose experiment was first published in *Immunity*, speculated that RA patients most likely have another gene to account for the T-cell difference.

[43] Ewald, Paul W. "The Evolution of Virulence." *Scientific American*, April 1993.

[44] Transposons were discovered and named by Dr. Barbara McClintock, for which she received the 1990 Nobel Prize in Medicine.

---

[45] Garrett (1995) p. 432.

[46] Remarks by bacteriologist Alexander Tomasz, "Disease Causing Bacteria Resistant to Antibiotics," at the annual meeting of the American Association for the Advancement of Science, San Francisco, February 19, 1994.

[47] Garrett (1995) p. 413.

[48] Some estimates now put this figure at nearer 40 million.

[49] *Streptococcus pneumonia* also has so many different strains that one exposure does not immunize against the dozens of others.

[50] Ibid., p. 160.

[51] All quotes attributed to Drs Baseman and Tully in this chapter may be found at www.medscape.com/other/EID/1997.

[52] Appendix "Antibiotics: Efficacy Against Susceptible Pathogens." *Physician's Drug Handbook* (1993), pp. 1139-1145.

[53] Ibid., Drs Baseman and Tully.

[54] Ibid., Drs Baseman and Tully.

[55] The following websites are very informative about PCR and a wide variety of case studies: www.gene.com, www.vindae.com, www.mit.edu, and http://rap.nas.edu/lab.

[56] Garrett (1995) pp. 582-6.

[57] See Dr. Baseman's and Dr. Tully's excellent overview and their study results at www.medscape.com/other/EID/1997 obtained from the Medline Medscape site. Also, a small group of immunologists contend that the human immune system can respond to cancer, and provides evidence leading to this nontraditional conclusion. Rosenberg (1992) pp. 57-58 and chapters 6-11. Another fine overview entitled "The Pathogenesis and Treatment of Mycoplasmal Infections" can be found at www.immed.org/illness/autoimmune_illness_research.html. This article appeared in the *Antimicrobics and Infectious Disease Newsletter* (Elsevier Science) 1999; 17(11):81-88.

[58] Linker III, Joe B. and Williams Jr., Ralph C. "Tests for Detection of Rheumatoid Factors," in Rose (1986) pp. 759-761.

---

[59] Repeated stimulus of the immune system with TB test materials can significantly extend the life of melanoma patients. This treatment was given to a family friend whose life was saved as a result.

[60] Tully, Dr. J. G. "Reflections: Some Personal Impressions of Early Life and Forty Years of Mycoplasmology." Prepared for the Archives of the International Organization for Mycoplasmology upon his retirement from the National Institutes of Health in 2001.

[61] See www.thearthritiscenter.com/arthritis_info.htm#Anchor-Infections-11481.

[62] Orlock, Carol. "Of Germs and Genes." *Arthritis Today*, March/April 1995.

[63] Ibid.

[64] New York City Department of Health, Bureau of Communicable Diseases. October 2000.

[65] See http://edcenter.med.cornell.edu/CUMC_PathNotes/Female_Genital_Tract/FGT_2.html.

[66] Toivanen (1988) pp. 126-127.

[67] Yli-Kerttula, U.I. and Vilppula, A.H. "Rheumatic salpingitis?" *Clin. Rheumatol.* 1984; 3: 85.

[68] Written testimony of Dr. Garth L. Nicolson to the Congressional Committee on Government Reform (Subcommittee on National Security, Veterans' Affairs and International Relations), January 24, 2002.

[69] Hilborne and Golomb (2001) pg 9.

[70] See www.cdc.gov/ncidod/eid/vol8no1/01-0091.html. The study was co-sponsored by the U.S. Army Medical Research Institute of Infectious Diseases, Fort Detrick, MD and the National Cancer Institute-Frederick Cancer Research and Development Center, Frederick, MD.

[71] LaFee, Scott (Copley News Service). "Scientists Probe Autism Mystery as Number of Reported Cases Rises." Reported in *South Bay Daily Breeze*, January 28, 2002. Also see www.autism-society.org and www.cureautismnow.org for more information.

[72] Thornton D. "A Survey of Mycoplasma Detection in Vaccines." *Vaccine* 1986; 4:237-240.

---

[73] Nicolson, G.L.; Nasralla, M.; Franco, A.R., et al. "Mycoplasmal Infections in Fatigue Illnesses: Chronic Fatigue and Fibromyalgia Syndromes, Gulf War Illness and Rheumatoid Arthritis." *J. Chronic Fatigue Syndr.* 2000; 6(3/4):23-39.

[74] U. S. Congress, Senate Committee on Banking, Housing and Urban Affairs. "U. S. Chemical and Biological Warfare-related Dual Use Exports to Iraq and Their Possible Impact on the Health Consequences of the Persian Gulf War." 103rd Congress, 2nd Session, Report May 25, 1994.

[75] Gray, G.C.; Kaiser, K.S.; Hawksworth, A.W.; et al. No Serologic Evidence of an Association Found Between Gulf War Service and *Mycoplasma fermentans* Infection. *Am. J. Trop. Med. Hyg.* 1999; 60:752-757

[76] "Health Consequences of Service During the Persian Gulf War: Recommendations for Research and Information Systems." Testimony given by Dr. Garth Nicolson to the Congressional Committee to Review the Health Consequences of Service During the Persian Gulf War, Washington, DC, 1996.

[77] Hilborne and Golomb (2001) chapter 2.

[78] O'Dell, J.R.; Haire, C.E.; Palmer, W.; et al. "Treatment of Early Rheumatoid Arthritis with Minocycline or Placebo: Results of a Randomized, Double-blind Placebo-controlled Trial." *Arthritis Rheum.* 1997; 40:842-848.

[79] Nicolson, Garth and Nicolson, Nancy. Written Testimony to the Committee on Government Reform and Oversight, Subcommittee on Human Resource and Intergovernmental Relations, U.S. House of Representatives, Washington, DC, 1997.

[80] Personal communication with Dr. Nicolson, July 2001.

[81] U. S. General Accounting Office. "Gulf War Illnesses: Improved Monitoring of Clinical Progress and Reexamination of Research Emphasis are Needed." Report GAO/SNIAD-97-163, 1997.

[82] Dr. Nicolson is Chief Scientific Officer of the Institute for Molecular Medicine in Huntington Beach, CA. His wife Nancy assists him at the Institute and co-authors many of the Institute's pubications. Dr.Nancy Nicolson was president of the Rhodon Foundation for Biomedical Research and has been professor in the Department of Immunology and Microbiology at Baylor College of Medicine.

---

[83] Nicolson, et al. *J. Chronic Fatigue Syndrome* 6(3/4); 23-39, 2000.

[84] Interview comments to Dr. Roger G. Mazlen, host of the Chronic Fatigue Syndrome Radio Show, January 4, 1998.

[85] Op. cit., Nicolson, G.L., Nasralla, M.Y., et al. (1999)

[86] Berns, P.A., MD; Nicolson, G.L. and Rimland, B. "Molecular Hyperbaric Medicine Studies on Autism using Hyperbaric Oxygen Therapy and Antibiotics." Study in progress.

[87] Ibid.

[88] Nasralla M.; Haier, J. and Nicolson, G.L. "Multiple Mycoplasmal Infections Detected in Blood of Chronic Fatigue and Fibromyalgia Syndrome Patients." *Eur J Clin Microbiol Infect Dis* 18:359-365, 1999.

[89] Personal communication with Dr. Lindner, November 1996.

[90] Nicolson, G.L. and Nicolson, N.L. "Autoimmune Neurological and Rheumatic Diseases: Role of Chronic Infections in Morbidity and Progression." *Proceedings 13th International Symposium on Integrative Medicine 2001*; 13:104-112.

[91] Ablashi, D.V.; Lapps, W.; Kaplan, M.; Whitman, J.E.; Richert, J.R. and Pearson, G.R. "Human Herpes Virus-6 (HHV-6) Infection In Multiple Sclerosis." *Mult Scler* 1998 Dec;4(6):490-6. See also www.albany.net/~tjc/hhv-6.html.

[92] Sriram, S; Mitchell, W. and Stratton, C. "Multiple Sclerosis Associated with *Chlamydia pneumoniae* Infection of the CNS." *Neurology* 1998 Feb;50(2):571-2 and Stratton, C.; Mitchell, W. and Sriram, S. "Does *Chlamydia pneumoniae* Play a Role in the Pathogenesis of Multiple Sclerosis? *J Med Microbiol* 2000 Jan;49(1):1-3.

[93] Personal communication with Dr. Lindner, November 1996.

[94] Naubauer, R.A. "Protocol for the Treatment of Multiple Sclerosis with Hyperbaric Oxygen." *J. Hyperbar Med* 1990; 5:53-54.

[95] See www.lef.org/protocols/prtcl-077a.shtml. This is the Life Extension Foundation's website.

[96] For more information, contact the National Multiple Sclerosis Society, New York, NY. (800) 344-4867.

[97] Garrett (1995) pp. 513-522.

---

[98] Publication of the CDC Division of Bacterial and Mycotic Diseases at www.cdc.gov.

[99] See http://www.lef.org/protocols/prtcl-008.shtml for an overview of symptoms, tests, and treatments. Also, contact the ALS Association National Office, 21021 Ventura Blvd., Suite 321, Woodland Hills, CA 91364; (818) 340-7500; patient hotline: (800) 782-4747; e-mail, alsinfo@alsa-national.org. This association is a nonprofit, voluntary, national health organization committed solely to the fight against ALS through research, patient support, information, advocacy, and public awareness.

[100] Nicolson, G.L.; Nasralla, M.; Haier, J. and Pomfret, J. "High Frequency of Systemic Mycoplasmal Infections in Gulf War Veterans and Civilians with Amyotrophic Lateral Sclerosis (ALS). Eur. J. *Neurology* 2001. In process.

[101] Berger, M.M.; Kopp, N.; Vital, C.; Redl, B.; Aymard, M. and Lina, B. "Detection and Cellular Localization of Enterovirus RNA Sequences in Spinal Cord of Patients with ALS." *Neurology* 2000; 54:20-25 and Nicolson, G.L.; Nasralla, M. and Nicolson, N. "The Pathogenesis and Treatment of Mycoplasmal Infections." *Antimicrob Infect Dis Newsl* 1999; 17:81-88.

[102] See www.coleypharma.com/infectious.html.

[103] See www.nih.gov/sigs/aig.

[104] See www.lepra.org.uk/review/sept99/article1.html.

[105] See www.gatesfoundation.org/globalhealth/tuberculosis/grants/.

[106] See www.petevents.com.au/news_articles/55.shtml (Chlamydia), www.nau.edu/~fronske/gonorhea.html (Gonorrhea), www.cdc.gov/ncidod/dbmd/diseaseinfo/shigellosis_g.htm (Shigella), www.avcc.edu.au/news/univation/mar97/page14.htm (Salmonella), www.uti.ca/v6n3.htm (Giardia), www.aphis.usda.gov/vs/cvb/vich/formaldehydeFinal.PDF (Clostridium).

5. INFECTIONS OTHER THAN MYCOPLASMA

Long-term antibiotic treatment has been seen to inhibit mycoplasmal infection long enough for the body's natural immune system to destroy the invaders. Although Dr. Tully notes that physicians who treat chronic illnesses estimate that more than 25% of their patients benefit from a long-term, low-dose antibiotic regimen, this treatment is not guaranteed to work for all patients diagnosed with arthritis.[1]

Dr. Franco of the Arthritis Center of Riverside conducted a study of 255 of his RA patients. After long-term antibiotic treatment, 78% had a better than 20% improvement, and 53% had a better than 50% improvement; 22% of the patients did not improve.[2] His experience with lupus patients shows that some benefit from the antibiotic treatment, with improvement of their joints, skin, and pulmonary conditions. However, those patients who test positive for antineutrophilic cytoplasmic antibodies seem to have an increased likelihood of worsening with minocycline treatment.[3]

The point has been made repeatedly in this book that there is no single solution to healing arthritis. Despite thousands of documented success stories, there are still many individuals who do not respond to Dr. Brown's protocol.[4] This could be because they have additional serious medical conditions or coinfections, or perhaps their bodies harbor antibiotic-resistant microbes, or possibly because their symptoms have been misdiagnosed. As we have seen, food allergies can produce arthritis-like symptoms. Chronic illness individuals often have nutritional and vitamin deficiencies that must be corrected in parallel with any treatment against infection(s).

Physicians may be treating mycoplasmal, chlamydial, and other chronic infections but they are often not taking into account the intracellular persistent phases of these infections. During treatment, the microorganisms may be assuming a dormant phase within healthy tissues until they sense a more opportune time to emerge. The treatment may not address coinfections attributable to insect bites, myco-toxins, and/or bacteria.

Lyme Disease is one of a growing number of diseases exhibiting a full range of arthritis-like symptoms. These include other tick-borne illnesses such as Rickettsial disease, Babesiosis, and Ehrlichiosis.

Perhaps the best known example of disease caused by *Rickettsia rickettsii* in the United States is Rocky Mountain spotted fever. Nine strains found worldwide cause a variety of illnesses, including typhus.[5] Babesiosis is caused by tick-borne *Babesia mircoti*, which are malarial–like piroplasms. Ticks are also carriers of *Ehrlichia phagocytophila*, which causes Ehrlichiosis, a Lyme co-infection that can be fatal in about 10% of cases. At present it responds only to doxycycline.[6] Sometimes a wider range of antibiotics must be used; antiprotozoal and antimalarial drugs are needed to treat Babesiosis.

Bacterial infections involving the brain and central nervous system often do not respond to certain antibiotics because the biochemical structure of the drugs makes the molecules too large to cross the blood/brain barrier.[7] Minocycline can cross the barrier, but tetracycline cannot.[8]

This barrier acts protectively to limit the penetration of harmful substances to the brain. By blocking the transport of curing substances as well, this filtering mechanism acts as a limiting factor for brain treatments with drugs. These neurological conditions require high doses of antibiotics to raise serum concentrations to levels able to penetrate the blood/brain barrier, but at the risk of damaging other organs. Intensive international research efforts are underway to discover a selective penetration method that would guarantee the transport of drugs through the intact barrier.

VECTOR-BORNE ILLNESS

Lyme Disease (LD) will be used in this chapter as a representative and proven example of vector-borne (i.e., insect-transmitted) illness. Although formally recognized for over 15 years, Lyme Disease is still one of the most under-, over-, and mis-diagnosed diseases today. Some symptoms are common to all chronic illnesses like Fibromyalgia or Chronic Fatigue Syndrome: fatigue, muscle aches, joint pain and swelling. Neurological complications of LD may include meningitis, chronic neuroborreliosis, or Bell's palsy.[9]

Through diligent pest control measures, improved sanitation, and antibiotics, we have been lucky to prevent serious outbreaks of insect-borne disease in the United States. Lyme Disease remains a significant exception.[10]

Co-infections are very common. According to Dr. Nicolson, 60% of LD patients, 70% of those with Ehrlichia, and 20-25% of those individuals diagnosed with Babesiosis also test positive for mycoplasma. The Institute for Molecular Medicine has documented 125 symptoms related to co-infections.[11]

Lyme Disease (LD)

In 1975, 51 residents of Old Lyme, Connecticut were afflicted with a mysterious illness that resembled RA. By

1990, what has come to be called "Lyme Disease" was reported in all 50 States and parts of Western Europe. This is not because LD appeared as a new or localized disease spreading from the U.S. east coast; rather, it is because its bacterial origin had finally been recognized and a name given to the condition. LD is as ancient as the insect that carries it.

LD Carriers

The disease was traced to a little-studied spirochete bacterium, *Borrelia burgdorferi*, which is transmitted to humans by a tick *(Ixodes scapularis)* carried on rodents, deer, and birds.[12] Recent studies are investigating potential benevolent hosts—those species that don't infect ticks with Lyme during the nymph stage of the insect's life cycle. If these hosts can be identified, measures can be taken to reduce the numbers of those that do carry the disease, thus diluting the LD-carrying population.

According to ecologist Rick Ostfeld, ticks are born without the bacteria but many pick it up from the blood of the animals they feed on as larvae. White-footed mice seem to be the worst of the carriers, carrying some 70 larval ticks at a time and infecting them with Lyme at a rate close to 95%.[13]

International Ecology Society researcher Kathleen LoGiudice proposed that the opossum may be a benevolent host for two reasons: (1) each feeds an average of 400 larval ticks at a time, most of which died before molting into nymphs, and (2) of the survivors, only about 2% were infected with the bacteria.

Deer are considered prime carriers of adult ticks, which feed on the deer's blood, then drop from their host to lay their eggs. Little research has been done to quantify the number of larval ticks the deer carry or whether they are actually benevolent hosts.

Known disease carriers like white-footed mice thrive in a fragmented forest environment where their natural predators (coyotes, weasels, and foxes) have migrated away to larger areas or have been killed as pests in urban areas. Knowing more about animal hosts as LD carriers is essential to limiting the spread of the disease. Policymakers should use this knowledge as they plan land use, forest management, and urban development.

At present there are five subspecies of *B. burgdorferi*, with over 100 strains in the United States and 300 strains worldwide.[14] *B. burgdorferi* exists in at least three different forms: bacterial (spirochete), spheroplast, and cyst form. Only the spirochete can be killed by beta lactam antibiotics. Tetracyclines and erythromycins can kill the spheroplasts, but only metronidzole is effective against the cysts.[15]

During their two-year life cycle, ticks use a variety of carriers—mostly large mammals such as deer and humans, but also migrating birds—who can be counted upon to disperse them over a wide geographic area as they mature. Some 50 species of birds and 30 species of mammals, including household pets, have been identified as incidental hosts.[16]

The adult ticks fall from their hosts in the spring to lay their eggs on the ground and in forest floor debris. The eggs develop into larvae during the late spring and summer. The larvae attach themselves to small mammals and birds foraging close to the ground. The larvae grow into nymphs over the fall season; many die during the winter, but those who survive seek out birds and large and small mammals as carriers as the weather warms in the spring. The nymphs reach the adult stage in the fall, over-wintering on large mammal hosts until the spring cycle begins again. Most cases of Lyme infection begin in the spring and summer. This cycle is portrayed in Figure 6.[17] The drawing is over-simplified since it does not show very small rodent carriers.

Figure 6. Life Cycle of Lyme Disease Ticks

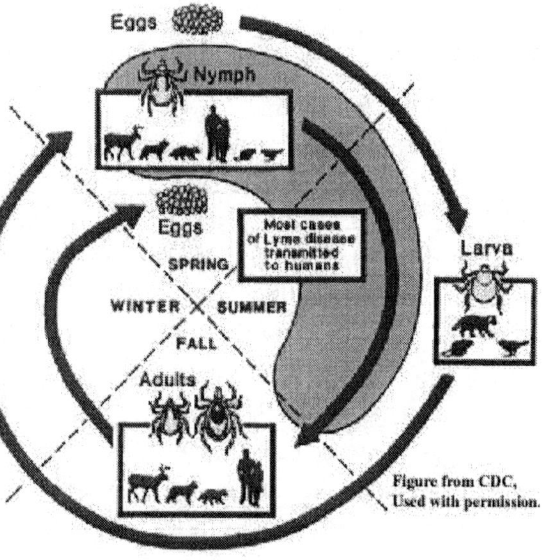

Mice are also carriers of another serious disease, the hantavirus, a potentially lethal respiratory illness that re-emerged in 1993 in the American southwest. It is similar in DNA profile to a rodent-carried virus that caused fatal kidney dysfunction among a group of veterans returning from the Korean War in the 1950s. An outbreak in the 1970s was reported in Eastern Europe and Asia. The CDC and the U.S. Army collected and tested rats for the virus in all major port cities of the United States, finding the Seoul hantavirus to be endemic. According to the CDC, hantavirus was reported in Argentina in June 1997, spread from person to person. Until then, scientists believed it was transmitted only by contact with airborne particles of dried rodent excrement.

Hantavirus is not a new illness; it has just been formally recognized and given a name after millennia of microbial evolution, adaptation, and distribution.

Motility of the Tick Spirochete

The disease-bearing tick punctures the skin, introducing the *B. burdorferi* spirochete. As the tick feeds it transmits the disease. About 70-90% of those who contract LD are bitten by nymphs.[18] The resulting circular red rash may expand to 12 inches or more in diameter over the next several weeks. By then the bacteria has pervaded muscle, tendons, organs, heart, and even the brain.[19]

Since the rash does not itch, it may not be noticed if the tick bite is on one's back or other area not normally viewed daily. The chronic illness symptoms occur later, after the infection has spread. Dr. Mark Klempner theorized that the bacteria must contain special enzymes capable of dissolving proteins, fats, and collagen for it to be able to travel so freely around the body in such a short time.

Presenting his research to the Lyme Disease Foundation's annual meeting in 1996, Dr. Klempner described the spirochete as having an internal bundle of flagella that could expand and contract, propelling it along, especially through thick fluids. The tips of the bacterium bind not only to the different tissues but also to a blood-borne chemotactic enzyme called plasminogen.

According to Dr. Klempner, the bacterium uses this enzyme as a sort of battering ram to breach blood vessel walls. This action in turn causes other enzymatic reactions that weaken tissues and allow further, deeper invasion. The bacterium eventually seeks out a hiding place outside the blood stream, e.g., between tendon fibers or in the brain where the immune system's killer cells are unable to reach it.

This explains the behavior of moose sometimes observed wandering city streets in the far north. They may seem comical but their disorientation is likely due to the brain damage caused by a Lyme spirochete infestation.

LD-infected humans can experience a wide range of neurological, cognitive, and psychiatric symptoms. In the later stage of the disease, patients exhibit memory deficits, loss of fluency of speech, and difficulty recalling motor sequences. Noting that fellow psychiatrists are reporting an increasing number of patients who test positive for neuroborreliosis, Dr. Robert Bransfield has developed a psychiatric diagnostic and tracking system.[20] This technique goes far beyond the standard medical approach. It combines the results of laboratory tests with a very thorough history, physical, and mental status examination to obtain a more accurate diagnosis.

Dr. Bransfield points out that co-infections with other agents leading to interactive infections pose a significant issue. He has also found that effective treatment consists of intramuscular and intravenous antibiotics, sometimes for an extended period of time. Hyperbaric oxygen treatment also shows increasing potential.[21]

The *Borrelia* organism can go dormant for years, then re-emerge as a cell-wall-deficient form, making it extremely difficult to detect and culture.[22] Experiments show that healthy, normal human B-cells placed in a culture with live *Borrelia burgdorferi* are penetrated and overtaken within a few minutes. The B-cells' lysosomal enzymes should be expected to dissolve the bacteria, but surprisingly the bacteria actually thrive, and eventually destroy the lymphocyte.[23] By taking over B-cells, the pathogen is able to cloak itself, camouflaged to its normal enemies in the blood—

complement, enzymes, macrophages, and killer T-cells that would otherwise destroy it.

The genus *Borrelia* includes two human pathogens: the agent causing relapsing fever (found in tropical and subtropical areas) and *B. burgdorferi sensu lato* (found in Europe and North America). A few region-specific strains of tick nymph-borne spirochetes have been identified.[24] At least four additional species play a role in Europe:

B. burgdorferi sensu strico (ss)
B. garinii
B. afzelii
B. valaisiana

Studies in the late 1990s examining small infected mammals found additional vectors for *Borreliae*: fleas, flies, mites, mosquitoes, and spiders.[25] Several diseases exhibiting microbial colonization similar to Lyme Disease have been traced to specific strains of *B. burgdorferi*.[26] Many other instances of microscopic insect-borne inflammations have been documented, e.g., those associated with chiggers.[27]

Tests for Lyme Disease

All testing methods currently available for LD have serious limitations.[28] The commonly used blood, urine, and spinal fluid tests have a significant rate of false negatives. Some tests (e.g., *in vitro* culture) may be inadequate for clinical purposes, while others provide results needing skilled interpretation.[29] *B. burgdorferi* can be detected by culture in BSK II (modified Barbour-Stoenner-Kelly) but culture is not reliable for routine testing. There are also problems with blood sample stability during transport to the testing lab.[30]

Those who test negative after the usual set of LD tests may wish to consider a new blood culture test. The Bowen

Research & Training Institute, North Palm Harbor, FL, has developed research protocols to identify the causative agents of Lyme Disease, Ehrlichia and Babesia.[31] The Lyme Urine Antigen Test offered by IGeneX may also be useful.[32]

An estimated 2 million people suffer from LD.[33] Some 15,000 new cases of LD are reported annually. Others put the figure at ten times that, based on data extrapolated from vaccine studies and CDC lectures on diagnostic criteria to prevent false positives, while ignoring false negatives.[34] The CDC requires a positive test for surveillance purposes in reporting cases of LD, and requires a diagnosis based on a doctor's evaluation of symptoms with the tests providing support.

PCR may become the gold standard for LD testing, although a real problem is not the number of false positives but the number of false negatives. *Borrelia* organisms are rarely present in body fluids but are normally bound to tissue cells. Thus blood samples normally taken for LD diagnosis usually do not contain enough germs to generate positive results. Skin biopsies for Neuroborreliosis and *Erythema migrans* give results in 1 or 2 days compared to the 3-4 weeks needed for standard culture.

LD is characterized by high fever in its early stages. This elevated temperature is not the response to the invading organism, but rather the body's reaction to the spirochete's toxic waste product.[35] It is similar to the Jarisch-Herxheimer effect experienced by RA patients when the antibiotic is working effectively to suppress mycoplasmas. Arthritis-like symptoms reflect the body's battle with toxins released by dead or dying microbes.[36]

The shape-shifting nature of an altered protein gene of *Borrelia afzelii* was reported after DNA examination.[37] A 1998 study found that *B. burgdorferi* DNA could be detected using PCR tests. The conclusion was that positive results of DNA bonding in the synovial membrane strongly suggest ongoing infection. In all patients studied, arthritis was completely resolved after long-term antibiotic treatment.[38] According to Dr. Nicolson, over 60% of LD positive patients also test positive for mycoplasmal infections and other bacteria.[39]

Two blood serum tests can detect antibodies produced to combat the spirochetes: immunofluorescence assay (IFA) and ELISA. Unfortunately, neither of these tests is highly accurate for this application. Even during the more advanced stages of the disease, these tests are particularly prone to false positives, so relying on these results alone is a mistake.[40] The diagnosis of LD must also include such factors as probability of exposure to ticks carrying the disease, timing of the characteristic *Erythema migrans* or "bull's eye" rash (usually during warm summer months), the patient's medical history, specific symptoms, and physical examination results. Recurrent *Erythema migrans* rash has diagnostic significance. Dr. Bransfield notes that chicken pox and other conditions can bring out the bull's eye rash around the pox lesions in LD-infected patients.

People who live in areas where the disease is endemic should consider vaccination, which is about 80% effective after a series of three shots.[41] When camping or hiking in wooded areas one should take precautions such as binding open trouser cuffs to the ankles with rubber bands, wearing light-colored clothing to spot ticks and remove them more readily, and regularly shaking out blankets, jackets and other items where ticks may hide. Not all insect repellents are completely reliable.

Treatment for Lyme Disease

LD can be treated with the usual short course of antibiotics but *only* if caught in the very early stages.

Antibiotic protocols for late stage LD must be much more intensive and complex than the relatively simpler treatment proposed by Dr. Brown for mycoplasma infection.[42] Most LD clinicians agree that steroids are contraindicated.

In the opinion of some researchers, LD may rival mycoplasma infection as the causative agent for rheumatoid arthritis.[43] One important but subtle difference between classical RA (mycoplasmal infection) and LD (vector-borne infection) is that LD affects the large weight-bearing joints, especially the knees) where RA prefers the small joints of the peripheral extremities, notably the hand. This may be because mycoplasmas migrate to the cooler areas of the body while spirochetes prefer warmer areas where the body temperature is relatively constant. LD can be as degenerative and crippling as classical RA.

Treatment for LD can be very expensive. Long-term IV therapy, for example, can cost $6,000 per month.[44] In the absence of the diagnostic tools required to identify LD, doctors have little data on which to form their diagnoses. Insurance companies are understandably reluctant to authorize coverage for treatments based on guesswork. However, they are inexcusably reluctant to invest in the tools and procedures required for accurate diagnoses.

In the words of Dr. Bransfield, "Lyme Disease is an illness that has proved managed care to be a catastrophic failure...Managed care short-term cost containment techniques have resulted in very expensive long-term direct and indirect costs. Most of the indirect costs have been shifted to the general public."[45] He is dismayed by seeing LD patients denied needed treatment early enough to prevent their increasingly deteriorating condition, which in some cases leads to lifetime disability.

Patients must be proactive in researching their condition, tapping the formidable resources available to them through Lyme-related foundations and their websites.

Because LD's forty-odd symptoms fit a number of medical conditions, it is important to find definitive tests and physicians who have the expertise to evaluate them. A good place to start is the Lyme Alliance Support Group network at www.lymealliance.org/resources/support.php. A list of LD-related websites appears in Appendix IV.

An Anti-toxin Treatment for LD

A new therapy developed by Dr. Ritchie Shoemaker[46] has received attention from physicians who treat Lyme Disease patients. The LD spirochete has been found to produce a toxin (a 37 kD protein) that has similar properties to botulinum C2 and other cytoskeletal toxins.

The therapy is the same as that given to Chesapeake Bay, Maryland, fishermen who suffered from "estuary disease" caused by the *Pfiesteria* neurotoxin. This treatment exploits the affinity of the toxins for the fatty tissues of the body. Because the toxins are low molecular weight and fat-soluble, they tend to be trapped in the adipose tissues. Although eventually broken down in the liver and routed to the bowel for excretion, the toxins are not completely eliminated. Some small fraction are reabsorbed by the colon as fats and proteins needed by the body.

According to Dr. Shoemaker's theory, the toxins accumulate and recirculate, affecting all systems of the body. However, a more plausible explanation may explain the cycle. What may actually be happening is that resident pathogens interact with the toxins and use them in some as-yet undetermined fashion for their benefit. This interaction is analogous to a feedback loop in electrical engineering, where gains (accumulation of toxins) and losses (elimination of toxins) must sum to a value greater than one to explain the resulting enduring/growing signal presence (sustained/ growing symptom severity). Only one factor in the feedback loop need be greater than one to sustain the loop.

Since toxins are relatively inert, it is natural to assume that there may be an infectious agent actively at work, contributing to the feedback cycle. This pathogen (or cluster of pathogens) may perhaps extract nutrients from the toxins it encounters and using these to generate replacements for the lost/excreted toxins. The original source of the toxins could be internal (e.g., microorganisms developed in the intestinal tract or in the blood) or external (e.g., inhaled pesticides, contact with water-borne pathogens that take up residence in the gut). This theory invites further research.

Dr. Shoemaker's therapy uses cholestyramine to bind the fat-soluble toxins into molecules that are too large for the colon to reabsorb, and thus they are preferentially excreted. The main side effect from the therapy is severe constipation, but this problem can be offset by taking inexpensive, readily available preventive measures. These include consuming pineapple juice four times per day, or taking magnesium citrate tablets plus extra Vitamin C, or OTC stool softeners

Cholestyramine is a cholesterol-lowering drug but it is much safer than others usually prescribed because the molecules produced do not find their way back into the GI tract or into the bloodstream. Thus some of the deleterious side effects associated with the newer drugs are avoided. Dr. Shoemaker's approach to LD is described in detail at www.chronicneurotoxins.com.

A more benign and less expensive approach than drugs and compensating measures could be equally effective. The well-known oatmeal and oat bran dietary elements, if consumed consistently, will facilitate the binding and removal of fat-soluble toxins. The added benefit is fiber for colon health. Psyllium, a natural supplement recommended for individuals with Irritable Bowl Syndrome, may also be helpful in reducing both fats and toxins as well as avoiding constipation.

MYCOTOXINS

Some 37 million Americans suffer from chronic sinus infections each year. Tens of thousands of unnecessary sinus operations are performed when the problem may actually be the result of a mold allergy that can be neutralized without surgery.[47]

A 1999 Mayo Clinic study cites mycotoxins from molds as the cause of allergic fungal sinusitis[48] Physicians are beginning to recognize that molds are responsible for allergies, asthma attacks, and negative impact on the immune system, leading to increased susceptibility to colds and flu. The prior prevailing medical view held that mold accounted for less than 10% of chronic sinusitis. The Mayo Clinic study found that number to be closer to 93%. This translates to over 34 million people seeking medical treatment and drugs for a condition that is easily prevented.

Molds are a subset of the fungi which are found everywhere on the earth. There are more than 100,000 species of molds. Some, like mushrooms and yeasts, are beneficial; others, like mildew and rust, are not. The majority of molds are not pathogenic. Molds are essential for the natural breakdown and recycling of organic matter. However, when molds lose moisture, they release spores because they sense death and in turn, the need to reproduce. The process also releases mycotoxins. Outdoor spores are not usually a source of toxicity but indoor molds produce toxins in higher concentration. These have the potential to cause illness. Since moisture plays such an important part in mycotoxin production, indoor humidity must be carefully controlled to prevent mildew, mold and mold spores.

Molds and spores themselves can cause allergy and/or infections but more harmful are the mycotoxins released by molds when their food source (moisture) is removed. There are over 200 recognized mycotoxins, but many more are unknown. The study of these substances and their effects on human health has barely begun. We do know that they can cause a variety of short-term responses such as dermatitis, cold and flu symptoms, headache, fatigue, diarrhea, and impaired immune system function, which may lead to more serious opportunistic infections. The long-term effects are potentially carcinogenic and teratogenic.

When spores enter the body through the nasal passages, the immune system sends eosinophils to attack the fungi. The eosinophils irritate the membranes in the nose. Antibiotics and OTC decongestants are widely used to treat chronic sinusitis, but antibiotics are not effective because they target bacteria, not fungi. The over-the-counter drugs may temporarily relieve symptoms, but they have no effect on the inflammation

Stachybotrys chartarum mold produces at least 170 known mycotoxins.[49] When this mold dries, mycotoxin production increases up to 40 thousand times.[50] The inhaled *Stachybotrys* mycotoxins accumulate in the body and are receiving increased attention as a phenomenon called "sick building syndrome." *Stachybotrys atra* toxic mold is the designated culprit in illnesses contracted at schools, homes, and office buildings and the focus of multimillion-dollar lawsuits. However, contamination by strains of aspergillus, chaetomium, and penicillium can be just as harmful. Mold has become big business in just the last six years since it has been shown to be associated with serious health problems.

Antipollution activists, lawyers, and support groups are suing construction companies, landlords, and insurance companies for damages to property and health.[51]

About 25% of the population is allergic to molds.[52] For people with asthma, ingesting foods containing mold may present a particular risk. Examples are: beer, wine, baked goods, sour cream, and cheeses.

Leftovers kept longer than 48 hours can pose a risk of food poisoning. Bacteria can begin to multiply in as little as 20 minutes when the hot food's temperature drops. The unsafe range of temperature is between 40-140 degrees Fahrenheit. The refrigerator thermometer should read between 35-40 degrees. High-fat foods such as meat and cheese tend to absorb plasticizing chemicals from containers not made of polyethylene.[53]

Practical Measures to Remove Mold

Mold can establish itself within 24 hours under the right conditions. When water penetrates walls, mold will form inside the wall space within 2-4 weeks if no action is taken. When mold growth is visible on interior walls, it usually means that heavy mold growth already exists in inner wall cavities. When a leak occurs, act immediately to determine the extent of wet materials through visual inspection and by using a moisture meter. If damage is extensive, enlist the help of a testing agency. Next, remove and dispose of wet or damp materials including wallboard, wallpaper, carpet, and padding. After thoroughly cleaning and disinfecting inner surfaces, dry all inner wall cavities and flooring thoroughly before installing new materials.

If mold has already formed, a restoration or abatement contractor must perform the above procedures. A professional is required because improper disturbance of infected wallboard will generate high levels of air-borne mold where none may have existed before. The contractor will seal off the work area with poly sheeting, install air filtration equipment, and will wear protective respiratory gear. An independent testing agency should inspect the cleared area before it is re-occupied. The worst course of action is to do nothing. Failure to adequately and aggressively address moisture problems at the time they occur invites environmental problems, health concerns, and increased costs later to remedy the situation.

There are preventive steps to take to protect one's home from molds, which require moisture plus a porous surface such as drywall, wallpaper, or carpeting to take hold. These are:

- Fix leaks immediately after a spill;
- Thoroughly dry out areas affected by spilled liquids;
- Keep bathrooms, basements, laundry rooms, and kitchens well-ventilated;
- Turn on fans after bathing, cooking, or washing;
- Regularly inspect closets and airtight or sealed-off areas for mold growth;
- Remove small mold patches immediately with a 3:1 solution of water to bleach. Add a little detergent to the solution to clean any dirt or oil on the surface that may retain mold. Do not add ammonia, since fumes released by mixing with bleach are dangerous. Boat/pool supply stores sell environmentally sensitive mildew cleaner;
- Persons cleaning mold should be free of cold/flu symptoms and allergies because mold spores can complicate existing conditions;

- Wear protective clothing while cleaning to avoid skin contact and inhalation of spores;
- Dispose of sponges or rags used to clean mold;
- Large patches (greater than a few square feet) require professional cleaning by a mold abatement company;
- If mold returns quickly or spreads, check for an underlying problem such as an unseen leak or water seepage.

Some molds compete for territory with other fungi by producing toxins directed at the invaders. These toxins are also harmful to humans when ingested, inhaled, or through dermal (skin) contact. These toxins are well known in food-borne illnesses. For example, *Fusaria* mold can grow on grain left in fields over the winter or in poorly ventilated silos. The disease resulting from ingestion of this mold is called alimentary toxic aleukia, with symptoms resembling a severe radiation overdose. Thousands died in the Soviet Union during World War II during a disease outbreak traced to consumption of *Fusaria*-contaminated grain.

The aflatoxins produced by *Aspergillus flavus* and *A. parasiticus* also commonly contaminate food grains before and after harvest, presenting a serious health problem for humans and livestock. In tropical regions, aflatoxins have been identified with the development of liver cancer.

MOSQUITO-BORNE DISEASES

Mosquitoes are sometimes called "flying hypodermic needles." One has only to imagine those needles filled with pathogens such as malaria and yellow fever to grasp the enormity of this problem. Malaria is endemic throughout the world, but fatalities occur most often in developing countries where wet, tropical conditions prevail. The disease kills more than a million Africans (mostly children) and an estimated one million in South America and Asia each year. Malaria-related deaths were at an all-time high in Africa in 1993 and the disease is spreading steadily worldwide.[54]

It is a mistake to believe that these tropical diseases are confined to faraway, emerging nations. An estimated one million soldiers suffered from malaria during the U.S. Civil War. A cargo ship from Japan docked at a Texas port in 1985 with a hold full of tires, many filled with puddles of stagnant rainwater and bearing untold colonies of Asian tiger mosquito larvae. These insects are known to transmit an especially virulent strain of Dengue Fever and several other viruses. The mosquito has become established in 17 southern states and has been found as far north as Illinois. This hardy insect is capable of withstanding cold winters.[55]

Only two of dozens of mosquito-borne diseases are described in the following subsections as examples: Dengue Fever and Filariasis.

Dengue Fever

The arbovirus Dengue Fever originated in ancient East Africa. It causes excruciating headaches and eye pain, along with bone pain and swelling in the joints. In 1780, this mosquito-borne disease swept Philadelphia and was called "breakbone fever" since the most frequent complaint was severe aching joints. By the middle of the nineteenth century the disease was endemic throughout the Americas. The Dengue virus is closely related to the yellow fever virus. In the 1940s, yellow fever vaccinations were thought to have eradicated the disease, but it thrived in the massive human migrations and refugee camps during World War II.

In the 1950s it emerged again, as an evolved and more lethal viral strain, Dengue-2, with an extraordinary ability to exploit human antibodies to its advantage. The microbe allows human antibodies to signal the macrophage cells to engulf it, but instead of being destroyed, the microbe takes control of the body's immune system's killer cells. It is then able to bypass all immune system defenses and enter every organ in the body. Macrophages, the body's primary defenders against infection, become "Trojan horses" for the virus.[56]

Dengue strains have reemerged every decade since the 1950s as serial infections that may cause little or no illness at first but which lie in wait, preparing the body's immune system for the next round. In hemorrhagic dengue, internal bleeding and shock can lead to death in 15% of cases.[57]

Filariasis

Filariasis is a debilitating blood-borne disease caused by nematode worms and initially transmitted by mosquitoes. The worm larvae circulate in the bloodstream of infected persons, and adult worms live in the lymphatic vessels. Filariasis is not life threatening, but it does cause extreme discomfort, swelling of the limbs and genitals, damage to the kidneys and lymphatic system, impairment of the immune system to fight infection, and general malaise. The toll in terms of emotional and economic impact and the disruption of family and community life is immense.

According to the World Health Organization (WHO), Filariasis is the world's second leading cause of permanent and long-term disability. Approximately 120 million people in 73 endemic countries worldwide are affected, primarily throughout the tropical and subtropical regions of South America, Asia, the Pacific Islands and Africa. The disease is termed "potentially eradicable" through drug therapy and vector control. However, infection rates are increasing for a variety of reasons: expansion of urban areas, political upheaval, and unavailable funds for insect control measures.

Arbovirus Resistance

Arboviruses like malaria are rapidly evolving and transmutating. Optimists tried to defeat parasitic malaria in the 1960s, and for a time it seemed that they had succeeded. However, by the 1990s, the efficacy of chloroquine—the best and most affordable of the antimalarials—was waning. Resistance to other derivative drugs such as mefloquine, quinine, trimethoprim, and quinidine was rising. Despite the existence of proteins on their surfaces that clearly should have signaled alarm to the host's immune system, these parasites could not be dislodged.

Another quinine derivative, quinolone AM-1155, has recently been investigated in Japan and suggested as a useful antimicrobial agent for the treatment of *Mycoplasma pneumoniae* infections.[58]

One theory,[59] based on British colonial experience in Africa for decades, asserts that chloroquine resistance can only get to a certain level before humans develop sufficient baseline immunity to keep the parasites in check. The theory was proposed by Kent Campbell of the CDC, who asked insightfully, "What *is* malaria?" By the late 1980s the CDC and their African colleagues were witnessing a dangerous new malaria mutation on the continent.

Efforts to maintain balance required higher and higher doses of chloroquine, causing significant damage to red blood cells as a side effect. A state of mutual tolerance developed between the antibodies and activated T-cells. As long as one did not overmedicate, it was beneficial to have some of these parasites in one's body at all times and to maintain a balanced condition. Chloroquine had little or no effect on the parasites, but was helpful in treating the fever and malaise associated with malaria.

This condition of imbalance is similar to the instance of mycoplasma infection asserting itself in an immuno-suppressed individual to produce symptoms of chronic disease such as arthritis. Here we see a classic example of engineering control theory applied to organisms rather than to the usual mechanical or electronic devices.

Treating patients to enable them to live with their parasites merely succeeds in providing a ready reservoir of increasingly drug-resistant organisms. This in turn is a recipe for disaster—a future epidemic catastrophe.

BLOOD-BORNE VIRUSES AND BACTERIA

The blood is a conduit for a wide variety of microorganisms to travel throughout the body, wreaking havoc along the way to their ultimate targets in tissues and/or organs. New research suggests that arterial inflammation producing an immune-system response contributes to heart attacks. The cause of the inflammation is under investigation but seems to be traced to a substance carried in the blood.[60] Some well known blood-borne illnesses are AIDS/HIV, Sepsis, and Filariasis.[61]

Human Immunodeficiency Virus (HIV)

HIV/AIDS is characterized by a reduction to 20% or less of normal in the numbers of CD4 helper T-cells, rendering the individual's immune system highly vulnerable to serious illnesses such as pneumonia. HIV has been found in blood, semen, saliva, tears, nervous system tissue, breast milk, and female genital tract secretions. HIV is most commonly transmitted in infected blood and bodily secretions, commonly during illicit intravenous drug use and/or sexual intercourse.

The HIV microbe hides deep inside the infected person's lymph nodes, often for years, before producing detectable symptoms. Unfortunately, the world view of HIV as a politically correct and privileged organism rather than a latent deadly disease requiring testing, detection, and quarantine has caused the global spread of the virus and the number of cases of infection to increase exponentially.[62]

The documented synergy between HIV and other microbial epidemics such as malaria, Epstein-Barr virus, tuberculosis, and others is a clear indication that immune system suppression gives rise to a wide variety of chronic diseases.[63] This calls into question all treatments that rely on immunosuppressing drugs and the widespread use of over-the-counter medications such as cold medicines and antihistamines.

Mycoplasmal infections have been found as cofactors in the progression of AIDS, leading to kidney lesions and respiratory complications.[64] Detection of infections in clinical specimens is frequently dismissed as "only mycoplasmas" even when they appear to be the primary pathogens.[65] Perhaps this is because they are believed to be untreatable by the conventional ten-to-fourteen-day dosage course normally prescribed for antibiotics. Another reason for the lack of scientific interest in mycoplasmas may be that they were initially linked to the detection of infections in AIDS patients.

Until recently, the moral judgment of those who fund medical research has politicized and stalled the investigation of this autoimmune disorder.[66] The pendulum has swung the other way, and now more funds are allocated to AIDS research with little going to investigate other infectious diseases. Fortunately, AIDS research is disclosing pathogenicity mechanisms generally applicable to other microorganisms including mycoplasmal forms.

Sepsis (Bacteremia)

This illness is an overwhelming and life-threatening bacterial infection of the blood and body organs caused by bacteria that has entered body tissue, most often through a wound or incision. The ensuing infection leads to the formation of pus, and/or to the spread of the sepsis bacteria throughout the blood stream.

Sepsis (bacteremia) is often caused by organisms that are resistant to most standard antibiotics. People with weakened immune systems are more susceptible than others. Commonly affected areas are the lungs, the genitourinary tract, the liver, the gastrointestinal tract, surgical wounds or drains, and skin eruptions such as bedsores.

Ultraviolet Light Treatment

Dr. Gordon Josephs belongs to IOMA, the International Oxidative Medical Association, a group of progressive group of doctors who utilize a variety of non-mainstream therapies. Ultraviolet Blood Irradiation (UBI) is one such treatment used since 1933 to kill viruses, bacteria, and fungi often with dramatic results. In the 1950s with the introduction of new wonder drugs, this technique was abandoned. IOMA and the Foundation for Blood Irradiation (FFBI) are working to regain recognition for this therapy. Researchers in Russia have used this process to treat HIV with impressive results.

UBI treatment is very inexpensive, does not subject the patient to risk, is non-toxic, has FDA approval, and results are observable within five weeks. UBI can be tried on any chronic illness such as RA, chronic fatigue syndrome,

Fibromyalgia—any disorder where a hidden pathogen like mycoplasma could be the cause.

Dr. Josephs admits that there must be some unknown infectious microorganism at work to cause RA, otherwise minocycline would not be effective. However, he notes that some patients may not be able to follow a long-term antibiotic regimen.

The UBI treatment can be performed in the doctor's office. The patient sits comfortably in a chair while a 19g needle is placed in a large vein. The patient's blood flows through the needle and through special plastic tubing containing a quartz section and which has been heparinized to avoid coagulation. The drawn blood is exposed to ultraviolet rays in a special UV light box and collected in a syringe to be reintroduced into the vein.

About 1.5cc per pound of body weight is so treated (usually 3-4 "syringe-fuls," never exceeding 300 cc). The procedure, called photopheresis, takes less than an hour. The treatment is not suitable for patients with small veins.

Photopheresis is currently undergoing clinical trials at more than 100 centers around the county for the treatment of graft-versus-host disease, myasthenia gravis, systemic sclerosis, systemic lupus erythematosus, multiple sclerosis, RA, HIV-associated disease, pemphigus vulgaris, and autoimmune insulin-dependent diabetes. Dr. Richard L. Edelson, Professor and Chairman, Yale University Department of Dermatology, leads perhaps the best known research in the area. His group has applied photopheresis to the immunobiology of normal and diseased skin, human T-cell physiology, and cutaneous T-cell lymphoma (CTCL).

The procedure does not remove the cause of the disease but has some temporary benefit by depleting surplus white blood cells that cause inflammatory and destructive enzyme action. The white cells gradually regenerate, so the procedure must be repeated.[67]

UBI therapy was used extensively and with excellent results during the 1930s, 40s, and 50s for the treatment of a wide variety of conditions. Published reports abound on its use in bacterial diseases, including septicemias, pneumonias, peritonitis, wound infections; viral infections including acute and chronic hepatitis, measles, atypical pneumonias, poliomyelitis, encephalitis, mononucleosis, mumps, and herpes; circulatory conditions including thrombophlebitis, peripheral vascular arsenal disease, and diabetic ulcer; overwhelming toxemias, non-healing wounds and delayed union of fractures, rheumatoid arthritis, and many others.

Applications of ultraviolet light are well known in medical dermatology. UV has long been known to inactivate viruses while preserving their ability to be used as antigens in the preparation of vaccines. The theory is that the viral genome is more sensitive to UV damage than viral surface antigens. Thus, the virus can be killed by damage to its nucleic acids while at the same time leaving antigenic surface components (proteins, glycoproteins, and/or fatty acids) relatively intact. This facilitates the learning by the immune system of the shape of the inactivated infectious agent much like a vaccine specific to the actual problem microbe.

Viral illnesses, given their comparative resistance to chemotherapeutic control, have emerged over the past several decades as a major challenge for medicine. In addition, immune system dysfunctions are increasingly recognized as playing a major "host factor" role in many disease processes, including cancer. Given the range of potential applications of UBI therapy and the ability to construct more sophisticated equipment, further research is warranted.

Physicians can learn this technique by contacting IOMA at FAX 405-634-7320. Details of the theory behind UBI treatment, and a bibliography of scientific references are given at www.biophoton.com.

AMOEBIC INFECTIONS

Parasitic infestations are estimated to affect about 150 million people in the United States and at least 40% of the world's population. Parasitologist Dr. Hermann Bueno asserts that parasites are the missing diagnosis in the etiology of many chronic health problems, including arthritis.[68]

Professor Roger Wyburn-Mason, M.D., Ph.D.—author of several important medical textbooks and a renowned specialist in nerve diseases, honored by having two nerve diseases named after him during his lifetime—claimed in 1970s that the cause of RA and other collagen-related degenerative chronic diseases was a pathogenic amoeba which infects every human being to some degree.[69] He called these microbes "limax amoebae," linking this microorganism not only to RA but also to certain cancers that involve the lymphatic system. He documented his work over 26 years in numerous British medical journal articles and in his book *The Causation of Rheumatoid Disease and Many Human Cancers.*[70]

Dr. Wyburn-Mason stressed that the Amoeba *chromatosa* was often confused with macrophages, and that they had the power of independent existence for an extended period of time. This observation seems to confirm Dr. Brown's theory of cell-wall-deficient, shape shifting mycoplasmas. These amoebae can attack any tissue in the body. The resulting illness depends on the area of the body assaulted. Dr. Wyburn-Mason called those diseases where the limax amoebae are detected the "Rheumatoid Diseases." A few examples are shown in Table 3.

Table 3. Area Infected vs Resulting Condition

Adrenal gland	Addison's disease
Small intestine	Crohn's Disease
Muscles	Dermatomyositis
Thyroid	Graves' Disease, Hashimoto's Thyroiditis
Red blood cell membrane proteins	Hemolytic anemia
Blood	Hemolytic Disease
Platelets	Idiopathic thrombocytopenic purpura
Pancreatic beta cells	Insulin-dependent Diabetes
Nerves, brain, spinal cord	Multiple Sclerosis (MS)*
Nerve/muscle synapses	Myasthenia gravis
Arteries	Periarteritis nodosum
Gastric parietal cells	Pernicious anemia
Skin	Psoriasis
Joints, connective tissue	Rheumatoid Arthritis
Heart, lungs, gut, kidney	Scleroderma
Salivary glands, liver, kidney, brain, thyroid	Sjögrens Syndrome
DNA, skin, platelets, organs, connective tissue	Systemic Lupus Erythema-tosus
Colon	Ulcerative Colitis

* This protocol must <u>not</u> be given to an individual with MS.

The suggested treatment was Clotrimazole, an anti-fungal medication usually prescribed in low dosage in the United States to treat Amoebiasis and Tricomonas Vaginitis.

Dr. Jack M. Blount, Jr. of the Philadelphia Medical School was nearly totally disabled by RA in 1974. He discovered Dr. Wyburn-Mason's work after trying all known conventional treatments in an effort to relieve his pain and retard the progress of the disease. Dr. Blount increased the recommended dosage of Clotrimazole and within two weeks noticed remarkable improvement in his RA condition. He convinced his patients to try the U.S. equivalent of Clotrimazole, Flagyl (known generically as Metronidazole). Since his recovery, Dr. Blount has treated over 16,000 patients with this antiamoebic approach with significant success.

Dr. Blount was so impressed with his own personal remission from RA and that of his patients that he founded the Rheumatoid Disease Foundation.[71] Sadly, his enthusiasm for this remarkable treatment was met with hostility from rheumatologists who ignored the many publications and scientific tests performed by Dr. Wyburn-Mason. They insisted on additional double-blind studies before they would listen. Dr. Blount was able to confer with other physicians, including Dr. Robert Bingham of Desert Hot Springs, CA and Dr. Paul Pybus, colleague of Dr. Wyburn-Mason, who achieved impressive results with their own rheumatoid arthritis and osteoarthritis patients.

The antiamoebic treatment consists of three primary prescription medications: Depot Medrol, Allopurinol, and Metronidazole. The treatment takes about 6-7 weeks under close supervision by the attending physician. The patient is also given methods to improve the immune system and lifestyle modifications very similar to those described in this book. Amoebacidal treatment does not correct the damage already done to the tissues, but the progress of the disease is usually halted and the painful symptoms decrease and in many cases disappear. Some patients may become reinfected and must repeat the treatment, depending on the severity of the infection.

Dr. Blount advises taking measures to limit amoebic infection by use of filtration and by making sure home water pipes are made of copper. Like biofilms, amoebae such as Cryptosporidium (*C. parvum*) and Giardia (*G. lambia*) grow quickly in swimming pools and spas, and chlorine does not effectively kill them. Copper algaecide is recommended at 4 ounces per 5,000 gallons of water. Copper plates can be placed in the pool.

Cryptosporidium and Giardia

These organisms are water-borne protozoan cysts that shed their protective shells when ingested. The organisms infect the intestines and cause illnesses Cryptosporidiosis and Giardiasis. The cysts are resistant to traditional disinfection agents such as chlorine and ultraviolet light, and thus they are extremely difficult for municipal water treatment processes to detect and destroy.

Cryptosporidiosis symptoms are diarrhea, nausea, vomiting, abdominal cramps, headaches, and low-grade fevers. Symptoms may persist for a few weeks before the body's immune system can stop the infection. The very young, the elderly, and those with weakened immune systems risk serious illness and possible death resulting from Cryptosporidiosis. The infection drew national attention in 1993 when Milwaukee, Wisconsin's water supply became contaminated. 400,000 cases of the disease and 100 related deaths were traced to Cryptosporidium cysts.

Giardiasis is one of the most common causes of diarrhea in North America, and results from ingestion of cyst-contaminated water. Infection is more common among children and may last several weeks. Giardiasis may be effectively treated with antibiotics.

Cryptosporidium and Giardia cysts are often spread through animal feces, including a leaky diaper or other pool-related "accidents." Thus the cysts are more typically found in surface water sources (lakes, rivers, and reservoirs) rather than in well water. Before entering a swimming pool or spa, check the color and texture of the water. You should be able to see clearly through about ten feet of water to the bottom. Foam or bubbles near the pool's edge indicate growth of organic matter and unclean conditions.[72]

Call your local water company for information about the source of your drinking water and whether there have been any recent problems with contamination.

To remove the cysts at home, install a 1-micron carbon block filter in an under-sink housing. There are several styles of filters on the market: for use with a separate faucet, in a countertop filter system, or as part of a chemical contaminant filtration system.

BLOOD SUPPLY CONCERNS

Since the advent of the AIDS epidemic, the blood banking industry has been undergoing a revolution of increased sophistication. With the increased public demand for guaranteed safety of blood products, many methods of sterilization have been examined intensively.[73] Among these, ultraviolet inactivation of viruses contaminating blood and blood products has been studied using the UBI technique described above.

Since 1985 the FDA has issued repeated warnings to the Red Cross of a "potential for harm" to patients based on failure of federal inspections and noncompliance with good manufacturing practice standards.[74] However, increasingly tough FDA actions and court orders have not succeeded in correcting problems in the collection, processing, and distribution of blood used in medical procedures. Dr. Bernadine Healy, American Red Cross President, admits that there have been "near misses." An FDA inspection in July 2000 found 25 violations in an Atlanta Red Cross center, and another 63 at Red Cross headquarters in Washington, D.C. FDA court documents report Red Cross recalls of blood jumped from 36 in 1988 to 641 in 2000.[75]

Activists such as Dr. Sidney M. Wolfe, director of Public Citizen's Health Research Group, are demanding that the FDA work significantly harder to protect the nation's blood supply. The FDA should insure strict compliance with U.S. laws and regulations in every agency that handles blood and blood products. The Red Cross collects about half of this supply, representing about 6.5 million units of blood.

Hepatitis C Transmission

A potential danger is transmission of hepatitis C, which is now a major epidemic in the United States. More than 70% of those who have hepatitis C display no symptoms and do not know they are carriers, so they unwittingly transmit the virus.[76]

Normal liver function is critical to good health. At least five liver viruses (hepatitis A through E) are now recognized:

- A is contracted from infected food and water. It causes jaundice and a brief illness. Complete recovery is typical and vaccine is available;
- B is transmitted by blood and can cause serious liver damage. Like hepatitis A, its effects appear in the short term. Vaccination is available;
- C was only identified in 1989. It is transmitted by direct blood contact (e.g., transfusions), through sexual inter-course, or via infected needles, and can

remain dormant for decades while the liver is slowly damaged;

- D and E are at the moment elusive and of unknown significance. Research needs to determine whether these are relatively harmless or if, like hepatitis C, they are latent pathogens.

Hospitals and blood banks are now able to screen blood routinely for the virus, but individuals who received a transfusion prior to 1992 should request a test for hepatitis C. A positive test result should prompt the doctor to try antiviral therapy with interferon-alpha and ribavirin. Do everything possible to avoid infecting others. Avoid alcohol, which increases the rate of liver damage, and request hepatitis A and B vaccinations to prevent additional liver problems. Antiviral therapy can reduce liver inflammation but cannot cure the disease.

Contaminated Blood: a National Health Problem?

Blood has been collected from donors for decades and not tested for pathogenic mycoplasmas. Transfusions are unwittingly passing this microorganism along in an iatrogenic manner. Blood sterilization for blood components and artificial blood are technologically feasible.

Rheumatic and heart disease population statistics, age, causative organism blood test positives, and death cause percentages should be relatable by a mathematical formula. In any given age group, infected-percentages should be approximately proportional to sample measures of the levels of blood infection for the causative microbes for these diseases in the general population.

However, these diseases take many years to develop and transfusions are not the most significant way the average person gets the disease, because there are other primary modes of infection. For example, those infected with AIDS typically do not get the disease through transfusion.[77]

Individual blood testing is expensive and there are too many organisms to test for. Only a limited number of microbes and viruses are tested for in practice Because mycoplasmas in blood do not immediately affect mortality statistics, these microorganisms do not seem to be viewed by the collectors as an important problem in the quality of the blood supply. However, the CDC takes the view that blood purity is still an important issue.[78]

Thorough sample testing of blood (for all organisms where a test is possible) would provide a good indication of the level of chronic infections in the general population and is a logical place to gather such data if the CDC and FDA were funded to monitor this data effectively. The FDA is responsible for purity of medicines and the CDC's charter is to keep epidemiological statistics.[79]

---

[1] Vergano, Dan. "Bacteria Tied to Chronic Illnesses." *Medical Sentinel* (1999;4:172-6).

[2] Details can be found at www.thearthritiscenter.com/arthritis_info.htm.

[3] Ibid.

[4] A study from the University of Nebraska focused on patients who had rheumatoid arthritis for less than one year. After three years on the antibiotic drug, 44% of the patients had improved by 75% or more. Improvement criteria included joint tenderness, stiffness and swelling. The study also found that those who experience significant improvement can expect their disease to flare again if therapy is stopped. See www.pslgroup.com/dg/44866.htm.

[5] For full details, see www.pedid.uthscsa.edu/Rickettsia.htm. This web site also provides additional and updated references for *Pediatric Infectious Diseases: Principles and Practice, 2nd Ed.* WB Saunders: Philadelphia, PA, 2002

---

[6] Ibid. Also see Zimmerman and Zimmerman (1996), pp.97-98.

[7] One of the major problems in treating patients with brain tumors is getting the large molecules of chemotherapeutic substances past the blood/brain barrier to reach the tumor.

[8] Chen, M., et al. "Antibiotics to Treat Huntington's Disease." *Nature Medicine* 2000;6:797–801.

[9] See www.lymenet.org for more information on Lyme disease, and http://www2lymenet.org/domino/abstract.nsf/CLD for a collection of medical journal abstracts. The website of the International Lyme and Associated Diseases Society (ILADS) is found at www.ilads.org. See also www.lymeinfo.net, www.LymeAlliance.org, and www.lyme.org. A comprehensive list of recent newspaper articles on Lyme Disease may be found at www.aero-vision.com/~cheryl/media.html.

[10] Zimmerman and Zimmerman (1996), p. 90.

[11] See www.immed.org.

[12] See www.cdc.gov/ncidod/eid/vol7no5/bjoersdorff.htm for details of a CDC study examining the role of migrating birds as benevolent hosts to Ehrlichia-infected ticks.

[13] Shapley, Dan. "Scientists Hope to Identify Benevolent Hosts for Ticks." *Poughkeepsie Journal*, March 25, 2001.

[14] International Lyme and Associated Diseases Society (ILADS) Position Paper on the CDC'S Statement Regarding Lyme Diagnosis. Full text at www.ilads.org/position.htm.

[15] Burrascano, Jr., Dr. J.J. "Advanced Topics in Lyme Disease." 13th ed. At http://library.lymenet.org/domino/file.nsf November 20, 2001. This is an excellent, comprehensive overview that is continually revised as new information is obtained.

[16] Zimmerman and Zimmerman (1996), pp.92-93.

[17] See www.cdc.gov/nicdod/dvbid/lyme/lyme_life_cycle.htm.

[18] Op cit., Zimmerman and Zimmerman (1996).

[19] Grier, Tom. "The Motile Menace." Article written for the Lyme Alliance, 1996. See www.lymealliance.org/research/grier/grier_3.php.

---

[20] Bransfield, Dr. Robert. "The Neuropsychiatric Assessment of Lyme Disease." See www.mentalhealthandillness.com/lymeframes.html for the full text of this excellent article, including supporting references.

[21] Ibid., Bransfield.

[22] Brorson, O. and Brorson, S.H. "*In vitro* Conversion of *Borrelia burgdorferi* to Cystic Forms in Spinal Fluid and Transformation to Mobile Spirochetes by Incubation in BSK-H Medium." *Infection* 26:144-150, 1998.

[23] Research results demonstrated by Dr. David Dorward from the NIH Rocky Mountain Laboratories. See www.lymealliance.org/research.

[24] See www.nixticks.com, www.aldf.com/DeerTickEcology.html, and www.cdc.gov/ncidod/dvbid/lyme.

[25] See www.geocities.com/HotSprings/Oasis/6455/insects-biblio.html for an annotated bibliography of recent research articles from NIH and NLM via Medline.

[26] See www.riaes.org/resources/ticklab/ticks.html and www.pasteur.fr/recherche/borrelia/Gene_index.html.

[27] See www.chiggaway.com/Biggest.htm.

[28] See www.labodia.com/reviewlymelabtests.htm for a comprehensive overview of current test methods and shortcomings.

[29] See Appendix IV for websites of testing laboratories.

[30] Dr. Klempner was criticized for publishing the results of a flawed study in which LD blood samples were contaminated. See Harris, Nick. "The Referee Calls Foul!" February 26, 2001Response to Phil Baker, NIAID, NIH, press release Re: Klempner paper in *Am.J. Med.* 110:217-219,2001. Details at www.lymealliance.org/newsletter/foul.php.

[31] See www.bowen.org for details. The Institute is a nonprofit corporation. They can be contacted at (727) 937-9077.

[32] For information, see www.IGeneX.com. This is the website of the IGeneX Reference Laboratory, Palo Alto, CA.

[33] Ramp, Stefanie. "The Dirty Truth About Lyme Disease Research." November 8, 2001. Article from the Fairfield County Weekly, San Francisco, CA. at www.fairfieldweekly.com/articles/lymedisease.html.

---

[34] Rosenfeld, Dr. Isadore. "How to Beat Lyme Disease." *Parade Magazine*. April 29, 2001. See also www.ilads.org/position.htm.

[35] Brown and Scammell (1988) chapter 16.

[36] Garrett (1995) pp. 553-555.

[37] Wang, J.; Masuzawa, T.; Li, M.; and Yanagihara, Y. "An Unusual Illegitimate Recombination Occurs in the Linear-Plasmid-Encoded Outer-Surface Protein A Gene of Borrelia Afzelii." *Microbiology* Dec 1997;143 (Pt 12): 3819-25.

[38] Priem, S.; Burmester, G.R.; Kamradt, T.; Wolbart, K.; et al. "Detection of *Borrelia burgdorferi* by Polymerase Chain Reaction in Synovial Membrane, but not in Synovial Fluid from Patients with Persisting Lyme Arthritis After Antibiotic Therapy." *Ann. Rheum. Dis.* Feb 1998; 57(2):118-21.

[39] Personal communication with Dr. Garth Nicolson, July 2001. See also www.immed.org.

[40] Tesar, Jenny E. "Lyme Disease." *Science Annual 1989*. H.S. Stuttman, Inc.: Westport, CN, 1989.

[41] Hensrud, Dr. Donald D., Director of the Mayo Clinic Executive Health Program. "This Won't Hurt a Bit." *Fortune*, November 26, 2001.

[42] The national Lyme Borreliosis Foundation in Tolland, CT provides a hotline (203-871-2900) with medical specialists available to answer questions regarding LD prevention, education, and treatment.

[43] Grier, Tom. *The Lyme Disease Survival Manual* (2nd edition forthcoming, Spring 2002). Contains 1200 medical references; documents similarities with MS and other chronic diseases. Describes the life cycle of the spirochete, LD diagnosis, treatment, prevention, and controversies associated with LD.

[44] Ramp, Stefanie. "The Dirty Truth About Lyme Disease Research." November 8, 2001. Article from the Fairfield County Weekly, San Francisco, CA. at www.fairfieldweekly.com/articles/lymedisease.html.

[45] Bransfield, op cit, www.mentalhealthandillness.com/lymeframes.html.

[46] Shoemaker (2001).

[47] Dr. Joseph Mercola, comparing unnecessary sinus surgery to routine gallbladder removal as "another major tragedy in medicine." For proposed alternatives to sinus surgery see www.mercola.com.

---

[48] Sherris, et al. *Mayo Clinic Proceedings* (1999).

[49] When aerosolized they have the potential for use as biological warfare toxins of the type called "yellow rain" allegedly used during the late 1970s in Laos, Kampuchea, and Afghanistan.

[50] Sherris, et al. *Mayo Clinic Proceedings* (1999).

[51] Hamilton, Anita. "Beware: Toxic Mold." *TIME*, July 2, 2001 and Nix, Denise. "'Stuff' on Wall Spurs Lawsuits." *South Bay Daily Breeze*, December 12, 2001, p. A3.

[52] Dr. Ghosi Madani, an allergist at Little Company of Mary Hospital, Torrance, CA.

[53] Wagner, Eliza. "The Lowdown on Leftovers." *Natural Health*, October 1999.

[54] Zimmerman and Zimmerman (1996), pp. 177-188.

[55] Zimmerman and Zimmerman (1996), pp.146-7

[56] Garrett (1995) pp. 254-5 and 588.

[57] Zimmerman and Zimmerman (1996), pp. 145-151.

[58] Ishida, et al. (1994) via Medline.

[59] Garrett (1995) pp. 440-456.

[60] Mutating pathogenic microbes such as mycoplasmas, perhaps? See Alice Park's "Heart Mender," describing Dr. Paul Ridker as one of American's Best in Science and Medicine, a special feature in TIME, August 20, 2001.

[61] See www.bloodbook.com for details on a variety of blood disorders.

[62] For an excellent account of the politicization of the HIV epidemic, see Garrett (1995) chapter 14.

[63] Nicolson, G.L., Nasralla, M.Y., Haier, J., Erwin, R., Nicolson, N.L., and Ngwenya, R. "Mycoplasmal Infections in Chronic Illnesses: Fibromyalgia and Chronic Fatigue Syndromes, Gulf War Illness, HIV-AIDS and Rheumatoid Arthritis." *Medical Sentinel* 4:172-176, 1999.

[64] Nicolson, et al. (1999). Text at www.immed.org. Also see Vojdani, A. and Choppa, P. C. "Sensitive Method for the Quantitative Detection of Mycoplasma Infections." At www.immuno-sci-log.com/pcr.html.

[65] Baseman and Tully, at www.medscape.com/other/EID/1997.

---

[66] For an excellent overview of AIDS as an "equal opportunity destroyer," see Fumento, Michael. "AIDS: The Truth At Last?" *Reason*, December 11, 1995.

[67] Clark (1997), p. 88.

[68] See www.webhealth.co.uk. Use the site's search engine with the term "arthritis giardia".

[69] See www.garynull.com/Documents/Arthritis/Antiamoebic_treatment.htm

[70] Wyburn-Mason (1983).

[71] The Foundation's website is www.arthritistrust.org.

[72] Smith, Dr. Ian K. "A Quick Dip in a Dirty Pool." *TIME*, July 23, 2001.

[73] Horowitz, B. "Inactivation of Viruses in Blood Derivatives." *Transfusion-Transmitted Viral Diseases*, American Association of Blood Banks, Arlington, VA, 1987. Also see Fratantoni, J. and Prodouz, K. "Viral Inactivation of Blood Products," *Transfusion*. Vol. 30, No 6, 1990: pp. 480-81.

[74] Associated Press (unattributed). "Bad Blood Between FDA, Red Cross." CBS/AP News online, Washington, D.C., December 1, 2000. See www.cbsnews.com/now/story/0,1597,254190-412,00.shtml.

[75] Neergard, Lauran (AP). "Senate Will Look Into Handling of Blood by Red Cross." Reported in the *South Bay Daily Breeze*, January 2, 2002.

[76] Rosenfeld, Dr. Isadore. "Do You Have Hepatitis C? Are You Sure?" *Parade Magazine*, January 24, 1999.

[77] See www.thedailyapple.com/target/cs/article/cs/100250.html.

[78] See http://text.nlm.nih.gov/nih/cdc/www/99txt.html.

[79] This is according to each agency's mission statement. See the home pages of the FDA and the CDC on the Internet.

6. DIAGNOSTIC TESTS

In this chapter, several testing methods are described to help the arthritis sufferer work with his/her physician to determine the presence and extent of infection. A typical routine physical examination will involve blood, urine, or tissue samples. A urine test offers particularly valuable data to identify potentially infectious agents. A doctor analyzes the test values to see whether they fall between acceptable ranges. All laboratory test results must of course be interpreted in the context of the patient's overall health.

Other factors influencing test results may be drugs the patient is taking, foods ingested before the test, how strictly the patient followed pretest instructions (e.g., fasting), and variations in laboratory procedures and techniques. Some fundamental questions arise concerning the reliability of any diagnostic test involving organic samples, which may be collected exactly according to procedure at the doctor's office, but may suffer damage in transit to the lab. Sensitivity to time, temperature, humidity, altitude, and other factors may influence test results by altering the sample before the lab technician begins to examine it. False positives or out-of-range values may result. Several tests may be required to obtain an average. Internet resources can help interpret test results and augment the physician's assessment.[1]

Since disease often begins when the immune system is dysfunctional or weakened, a nutritional analysis should be a starting point.

NUTRIENT DEFICIENCY TESTING

By the U.S. Department of Agriculture's Center for Nutrition Policy and Promotion's own measure, 70% of Americans are not getting the nutrients the department claims are required to avoid major diseases.[2] For example, diets deficient in seafood, meats, and poultry will reflect low vitamin B_{12} values. A nutrition-oriented health care professional can assist with determining deficiencies and help tailor a personalized dietary profile. The patient will likely be required to keep a daily journal of not only food and liquid intake, but also environmental factors, such as workplace conditions, and lifestyle factors such as smoking, drug use, hygiene habits, and hobbies.

Hair Analysis

The Journal of the American Medical Association's 2001 study of this controversial clinical test to determine nutrient (mainly mineral) deficiencies and excesses from hair samples concluded that test results vary so widely that the procedure should be considered worthless.[3] Dr. Joseph Mercola and other physicians took exception to this study[4], characterizing it as flawed and pointing out that hair analysis is a useful diagnostic tool if, and only if, the hair sample is not washed prior to laboratory analysis. This important step is essential to preserve the essential mineral ratios, but has minimal effect on toxic metals. Other studies confirm the validity of hair analysis, if done properly. On his website, Dr. Mercola provides data on two recommended laboratories—Trace Elements and Analytical Research—for accurate, reliable analysis and high standards.[5]

It is advisable to check whether the facility doing the testing is affiliated with a drug/vitamin supply company. If so, the tests may reveal, not surprisingly, that the test subject has deficiencies in those particular supplements sold by the lab's commercial affiliate and sponsor. This association has probably led to the prevailing prejudice against hair analysis that still characterizes the medical community's opinion of this test.

Thyroid Testing

According to the Thyroid Society, twenty million Americans have some form of thyroid dysfunction but many are undiagnosed or misdiagnosed.[6] The thyroid gland controls the body's metabolism by producing hormones that regulate energy, control heart rate and body weight, and determine how the body uses nutrients. Thyroid test results, therefore, can be a valuable indicator of nutritional balance and efficient use of hormones.

Thyroid dysfunction, notably Hashimoto's Thyroiditis and Grave's Disease, has been shown to be linked to mycoplasmal infection.[7] One of two types of antibodies—thyroperoxidase or thyroglobulin—is found in nearly all patients with hypothyroidism (Hashimoto's thyroiditis) and in approximately 50% of those with hyperthyroidism (Grave's Disease). Mary Shomon has coordinated an excellent Internet resource[8] for those who wish to know about thyroid conditions and to find a qualified practitioner for diagnosis and treatment. This comprehensive overview is called "Thyroid Disease 101: Basic Information on Hypothyroidism, Hyperthyroidism, Nodules, Goiter, and Thyroid Cancer."

ALLERGY TESTING

There is a tendency to call any joint pain "arthritis" when in fact the cause may be something else: food allergy, crystalline/calcium deposits, muscle spasm, sports injury, or repetitive injury. Inflammation and stiffness are not reliable indicators. Many chronic diseases mimic arthritis so appropriate testing and constant detective work on the part of both patient and physician is absolutely essential.

A causal relationship between RA and a currently active state of food allergy and/or chemical sensitivity has often been reported.[9] The presence of multiple allergens heightens the histamine reaction.

Enzyme Linked Immuno-Sorbant Assay (ELISA) Tests

The cause of food sensitivity is undigested protein components that the immune system does not recognize as beneficial. It responds defensively by producing antibodies and starting an allergic reaction that can result in pain and inflammation. While food allergies usually cause an immediate reaction, food sensitivities may take a few hours or even a few days to develop.[10]

Delayed food allergy tests have been associated with over 65 medical conditions, including arthritis and Candidiasis, and over 200 symptoms such as headaches, fatigue, gastritis, fluid retention, joint pain, aching muscles, sinus pressure, depression, mood swings, constipation, and skin rashes.[11]

Although one can request food allergy testing from one's doctor, insurance typically does not cover such tests. The physician or allergist may insist on performing standard scratch tests or other diagnostic test. Fortunately, some laboratories in the United States offer ELISA tests to individuals in the form of IgG food sensitivity tests and IgE airborne, mold, and food allergy tests. One such resource is Immuno Laboratories, Inc.[12]

Food allergy tests are of two types:

1. The IgG ELISA Delayed Food Allergy Assay is the Immuno 1 Bloodprint. Allergic foods are commonly favorite foods, frequently eaten, and eaten in larger amounts. Virtually any tissue, organ, or system of the body can be affected, including the so-called "classical" allergic areas. Symptoms often disappear following 3-6 months of avoidance coupled with nutritional therapy.
2. The IgE Immediate Allergy Assay is the Immuno 3 Bloodprint. Small, even trace amounts of food can trigger an intense allergic reaction. In the worst case, anaphylaxis occurs leading to fatal results within minutes. The allergic food is rarely eaten, but the effect is severe. These allergies affect the skin, airway, and digestive tract triggering symptoms of asthma, rhinitis, urticaria, eczema, vomiting, diarrhea, angioedema, and anaphylaxis.

Self-Testing for Allergy Factors[13]

Undiagnosed allergies may be causing a variety of symptoms that contribute to arthritis. In 80-90% of arthritis with an allergic component, such as RA, removing the external allergen, either by avoidance or through kinesiology, results in dramatic relief of the arthritis inflammation as well. Microbial infection may still be present, but the immune system will be better able to deal with it.

Some questions to ask as a self-test that may indicate the presence of rheumatoid arthritis in one of its many allergic forms are:

- Do you have any of the most common symptoms of arthritis:
  - o pain and stiffness in one or more joints, especially on arising?

  - o persistent swelling, tenderness, and limited motion in one or more joints?
  - o pain and stiffness in a joint, tendon, or bursa that was once injured?
- Do these symptoms come and go, apparently with no reason?
- Do these symptoms appear to correlate with changes in the weather or at high altitude?
- Do you experience unexplainable night sweats, or a low-grade fever that comes and goes?
- Do you/did you have any allergies like eczema, hay fever, asthma, rashes, rosacea, or hives?
- Do any close relatives have a history of allergies?
- Do you/did you suffer from frequent strep throat, bronchitis, pneumonia, or ear infections?
- Have you ever had mononucleosis?
- Do you have a history of taking prescribed antibiotics?
- Do you have frequent "indigestion," heartburn, recurring diarrhea, or constipation?
- Are you more than 20 pounds overweight?
- Do you seem to suffer colds or flu more often than other people?
- Do your cold or flu symptoms seem to be more severe than others'?
- Do you have other chronic health problems like migraine headaches, sinus/nasal congestion, colitis, unexplained fatigue, or body-wide complaints?
- Do you experience chronic depression, anxiety, or mood swings?

Affirmative answers to five or more of the above questions should prompt consultation with one's physician about the possibility of allergy and/or infection as the root cause of the complaints.

The survey above is a composite of several questionnaires routinely given to allergy patients. However, it reflects a single-minded view regarding the cause of sensitivity to be allergens from food or environmental sources, not from resident mycoplasmic pathogens. The insertion of the questions regarding a history of illnesses such as strep throat, bronchitis, and mononucleosis are the author's attempt to round out the list of probable causes, namely mycoplasma remnants of early infection.

A recent posting on the Internet regarding Epstein-Barr virus illustrates the gaps in conventional allergy testing. The article, published by the Centers for Disease Control and Prevention on March 9, 1995, said, "Although the symptoms of infectious mononucleosis usually resolve in one or two months, the Epstein-Barr virus remains dormant in cells in the throat and blood for the rest of the person's life...[the virus] also establishes a lifelong dormant infection in some cells of the body's immune system." To which one might add: as it does for pathogens associated with AIDS, chicken pox, and shingles.

Allergen(s) may be found in foods, cosmetics, chemicals, and/or airborne substances. Of course, it is impossible to discover and remove *all* the dietary and environmental triggers to allergic arthritis, but it is feasible to identify enough of them to reduce the total load on the body's systems and relieve suffering. Joints and muscles must be given a chance to rest and repair as allergy-induced stress is decreased by elimination, reduction, or control of important offending substances.

Food allergies can also be a factor in weight gain. When one consumes a food that causes mild irritation in the form of headache, bloating, or gas, the body tries to counteract the discomfort by releasing endorphins. The pleasurable sensations these natural opiate-like painkillers produce are an inducement to eat more of the offending food. This explains the counterintuitive reason why people crave and seek out those foods that cause allergic reactions. They unwittingly become somewhat addicted to these pleasurable chemicals, so more of the so-called "comfort food" is consumed than would normally be eaten, and weight gain is often the result. Appetite can also be driven by powerful mood swings and stress.[14]

A yeast overgrowth (Candidiasis) in the digestive tract will prompt cravings for sweet and starchy foods the yeasts thrive on, causing overeating and associated weight gain. The hormones in birth control pills promote yeast growth. A yeast infection can also cause chronic irritation of the intestinal lining, and resulting swelling appears to be excess weight. Kits for self-testing are available,[15] or ask for a detailed stool analysis from your physician.

Applied Kinesiology

Techniques using applied kinesiology (muscle testing) in skilled hands can have significant positive effect in reversing chronic disease by identifying and eliminating allergens. The Total Body Modification (TBM) method and its derivative, the Nambudripad Allergy Elimination Technique (NAET), not only work, they are superior to ELISA, and less expensive.[16]

TBM and NAET represent an unusual and still controversial approach that employs muscle testing to diagnose allergy, followed by acupressure, acupuncture, or chiropractic methods to eliminate the specific irritating allergen. The goal is to retrain the brain and nervous system to deal with the allergen not as a poison to be attacked but as a benign substance temporarily present in the body. Dr. Joseph Mercola employs three TBM-trained therapists in his practice.

NAET's inventor, Devi Nambudripad, Ph.D., D.C., L.Ac., R.N., a chiropractor, acupuncturist and registered nurse has been practicing this technique since 1983. After curing herself and her family of intense and debilitating allergies, she extended her method to her patients with equal success. She has taught NAET to over 1,000 licensed medical practitioners, including medical doctors at her training center in Los Angeles, CA.[17]

At the 1998 Conference of the American Holistic Veterinary Medical Association, Dr. Deva Kaur Khalsa, presented "NAET, Allergies, and the Immune System." Dr. Khalsa offered numerous case studies on successful allergy identification and treatment for dogs and cats. Her clinical experience showed that many other problems such as irritable bowel disease, arthritis, and autoimmune disease have as their root cause an exaggerated immune reaction (i.e., an allergy). Once the allergies have been eliminated, the disease can then be cured.

Dr. Khalsa explains that when the immune system is busy dealing with the reactions to food and environmental allergens, it cannot summon the resources to fight bacterial infections, cancer, and other insults to the body. Food is the primary basis for all allergies, because many of the items found in food are also in the environment. Farm animals as well as household pets are also commonly allergic to grasses, weeds, pollens, molds and dust.

Vaccines given to livestock animals are another common cause of allergies. The viruses are incubated in beef kidney and beef serum, egg or chicken and thus are related to food allergies.

A veterinarian will often prescribe Prednisolone for an animal displaying allergy symptoms. This drug simply depresses the immune system further and disrupts the healthy functioning of the hepatic system, which is needed to cleanse the body of toxins and allergens. One of the bonuses of NAET is that it is effective even if the animal is being given Prednisolone or a similar steroid.

The theory behind TBM and NAET is that an allergic response is not only a physical problem but also an indication of energy flow dysfunction. In a healthy body, neurological communication channels are unblocked and energy is free flowing. When there is a blockage or imbalance in the body, such as an allergic reaction, the energy flow is disrupted and the ideal operating procedures of the immune system are distorted. TBM and NAET kinesiology techniques go to the original source of the imbalance, starting a corrective flow of energy through the body to reprogram sub-optimum immune system functions. The reprogramming usually is permanent. Overall energy flow is restored, the harmony of the body is balanced, and illness and disease are overcome.

TESTS FOR MICROBIAL INFECTION

Early detection and treatment of rheumatoid arthritis is possible. Tests are available for the informed patient who asks for them, but they are not routinely performed and marginal results are not considered significant. RA and other chronic diseases are linked in that they can be traced to the activity of pathogenic microbes and lack of cellular immunity. Unfortunately, the RA tests show low values even when infection is active. This is also true of a sizable group of diseases that manifest as “fever of unknown origin” or FUO. Members of this category include lupus, rheumatic fever, hypersensitivity angiitis, and Still’s disease.

Tetracycline as a Test

Physicians should use tetracycline as a probe to test RA patients since it targets mycoplasmas specifically and does not have an effect on other bacteria if given only once every two weeks or even once per month. A Jarisch-Herxheimer reaction would be evidence that antigens or toxins were being released, rather than the more common disease process associated with a broad-scale bacterial invasion such as pneumonia.[18] The dosage is tailored to the individual patient. Details are found in Appendix II.

Interferons

Interferons constitute a class of natural cell products from the immune system that stimulates antiviral resistance in cell cultures and in the body. These soluble, hormone-like proteins are produced in response to viral infections or to stimulation of immunocompetent as well as other somatic cells by a wide variety of distinct nonviral materials. These materials are for the most part protein or cell wall-related organic molecules/shapes. Interferons can also have significantly diverse biological activities. Measurement of levels of specific interferons in blood analysis provides quantitative evaluation of immune function in immune-related diseases such as AIDS, lupus, and RA.[19]

C-reactive Protein (CRP) Testing

In the 1930s, when Dr. Brown was developing his mycoplasma theory, researchers at the Avery laboratory of the Rockefeller Institute in New York were convinced that rheumatic fever was associated with streptococcal infection. By 1946, procedures were established to apply the measurement of CRP as a test for rheumatic activity. Results indicated that CRP detection could also be clinically useful as an index of polycyclic infection activity in such diseases as rheumatic fever and tuberculosis.[20]

The CRP test indicates inflamed arteries and has been linked strongly to a propensity for heart attack or stroke. The test is inexpensive but it is not routinely performed unless specifically requested.[21]

In the late 1980s, experiments binding CRP to the surface of *Pneumococcus* showed that alternative pathway activation could be blocked. CRP affixed to such invader cells serves as a protective mechanism for the host to ward off potential antigen-reactive cells, thus modulating the severity of the autoimmune reaction. However, it was found that CRP cannot bind to the strain of streptococci that cause acute rheumatic fever and therefore cannot protect the individual from this particular pathogen. Patients with immune deficiency who have no immunoglobulin will nevertheless have a normal CRP response to infection.[22]

It is important to test for binding indications and levels of CRP to obtain a correct diagnosis for the anti-antibody called the Rheumatoid Factor, or R-factor. A Bentonite flocculation test and a latex fixation test will also indicate the presence of the R-factor.[23] Testing for the R-factor is most useful in severe or fairly mature infections. It may take months for it to rise to levels deemed significant. Even after a positive test result, the R-factor's discovery may lead simply to an acknowledgment by the doctor that the patient has RA, but yield no definitive advice about how to cure the condition.

Erythrocyte Sedimentation Rate (ESR) Testing

The ESR test, often called "sed rate," is a nonspecific screening test for various inflammatory diseases and suspected rheumatologic disorders such as RA and lupus. The test measures the distance in millimeters that red blood cells settle in unclotted blood toward the bottom of a specially marked test tube in one hour. Although ESR is a screening test, not a diagnostic test, it can help detect and monitor inflammatory or malignant disease, tissue necrosis, rheumatic fever, tuberculosis, connective tissue disease, anemia, and acute myocardial infarction. It is useful in cases where symptoms are vague or physical findings are minimal. Test results and interpretations depend on a patient's age and sex.[24]

The advantage of this blood test is that readings will frequently be high when the patient is without symptoms. This is an alert to the physician that the disease is still active. The test must be done in the doctor's office, not in a commercial laboratory, since analysis within one hour of drawing the blood is critical to an accurate diagnosis. This is the blood test Dr. Mercola depends upon to monitor his RA patients.

Neutrophil Testing

Neutrophils constitute over 90% of cells found in synovial fluid of RA individuals. Electron microscopy reveals that neutrophils degranulate when they encounter cartilage with immune complexes entrapped; neutrophils first degrade and then invade the tissue. The connection between stimulus and secretion of enzymes from neutrophils can be measured during a histamine reaction, and the triggers to infectious bacterial allergy can then be identified.[25]

Animal experiments using *Mycoplasma arthritidis* have resulted in the development of chronic arthritis resembling RA in humans. The disease is characterized by swelling, an influx of neutrophils into the periarticular region, and a mild increase in the numbers of synovial tissue cells. The disease settles in the synovial membrane and adjacent tissues. In the later stages, collagen deposition and destruction of cartilage becomes apparent. Experiments with *Mycoplasma pulmonis, M. bovis, M. mycoides, M. capricolum, M. hyorhinis, M. alkalescens, M. meleagridis, M. gallisepticum,* and *M. hynosynoviae* also resulted in arthritis.[26]

PCR Testing

According to Drs. Baseman and Tully, "Sufficient evidence has accumulated recently to establish an important and emerging role for *Mycoplasma fermentans* in human respiratory and joint diseases. For example, *M. fermentans* has been detected by specific gene amplification techniques such as PCR in the synovial fluid of patients with inflammatory arthritis, but not in the joints of patients with juvenile or reactive arthritis. In two other studies using PCR, *M. fermentans* was identified in the upper respiratory tract of 20-44% of both healthy and HIV-infected patients and was associated with acute respiratory distress syndrome in non-immunocompromised persons."

A wide variety of PCR tests are available through the Institute for Molecular Medicine in Huntington Beach, CA. These tests are specific for four pathogenic mycoplasma species (*M. fermentans, M. pneumoniae, M. hominis, and M. penetrans*), *Chlamydia pneumoniae*, *Brucella* species, *Borrelia burgdorferi* (Lyme Disease), cytomegalovirus[27], and Human Herpes Virus 6 (HHV-6). Full details are found on the Institute's website, www.imd-lab.com.

The Mycoplasma Registry describes several types of mycoplasma tests, recommended preparations one should take before having the blood sample drawn, and a list of laboratories in the United States where tests can be ordered.

http://groups.yahoo.com/group/MycoplasmaRegistry is the website of a nonprofit organization based in San Diego, CA. They will provide a printed version of the brochure "How to Get an Accurate PCR Blood Test for Mycoplasmal and Other Infections" for a donation. Phone/Fax: 619/266-1116.

It is important not to take any antibiotics, colloidal silver, flax seed oil, or fish oils for at least one month prior to the PCR test. These substances will remove most of the infection from the blood, precluding accurate test results. Suspend intake of immune system-enhancing vitamins, herbs, or supplements since these may reduce the mycoplasma count. The optimum time for testing is when the patient exhibits symptoms and before antibiotic treatment has begun. Re-testing should be done if test results are negative but the symptoms persist. This organization also provides a list of laboratories that offer tests for Lyme Disease, Candidiasis, Chlamydia, HHV-6 Virus, and Rickettsia.

Joint Scan[28]

A gamma camera is used to determine how technetium 99, a rapidly degradable radiopharmaceutical, concentrates in areas of arthritic activity. The radioisotope targets the calcium nodules surrounding sites of infectious activity. These nodules show as "hot spots" in the picture. It appears that the calcium may be the body's natural mechanism for walling off the microorganisms to keep them from obtaining nutrients and stop them from spreading.

Genetic Marker Testing

HLA-B27 is a genetic marker found on the surface of white blood cells of about eight percent of the population. In general, people with either Ankylosing Spondylitis (AS) or

Reiter's Syndrome, one of the more common types of Reactive Arthritis, test positive for HLA-B27. Of Caucasians who develop AS, 95% have this marker. The percentage is not as high among other races, but is still strong. More than 50% of adults who have rheumatoid arthritis also have the inherited marker HLA-DR4. Having this marker increases one's risk of developing RA four fold.[29] Furthermore, research indicates that these genetic markers may predispose individuals to contract arthritis after particular infections, such as gastrointestinal infections, urinary tract infections, or diarrheal food poisoning.[30]

AS is often called rheumatoid arthritis of the spine because of the synovial inflammatory reaction observed in that area. The high level of lymphoctyes and plasma cells in the synovial membrane suggests an important immune system involvement. A substantial body of research details cellular interactions that occur in chronic synovitis, however, the researchers admit that they know only a little about the influence of genetic factors and the nature of the inciting stimuli. What is known is the highly associated genetic background signified by the frequency of the HLA-B27 marker.

There are tests that measure the B27-positive lymphoctyes of the RA patient compared with the antigens of Gram-negative organisms. Results can be used to see microbial interaction in relation to HLA background and thus develop a course of treatment that avoids the infectious trigger(s) for arthritis. The trigger(s) can be an episode of intestinal disease such as salmonella or dysentery, or an instance of venereal disease.[31]

Some progress is being made to discover genetic predisposition to RA, specifically, investigation of the linked cluster of genes, HLA-D4, that occurs more frequently in people with RA.[32]

Antibody Tests

Antibody tests are usually given for yeast infections. *Candida albicans* fungi stays benign in the gut until a dysfunctional immune system permits it to flourish or strong use of antibiotics kill off normal intestinal bacteria that keep *Candida* in check. Yeast infections, especially among women (but not limited to women) in Western societies, are common today. The related symptoms of fatigue, muscle ache, and joint pain overlap those of RA, but *Candida* arthritis is designated a separate form of fungal arthritis that may be mistaken for acute bacterial arthritis. Diagnosis depends on synovial fluid analysis.[33]

A yeast infection is sometimes misdiagnosed as a bladder infection or Irritable Bowel Syndrome (IBS). *C. albicans* thrives in a sugary environment. Yeast sends tendrils through the gut wall allowing leakage of larger protein food-molecules into the blood where they stimulate the Ig reaction to the food protein.

Anti-*Candida* antibody tests are extremely comprehensive and can indicate the level to which one's body is producing antibodies to fight off bacteria and food-molecules gone astray. An amino acid chromatography test is another method to test *Candida* status.

For patients already on antibiotics whose PCR test results show a false negative for mycoplasmal infection, antibody tests offer an alternative. Although these tests are not as accurate as PCR, they can reveal whether the patient has developed antibodies to mycoplasmas. The longer the individual has taken antibiotics, the more accurate test results may be.

BLOOD TESTS

Blood tests, particularly immunoglobulin tests, can determine the presence or absence of anemia, infection, and/or allergens. A chemical analysis for trace minerals, properly performed, can offer clues to health problems since toxic minerals such as lead and mercury can interfere with proper functioning of the body. The size, shape, and number of blood cells can offer excellent diagnostic data.

Dr. Brown's Recommendations

The following four specific tests are recommended by Dr. Brown:[34]

(1) Mycoplasma complement fixing reaction. This test measures the level of differential white blood cells (lymphocytes, monocytes, granulocytes, basophiles, and so forth). If rheumatoid disease is very active, the lymphocyte level rises, indicating that the differential white cells are under attack.

(2) Sedimentation rate. This is a simple blood test that shows the rate of activity of white blood cells. The speed at which these cells settle out of solution correlates with the rate of activity of the rheumatoid process.

(3) Sequential Multiple Analyzer Computer (SMAC). This is a total blood appraisal, including a variety of chemical tests for liver and kidney function, as well as cholesterol, albumin, and triglyceride levels. Albumin levels are depressed if arthritis is very active and return to normal as the patient improves. Chemical proportions that change under conditions of arthritis activity are phosphorus, sodium, potassium, calcium, and uric acid.

(4) Kunkle test. This standard diagnostic procedure uses a gamma globulin measurement to determine the body's ability to fight against the infection.

Darkfield Microscopy[35]

This instrument is used by blood-imaging and specialty diagnostic laboratory scientists to observe living whole blood cells. The microscope projects the dynamic image in high contrast, magnified 1,400X onto a video screen. The object appears bright against a dark background. The skilled physician can detect early signs of illness by looking for microorganisms known to cause disease. The length of time the blood stays alive is also an indicator of the overall health of the patient. Distortions of red blood cells indicate nutritional status, possible bacterial or fungal infection(s), and blood ecology patterns offering clues to illness. Routine blood tests and cultures do not show the rich detail necessary to make these diagnoses.

Dr. Philip Hoekstra, director of ThermaScan, Inc.,[36] has found that the blood samples of virtually all RA patients studied contain significant amounts of *Propioni bacterium acnes* in an altered state—the bacteria are cell wall deficient.[37] Dr. Lida H. Mattman, professor emeritus of biology at Wayne State University and Dr. Hoekstra's mentor, extracted this bacteria from the synovial fluid of RA patients, injected it into chicken embryos, treated the hatched chicks with antibiotics, and observed the RA disappear.[38] Dr. Hoekstra has tested blood samples of multiple sclerosis (MS) patients, finding another stealth pathogen, *Borrelia mylophora*, a bacterium resembling *B. burgdorferi* that is believed to cause Lyme Disease.

Borrelia mylophora has a special affinity for the myelin sheath covering nerves. White blood cells and their antibodies attack and destroy the myelin sheath in their efforts to get at the bacterium as it skillfully cloaks itself. Treatment of MS patients over several weeks with doxycycline has met with considerable success in subduing this bacterial infection.[39]

Although useful in some applications, one serious deficiency with darkfield microscopy is that it is unable to find intracellular infectious agents.[40]

Phase-Contrast Microscopy[41]

A specialized microscope allows the physician to examine blood cells as a diagnostic test of the performance of the immune system. The following are a few examples of observable indicators:

- Platelet aggregation and adherence to damaged blood vessels causing impaired circulation, high cholesterol, or Candidiasis;
- Protein linkage, a condition that shows improper digestion of protein;
- Rouleau, an aggregation of red blood cells caused by physical or mental stress, leading to poor circulation, fatigue, and depleted oxygen;
- Plaque, a sign of poor circulation, calcium imbalance, and fatigue;
- Eosinophils, large white blood cells found under conditions of allergy, parasite infestation, and edema;
- L-Forms, indicating a condition of immune system dysfunction, high blood sugar, or bacterial infection;
- Spicules or Fibrin, showing toxicity of the liver and/or bowel; and
- Neutrophilic viability, a measure of poor immunity, infectious state(s), and malabsorption of nutrients.

19TH CENTURY TESTING STANDARDS

Researchers have for decades determined whether there is a relationship between a specific microorganism and a disease by using a method developed by microbiologist Dr. Robert Koch in the late 1800s. The criteria have expanded over time, but the basic principles remain the same. The microorganism must be:

- observed in every case of the disease;
- isolated and grown in pure culture;
- reproducible when the pure culture is inoculated into a susceptible host animal; and
- observed in, and recovered from, the experimentally diseased host animal.

The question is: how does one apply these rules to an organism like *Mycoplasma* that is capable of shape shifting and mutating to avoid detection, and cannot be grown successfully *in vitro*? It would seem that relying on these outdated criteria offers a convenient and simplistic way for physicians to ignore a pathogen that is extremely difficult to culture, detect, and treat. It is easier for the physician to assume that the patient is imagining or faking symptoms of pain or fatigue, or ascribe the complaints to a known common disease like arthritis, unless the disease has other obvious symptoms, such as AIDS.

As long as some influential scientists still think of mycoplasmas as having standard bacterial or viral properties and force-fit outdated criteria on these elusive micro-organisms, no progress will be made to understand their true etiopathogenic role.

HOW WE THINK

Scientific progress depends on the validity of our model and how we think about it. Two ways of thinking are given in the table below. They are not mutually exclusive, but are complementary. Each way of thinking is useful in its own proper place. One way applies to medicine as a science the other is more applicable to medicine as an art.

Validity and certainty can sometimes be the enemy of discovery. The way leading to discovery and insights is akin to brainstorming, which leads to many wild and bizarre hypotheses and possible associations. One must then apply analytical constraints in order to validate or invalidate the hypotheses. A problem arises when analysis is applied too early in the process, curtailing discovery.

The website www.quackwatch.com written by Dr. Stephen Barrett is characterized by his attempt to apply standard validation criteria to some of the unconventional medical concepts disseminated on the Internet. Some, but not all, discussions on this website are thoughtfully written and collect a wide range of material from many different authoritative sources on a diverse assortment of topics. These are worth reading and thinking about in order to understand how traditional medical scientists view non-traditional medical concepts.

The denigrating manner in which Dr. Barrett presents some alternative medical treatments or procedures offends many who promote those concepts. For a balanced view, search the Internet using Google with keyword *iatrogenic* for some of the failures of conventional medicine.

Truth seems to lie somewhere in between the conventional view and the non-traditional approach, as shown in the following comparisons:

Way Leading to Validity and Certainty	**Way Leading to Discovery and Insights**
-Aristotelian logic	-Fuzzy Logic (Calculus of)
-Truth is absolute	-Truth is a function of time, place, and situation.
-Propositions are T/F 0=F 1=T	-Probability of truth 0< F < .5 <T < 1
-No Exceptions, or the rule is false	-Explore exceptions and expand the model.
-Look for single cause (Occam's razor)	-Look for multiple factors, correlations, and interactions
-Exclude anecdotal data	-Collect, correlate, validate, extrapolate toward a theory, postulate, test, abstract, look for patterns in anecdotes
-Use constrained searches on the Internet	-Use open searches, seek correlations and causes

---

[1] An explanation of laboratory tests and ways to interpret test results can be found at www.nlm.nih.gov/medlineplus/laboratorytests.html and at www.rheumatic.org/tests.htm.

[2] Coco, Donna. "The Numbers Game." *Natural Health*, May, 1999.

[3] Seidel S., Kreutzer, R., et al. "Assessment of Commercial Laboratories Performing Hair Mineral Analysis." *JAMA*. 2001; 285:67-72.

[4] Mercola, J.M. and Watts, D.L. *JAMA* Letter to the Editor. 2001; 285(12):1576-7.

[5] See www.mercola.com for full details and references.

---

[6] See www.the-thyroid-society.org.

[7] Briggs, Sharon, R.N. "Mycoplasma Infection: From GWI to Chemtrail Illness." Presentation to SHASTA CFIDS, California, August, 2000. See www.shasta.com/cybermom/mycoplasma.htm. She discusses work done by Dr. Garth Nicolson and other chronic disease experts.

[8] See http://thyroid.about.com/library/weekly/aa042100a.htm.

[9] The author has experienced severe bursitis symptoms within four hours of eating shrimp.

[10] Baker, Dr. Sidney M.; McDonnell, Maureen; and Truss, Carroll V. "Double Blind Placebo-Controlled Crossover Study Proves Effectiveness of IgG Food ELISA Testing." Paper presented at American Academy of Environmental Medicine Advanced Seminar, Virginia Beach, VA, October 1994.

[11] Interview with Dr. Sidney M. Baker, M.D. by Dr. James Braly, M.D. in *The Immuno Review*, Summer 1995. See also Baker (1994).

[12] Immuno Laboratories, Inc., 1620 West Oakland Park Blvd, Ft. Lauderdale, FL 33311. 1-800-231-9197.

[13] At the Institute for Molecular Medicine, a comprehensive Chronic Illness Survey Form is given to all family members of applicants for laboratory testing. See www.imd-lab.com.

[14] Ott, Chris. "Surprising Obstacles to Weight Loss." *Natural Health*, October 1999.

[15] Saliva test kits sold by Bio Health Diagnostics, (800) 570-2000.

[16] Personal communication with Dr. Joseph Mercola, July 2001.

[17] Weber, Lina. "The Man Who Couldn't Lift a Pea." *Natural Health*, July/August 1998; Letters to the Editor of *Natural Health*, September/October 1998; Tsering, Lisa and Maher, Timothy. "There's Something in the Air." *Natural Health*, July/August 1999; Nambudripad, Devi. *Say Goodbye to Illness*. Delta Publishing: 1993. See website www.naet.com.

[18] Brown and Scammell (1988) pp. 196-7. Estimating that 20,000 lives per year could be saved, the CDC recommended in June 1997 that older adults get the pneumococcal vaccine.

[19] Sidney E. Grossberg; Jerry L. Taylor; Ruth E. Siebenlist; et al. "Biological and Immunological Assays of Human Interferons" in Rose (1986) pp. 295-299.

[20] McCarty, Maclyn. "Historical Perspective On C-Reactive Protein" in Kushner (1982) pp. 1-8.

[21] *NEJM* 3/23/00 study reported in *TIME*, April 3, 2000, p. 94.

[22] Mold, Carolyn, et al. "C-Reactive Protein Reactivity with Complement and Effects on Phagocytosis" in Kushner (1982) pp. 260-261.

[23] Brown and Scammell (1988) pp. 82-3.

[24] Illustrated Health Encyclopedia, at www.pittsburgh.com/shared/health/adam/ency/article/003638.html.

[25] Weissman, Gerald, et al. "Neutrophils: Release of Mediators of Inflammation with Special Reference to Rheumatoid Arthritis" in Kushner (1982) pp. 11-18.

[26] Simecka, J. W.; Davis, J. K; Davidson, M.K; et al. "Mycoplasma Diseases of Animals" in Maniloff (1992) section V, chapter 24.

[27] Many CFS and Fibromyalgia patients have this systemic viral infection. Dr. Nicolson recommends testing for cytomegalovirus infection in any instance of autoimmune illness.

[28] Maniloff (1992) section V, chapter 24.

[29] Orlock, Carol. "Of Germs and Genes." *Arthritis Today*, March/April 1995.

[30] Dr. Robert D. Inman, rheumatologist and professor of medicine at the University of Toronto, Canada.

[31] Toivanen (1988) pp. 21-2.

[32] Samuels (1991) pp. 26-8.

[33] Yoshikawa, et al. (1980) p. 218.

[34] Brown and Scammell (1988) pp. 81-84.

[35] Leviton, Richard. "The Cause May Be in the Blood." *Alternative Medicine Digest*. Issue 18, 1997.

[36] ThermaScan, Inc. is affiliated with the Hematologic-Physiologic Research Institute, P.O. Box 1850, Royal Oak, MI 48068.

[37] Op. cit., Leviton (1997).

[38] Mattman (1993).

[39] Op. cit., Leviton (1997).

---

[40] Personal communication with Dr. Garth Nicolson, January 2002.

[41] See http://ally.ios.com/~drheal19/livecell.htm.

7. NATURAL METHODS TO REVITALIZE THE IMMUNE SYSTEM

A well-known relationship exists between poor health among Americans and our sugar- and starch-laden diet combined with a sedentary lifestyle. However, the medical community asserts that if poor diet and lack of exercise were causative factors of disease, they would have discovered it a long time ago.[1] In fact, some of the causes of poor health are known, but there are too many of them. Prevailing medical philosophy tends to prefer the single solution and simple answer to the complex one. This Occam's Razor[2] approach will not work for problem as complicated and intricate as a dysfunctional immune system.

Because the orthodox medical community as a whole does not take a holistic view of their patients, the result is a simple one-pill treatment of symptoms with the aim to relieve pain. This is often accomplished with drugs that provide relief in the short term but which have long-term negative effects.

While no vitamin, mineral, or supplement can fulfill all the advertising promises made by their suppliers, scientific studies are increasingly showing that arthritis sufferers can benefit from certain nutrients. In some cases, because the individual cannot absorb or use nutrients directly from natural foods or may be taking a medication that interferes with normal nutrient absorption, supplements may be necessary.[3]

Veterinary studies of animal (pet) nutrition sometimes contain references to the nutritional content of commonly available vegetables and cereals that are also part of the human diet.

AEROBIC EXERCISE

Jogging and running are not helpful to arthritics since these exercises increase the pressure of gravity, compressing vertebrae and leading to wear and tear on ankle, knee and hip joints. Jogging and running consist of a series of sudden downward shocks to the joints. Brisk walking and tai chi can be just as effective without the danger of impact damage. For those arthritics whose lower limbs are affected, the gentle stretching of yoga, accompanied by deep breathing, can provide significant aerobic benefit. Movement, but not vigorous exercise or strain, is what is important.[4] Exercise also produces endorphins, which improve pain tolerance.

Fatigue is a common symptom of chronic disease. Taking a nap may be tempting, but gentle exercise in conjunction with deep breathing may have the same restful effect while simultaneously reviving energy.[5] Deep breathing exercises while lying prone on a slant board can enhance circulation, oxygenate cells, and relieve gravitational pressure on joints. By oxygenating cells, we make it more difficult for harmful anaerobic organisms to live and grow. Oxygen is catabolic (destructive) as well as cleansing by breaking down complex substances into more simple compounds. Oxygen destroys the by-products, or metabolites, of anabolism, the constructive processes of the body. The body is a dynamic balance of anabolic and catabolic processes.

Great benefits can also be found in range-of-motion exercises done in the buoyancy of water. Swimming is an excellent way to loosen stiff joints and to stop muscles from becoming weak. Daily exercise in a heated pool or spa will provide remarkable relief. Others find that alternating heat treatment with cool compresses or ice packs keeps pain and swelling symptoms in check.

Strength training to increase muscle tone in order to support the skeletal system may require specific gymnasium equipment, but can also be done with simple isometric exercises. Although joint movement is often accompanied by pain, arthritics must learn to do gentle and gradual exercises with joints lightly loaded in order to keep them limber, lest their joints become immobilized and muscles atrophy from disuse. A strength training exercise regimen is also helpful in preventing osteoporosis.

STRESS REDUCTION AND PAIN MANAGEMENT

Short-term stress is actually beneficial for arthritics. During stressful times, the adrenal glands produce more steroids (natural cortisone), which temporarily help reduce inflammation. Dealing with a stressful event can be challenging and can provide some measure of distraction from the symptoms of joint pain and stiffness. However, long-term mental stress without compensatory physical exercise can be taxing on the heart and immune system. Stress triggers a wide-ranging set of bodily changes, called the general adaptation syndrome, designed to gear up the body to meet an emergency. Continuous stress to the point of misery causes mental despair, depression, and lack of motivation to make positive changes to change a downward emotional spiral.

Stress can be dangerous for those taking corticosteroids such as prednisone (synthetic cortisone). Long-term use of steroids also has a degenerative effect. When the body is stressed, the pituitary gland releases a chemical called ACTH (adrenocorticotropic hormone), which signals the adrenals to produce more cortisol. Cortisol plays an important role in the body, controlling one's salt and water balance as well as regulating carbohydrate, fat, and protein metabolism. Stress-induced cortisol levels may rise to as much as five times the body's normal daily production. If one becomes accustomed to supplemental synthetic cortisol in the form of a drug like Prednisone, the body will become lazy about producing cortisol on its own and become addicted to the supplement. Deficient cortisol levels during stress could lead to fever, low blood pressure, mood swings, or depression.

Reducing stress can be done in a variety of ways, some simple (taking a few minutes each day for quiet meditation), or comparatively extreme (finding a new, different career or relocating to another geographic area). Studies have shown that quiet activities such as knitting or listening to soothing music can trigger a "relaxation response" manifested in the release of endorphins, the body's natural painkillers. Measurably high levels of endorphins in synovial fluid have been found in RA patients who had a joyful outlook on life and coped well with their symptoms compared to those patients who complained about joint pain.[6]

Since the 1960s, there has been an increasing rise in chronic pain complaints. An average of 70% of applicants for Workers' Compensation benefits indicate the back as the primary pain location. Osteoarthritis is second only to heart disease as the most common diagnosis leading to long-term disability from work.[7] Chronic pain is an enormous national epidemic, reflected in the numbers of pain control facilities springing up across the country. The cost, in terms of physical suffering as well as burden to taxpayers, is staggering. These facilities are able to deal with patients more effectively and at lower cost than hospitals because nearly all features of treatment are performed in one place, reducing the patient's work time loss and travel time. Also, a comprehensive approach is taken to the patient's health problems.[8] However, it is difficult to obtain valid assessments and accurate diagnostic data when many patients submit bogus claims.

Studies have revealed learned pain syndromes, where the single most common reinforcing factor for illness behavior was the excused escape from everyday responsibilities.[9] This explains why individuals suffering from CFS are often seen as "faking it" or "lazy."

Most acute pain involves tissue damage traced to an etiological (infection, allergy) or mechanical (injury, repetitive stress) cause. Neurophysiologists typically use duration of pain as a way to differentiate between etiological and mechanical causes. However, determining this distinction can be difficult, especially in cases of recurrent acute pain experienced by arthritics during flare-ups. Patients may become depressed and emotionally disabled by the chronic pain they experience, and develop an inability to cope.[10]

Meditation and Self-Hypnosis

Using the mind's own ability to focus on positive goals and imagine peaceful settings is a powerful tool in pain control and stress management. There are many self-help guidebooks and audiotapes available to aid in learning meditation techniques.[11] A few sessions with a professional hypnotherapist can teach any highly motivated individual how to achieve relaxation and manage pain. The author attests to the value of self-hypnosis from personal experience. Guided imagery has been proven to be very effective in combating stress, coping with the discomfort of

RA symptoms, helping to get a full night's sleep, and promoting a general feeling of well-being. Self-hypnosis—a form of deep meditation—is a drug-free method of distraction therapy with no harmful side effects.

It is unlikely that an insurer will reimburse for lessons in self-hypnosis because it is not viewed as a "real procedure" and is considered a nonscientific approach. However, documented evidence[12] shows that hypnosis has great value as a therapeutic tool to control self-destructive habits, cope with pain, conquer fear, manage anxiety, overcome depression, and deal with emotional loss. Hypnosis is most often valuable not as a treatment but as a facilitator of other therapies. Hypnotic analgesia, or mastering pain, works by disciplined control of attention. The technique has been used as general anesthesia for surgery on patients who are unable to accept traditional anesthetics.

Researchers at the University of Massachusetts Medical School completed a study in 1998 evaluating the effects of meditation on psoriasis.[13] Patients practiced guided imagery while listening to relaxation tapes and visualizing the ultraviolet (UV) light healing their skin. The control group received regular UV treatment without the tapes. The meditating group's lesions healed four times faster than the control group's, illustrating the mind's influence on the healing process. The study was repeated with two different groups to confirm the dramatic results.

One can find a qualified hypnotherapist through the American Society of Clinical Hypnosis in Des Plaines, IL (312-645-9810) or the Society for Clinical and Experimental Hypnosis in Pullman, WA (509-332-7555).

Energy Psychology

Under this broad heading are those techniques combining needle-less acupuncture with psychology to obtain some of the most profoundly powerful tools in combating stress. Of these, the most popular method is called Emotional Freedom Technique (EFT). Dr. Mercola asserts that this is one of best ways to overcome stress and in turn, physical discomfort. It is one of the first things he prescribes for new patients with mild rheumatoid arthritis. The fundamental premise is that all negative emotions are disruptions in one's bioenergy system. These stress-induced imbalances often manifest themselves as physical symptoms such as joint pain, fatigue, headache, and other characteristics of chronic illness. More information is available at www.emofree.com.

Massage

Massage is not only soothing to the psyche, but has tangible effects in stimulating the activity of the lymphatic system, approximately thirty percent of which lies near the surface of the skin in some areas of the body. Massaging the affected joints will facilitate the natural breakdown process that is needed before cell rebuilding can occur. Massage can improve circulation and reduce pain and swelling. Always massage in the direction of the heart, using the fingertips or the heel of the hand, using a little cream or oil as a lubricant. Rolling a clean tennis ball over the affected area provides the same effect. The same funds otherwise paid for pain-killing drugs can instead be spent on a professional massage without the deleterious side effects. Basic techniques can be learned from self-help books.[14] Massage is very helpful for arthritic pets. It also works for arthritic spouses.

Neurostructural Therapy (NST)[15]

Also called Neuro-Structural Integration Technique, NST is performed by a trained practitioner in a sequence of movements designed to realign muscles, nerves and connective tissue. It is not strictly massage, acupressure, or chiropractic, but draws on key elements of these techniques for a gentle method of noninvasive healing. Originally developed in Australia by the late Tom Bowen in the 1950s, the method was called "Total Body Modification" (TBM). Several TBM websites provide detailed descriptions, lists of practitioners, and success stories.[16]

This technique has provided pain relief for many thousands of patients of all ages. Proponents, including Dr. Mercola, claim that after just a few NST sessions normal lymphatic flow is restored, the neuromuscular system resets tension levels, and scar tissue softens and shrinks.

Tai Chi

This gentle, rhythmic exercise teaches balance, reduces stress, aids in blood circulation, and assists in cell building since it is an aerobic exercise. Tai chi has been practiced in China for centuries as part of a daily physical fitness regimen. Groups of people can be seen early in the morning in public squares and parks, performing the specific sequence of moves called "forms." It is this intense concentration on exact body position and steady breathing while moving slowly that give a meditative aspect to the exercise. This exercise technique has recently become popular in the United States. Because movement is slow and not strenuous, people of all ages can perform the exercise. Tai chi is the counterpart to the fast-moving martial art form of kung fu. Classes are usually offered as part of city-sponsored adult education curricula. Books and videotapes can assist with home study.[17]

Pilates Method

On a par with Yoga and Tai Chi is the Pilates Method for strengthening weak muscles and stretching tight ones.

Pilates moves can correct muscle imbalances, increase range of motion, reduce pain, and improve mobility and joint stability by building up supporting muscles.[18]

Minimal movement therapies

When even the thought of exercise is painful, consider programs such as the Alexander Technique, the Feldenkrais Method, and the Trager Approach. Each of these is named for its developer, and each offers maximum benefit for minimal movement. They offer relief of joint stress by retraining the body to balance and distribute weight more evenly, thus reducing wear and tear on the joints. Physical therapists who work with stroke patients and those recovering from joint replacement surgery recommend the techniques, but are quick to say they are popular with athletes and performers at the peak of physical health.

Poor posture is an important contributing factor to pain as certain muscles tighten, spasm, or put pressure on nerves. Correcting the position of the head and neck can dramatically influence pressure on the spine and the nerves associated with it. As posture, mobility, and flexibility improve, organs realign and breathing capacity increases, in turn oxygenating cells throughout the body.

These techniques do not rebuild damaged cartilage, reverse joint deformities, or remove the disease, but they can decrease the need for medication. They can reduce pain while increasing mobility, personal confidence, and comfort. One's doctor is the best judge of the particular exercise therapy tailored to the patient's condition. Cost for treatments is comparable to physical therapy, but may not be covered by insurance unless a doctor recommends them. Some HMOs offer one or more of these methods in the form of low-cost classes for patients with chronic pain. Kaiser

Permanente in California, for instance, sponsors Feldenkrais exercise classes.[19]

DIET ADJUSTMENTS

After prescribing powerful immunosuppressive medication, the doctor may also suggest eating a "well-balanced diet high in fiber and low in saturated fats and cholesterol." This is a difficult task without consulting a nutritional expert and obtaining a personal health and lifestyle evaluation. The typical American diet is high in refined foods, fats, and sugars—all of which undermine the efficiency of our immune system's function. The practices of adding pesticides to fruit and vegetable cultivation and antibiotics to animal feed are designed to produce cosmetically appealing food products as they make their way from farms to grocery display shelves. These additives and chemicals may have long-term cumulative and detrimental effects as residues in our bodies.

To strengthen the immune system, one must make an effort to eat whole foods, i.e., not processed or refined, and reduce consumption of fats and sugars whenever possible.[20]

Simple refined carbohydrates are found in unexpected places, so it behooves the arthritic to read product labels to discover hidden sugar, honey, corn syrup, fructose, and other sweeteners in processed foods. This is difficult in American society where we are conditioned to ask, "Which pill can I take?" rather than "What should I eat?"

Maintaining a normal weight is also beneficial to the arthritis sufferer by allowing the circulatory system to function more efficiently. Body weight isn't a factor except for pain caused physical gravitational pressure upon inflamed, swollen joints in the lower extremities. In fact, underweight people have been reported to have a significantly higher risk of severe arthritis.[21]

The question of which diet is best for arthritis sufferers, found in many self-help books[22], has no reasonable answer. An arthritic may religiously follow a diet that has proved to help those similarly afflicted, only to find that s/he is worse off than before. What has been ignored is not only the concurrent removal of toxins but also the possibility that the proposed diet contains a substance that produces an allergic reaction in the individual. This allergy may be a food or pollen allergy or may be a particular substance that triggers the Jarisch-Herxheimer effect. Salmonella or botulism (food poisoning) can be such a trigger.[23] It is advantageous to obtain a food allergy profile developed by a qualified specialist in both allergies and nutrition. If arthritis symptoms are severe, the results of allergy testing may be the key to any progress in recovery. Allergy testing is discussed in Chapter 6.

Analysis such as in-depth immunoglobulin (ELISA IgE and/or IgG) testing and applied kinesiology techniques in the hands of a skilled practitioner will determine specific individual allergens. However, it may be difficult to convince some HMOs to pay for such tests and the medical staff may reject the request because they do not have the training to interpret the test results.

One size does *not* fit all when it comes to diet. For instance, a wheat, sugar, or milk allergy will cause a severe flare-up of arthritic symptoms in one person but will have no effect on another following the identical diet. An important personal step in countering arthritis is determining which particular foods are friend or foe. The typical physician's vague or no-comment stance on nutrition leaves the patient in a quandary.

The closest one can come to a comprehensive set of guidelines for diet and lifestyle changes is that developed by Dr. Mercola over nearly a decade of treating thousands of patients in his office as well as hundreds of thousands over the Internet. The latest detailed version of this regimen can be found at his website;[24] an outline appears as Appendix V of this book. A basic nutritional plan used successfully by Dr. Nicolson is given in Appendix III.

Some popular diets in self-help books advocate eliminating nightshade vegetables, which contain solanine, a natural toxin that is usually destroyed by a robust and healthy digestive system. A marginally functional digestive system cannot counter the toxins, and the residue remains in the body. Another reason for avoiding the Solanum genus is that potatoes are one of the worst crops for retaining pesticide and fungicide residues. It is best to shop for organically grown potatoes. Many people test positive for allergies to tomatoes. This is one of the first vegetables to try on an experimental food-elimination diet.

A "sure thing" part of any diet regimen designed to benefit arthritis sufferers is consumption of at least one quart of pure water (not tap water or distilled water) daily for every fifty pounds of body weight. Many people are chronically dehydrated. Hunger is often a signal that the body needs water.

Water lubricates the body, transports nutrients to cells, reduces constipation, improves digestion, reduces the risk of kidney stones and certain cancers, and assists the lymphatic system to excrete toxins. Pure water is essential for a healthy immune system. Unless your drinking water comes from a clean well or aquifer, invest in a good quality reverse osmosis filter to remove the fluoride in most cities' water supply.[25]

Arterial Plaque

There is one instance where nutritionists and medical professionals agree: that diet plays a major role in many cases of myocardial infarction (interruption of blood supply to the heart) since blockage may be due to an accretion of saturated fats taken from the bloodstream and deposited on the artery surface.[26] This build-up can become part of the plaque that blocks arteries but the mechanism is not fully understood. Infection may also play a part.

An atherosclerotic risk assessment panel recently concluded that atherosclerosis could have an infectious etiology requiring antibiotic therapy as a treatment option.[27] Their finding was based on observations of *Chlamydia pneumoniae* in the presence of oxidized low-density lipoproteins (LDL—the "bad" cholesterol) as macrophage engulfment of the pathogen creates a foam cell. Oxidized LDL, *C. pneumoniae*, and foam cells are major constituents of arterial plaque.

Another hypothesis is that plaque is formed as a result of bacterial L-forms adhering to healthy cell walls and building cholesterol coats to camouflage themselves from the immune system's hunter/killer T-cells.

Fiber[28]

In the United States, our diet often consists largely of processed foods and little fiber or roughage. For this reason diverticulosis is one of the most common colon conditions affecting Americans. Diverticula are pea-to-marble-sized pouches formed in weakened areas of the colon wall, usually in the sigmoid section on the left side of the abdomen. These diverticula develop as we age. They cause few problems—one is a vitamin B_{12} deficiency—unless they become inflamed or infected, at which point the condition becomes diverticulitis. If a pouch containing bacteria bursts, spilling its contents into the abdominal cavity, peritonitis can result. The bacteria seeps from the bowel through the pouch's thin cell walls and food molecules can enter the blood stream. Tetracycline antibiotics work to metabolize and destroy the pathogens in diverticula.

Too many diverticula can constrict the sigmoid even more than its normal narrow state. Constipation, diarrhea, or spasms are the result. Prevention is simple: drink lots of pure water daily and eat 25-35 grams of fiber per day—whole bran, whole grains, fruits such as apples and berries, and fibrous vegetables like broccoli, carrots, squash, and asparagus. If your body is unaccustomed to fiber intake, introduce it very gradually.

Individuals whose health profile is characterized by high insulin levels, high blood pressure, excess weight, high cholesterol, and/or diabetes should avoid all grains. They will likely benefit from eating some animal protein. The main issues with meat (i.e., fat content, antibiotics, hormones, and pesticides) are avoided if one uses only grass fed livestock.[29]

Fiber helps to lower cholesterol and to stabilize blood sugar levels. It provides a steady source of energy, gives bulk to stools, and speeds the passage of waste through the intestines. Since about ten percent of people past age 50 have diverticulosis, and nearly everyone does by age 85,[30] regular medical checkups should be scheduled to determine whether problems exist for people in the over-50 age group.

Because diverticulosis. is endemic to seniors, it is tempting to speculate that this condition may actually be infectious and that fiber is perhaps only palliative. Research should be done to explore the following connections:

- Diverticulosis implies a leaky gut condition;
- A leaky gut implies food particles in the blood;

- Food in the blood implies an immune system allergic reaction;
- An allergic reaction implies a flare-up of arthritis symptoms.

Hazards Lurking in Popular Foods and Drugs

We don't like to think that our government would allow harmful substances to appear in the foods and drugs we consume. However, these hazards are on our stores' shelves. The thoroughness of enforcement of FDA and USDA regulations, as well as the rules themselves, are far from complete. Let the buyer and consumer beware.

Processed Meats

Nearly all processed meats contain nitrates and nitrites. Both turn into carcinogenic nitrosamines during the digestion process. While these carcinogens can be neutralized by either drinking several cups of green tea with each meal or making sure that intestinal flora is adequate by using acidophilus supplements, it is doubtful that consumers take these conscientious measures. Processed meats, especially sausage, also contain oxidized (i.e., rancid) cholesterol, which can damage the cardiovascular system. In 1994 the National Cancer Institute's bulletin stated that hot dogs have been directly linked to childhood leukemia, yet hot dogs are routinely served in our school cafeterias.

Pickles, Anchovies, and Other Salt-cured Foods

These foods contain carcinogens. These toxins can be made harmless as with processed meats, but the best approach is severe limitation or complete avoidance.

Food Coloring

Dr. Andrew Weil's books target artificial coloring substances as cancer-causing agents. Caramel coloring is burnt sugar, a carcinogen, and an immunosuppressive substance.

Canned Fruit Juices

Here is a classic example of the consumer's need to read labels carefully. The list of ingredients usually begins with "water" followed by "high fructose corn syrup." Then we find the actual fruit puree. There is a 200-calorie price to pay for this sugared, fruit-flavored water. Vitamin C is usually shown as 100% because the manufacturer has added ascorbic acid to the ingredient list. Some add traces of other vitamins as a sales gimmick. Better to skip the sugar, eat a piece of fresh fruit (including the peel, if appropriate), and drink a glass of fresh water.

Parents and caregivers of very young children are quick to give fruit juice when water would be better for them. New recommendations offered by a panel of doctors speaking for the American Academy of Pediatrics recently set limits on the amount of juice children should consume.[31] The concern is that kids less than six months of age who drink too much juice run the risk of being too full to get adequate nourishment from breast milk or formula. There is also the risk of chronic diarrhea, since their intestines cannot digest so much sugar.

For older children given no-spill containers of juice with a small drinking spout, there is the danger of tooth decay as the juice's sugar washes over their teeth all day. The juice cups also train kids to turn to sweet food for comfort, leading to overeating and bad nutrition habits in future. Pure water flavored with a small amount of juice is an alternative.

The Academy's guidelines state that children aged one to six should drink no more than six ounces of juice per day. Those 7 to 18 should consume no more than 12 ounces per day. Whole fruits are better, since fruit contains nutrients and fiber in the form of pulp lost during juice processing.

Milk

For decades Americans have been conditioned by advertising to believe that pasteurized, homogenized cow's milk is the perfect food for humans, especially children. The United States dairy industry is a multi-billion dollar business, and milk is its chief product. Celebrities with "milk mus-taches" are paid for their endorsements.

Raw milk contains beneficial bacteria such as *Lactobacillus acidophilus*, which balances and controls the putrefactive bacteria that make milk curdle and turn sour. The pasteurization process destroys valuable enzymes and vitamins along with harmful bacteria. Some critics assert that pasteurization, like beef irradiation, allows the farmer to skirt FDA standards of cleanliness; the standards imposed on farms producing raw milk are considerably higher. Pasteur-ization offers another benefit to the industry—the extension of shelf life of dairy products.[32]

Consuming excessive amounts of meat and milk increases the body's need for calcium, the mineral necessary to neutralize the acid formed when digesting animal protein. Vitamin D is added to nearly all milk to enhance calcium absorption, but it is not a substitute for natural Vitamin D, which can be obtained simply from exposure to sunlight.

When calcium absorption is inhibited, mineral imbalances cause toxins to accrue in tissues and joints, further aggravating arthritis symptoms. Calcium inhibitors include[33]:

- alcohol;
- tobacco;

- marijuana;
- diuretics;
- caffeinated beverages;
- soft drinks with phosphoric acid;
- too much or too little exercise;
- refined sugar or an excess of any concentrated sweetener or sweet-flavored food;
- excess salt;
- meat and meat products; and
- dairy products.

Ironically, drinking Pasteurized milk does not increase calcium but instead depletes it. The body will take calcium from the bones in order to keep calcium levels in the blood within normal range and to be in balance with other minerals such as potassium and phosphorus. A 12-year Nurses' Health Study showed that of 80,000 women, those who drank two or more glasses of milk per day were 45% more likely to suffer hip fractures than women who drank one glass or less.[34]

Far from being the "perfect food," milk can lead to serious health problems. Consumption of processed milk and dairy products has been associated with iron deficiency anemia, allergies, diarrhea, heart disease, colic, cramps, gastrointestinal bleeding, sinusitis, skin rashes, acne, arthritis, diabetes, ear infections, osteoporosis, asthma, autoimmune diseases, arteriosclerosis, and possibly lung cancer, multiple sclerosis, and non-Hodgkin's lymphoma.[35]

The milk of mammals is species-specific, designed to protect the young of that species. Alteration of that milk by sterilization or pasteurization destroys that protection. Cow's milk contains up to 20 times more of the protein casein than human milk. This makes the nutrients in cow's milk difficult (if not impossible) for humans to assimilate. Processed milk and dairy products prompt the human digestive system to form unnecessary acid and mucous. Cows are usually injected with recombinant bovine growth hormone (rBGH) to artificially increase their milk production. Organic milk does not have rBGH.

Most individuals are unable to digest significant amounts of lactose, the predominant sugar in milk. This is because there is a genetically programmed decline in lactase levels after the first year or two of life. Lactase deficiency is not the same as lactose intolerance. Problems arise when undigested milk sugar is transported to the large intestine where it ferments under bacterial action, producing short-chain fatty acids and gastrointestinal symptoms such as gas, bloating, or diarrhea. A physician should be able to diagnose incomplete absorption of lactose.

According to a recent study[36], when total lactose intake is eight ounces or less per day, symptoms should be negligible. Lactose-intolerant individuals should be careful to read labels on processed foods to avoid those containing whey, milk solids, or other hidden dairy substances which may push the total past eight ounces. Nonfat milk presents no problems for the lactose-intolerant.

If the reason for drinking milk is to keep calcium at normal level, one should consider other sources containing zero lactose: sardines, tofu, salmon, and cooked collard greens, kale or broccoli. One ounce of processed cheese has 2-3 grams of lactose compared to one cup of milk, which contains 12-13 grams.[37]

Those who enjoy drinking milk should consider consuming nonfat milk, since milk containing any fat is typically homogenized. This process releases an enzyme that attacks the arteries, causing pits. The so-called “bad” cholesterol tries to patch these pits and help avoid internal bleeding. Heavy milk drinkers will have arteries covered by cholesterol patches and plaque.[38] If this buildup is too thick, the artery becomes too constricted to sustain blood flow, leading to heart attack or stroke. Avoid skim milk since it is lacks the fat and enzymes necessary for proper calcium absorption.

Reacting to cholesterol scare tactics in the media without knowing one's actual cholesterol level is a mistake. Lowering one's cholesterol level makes sense for those at risk for heart disease. For those not at risk, lowering cholesterol can in turn lower the level of serotonin in the brain and may lead some individuals to adopt risky and/or aggressive behavior.[39]

The National Heart, Lung, and Blood Institute estimates that 36 million Americans should be taking cholesterol-lowering drugs, up from 13 million in 1993.[40] They fail to point out that changes in diet, especially limiting saturated fats, and increasing exercise, will lower cholesterol without drugs. The Institute thus tacitly acknowledges that we Americans prefer to let pills do the work rather than give up our unhealthy living habits.

Fats

Not all fats are responsible for cancer; some, like olive oil, actually fight the disease. The popular view is that canola oil is harmless because it is monounsaturated. However, during processing, chemical residues leach into the oil. Cold-pressed canola oil is much better, but it is prohibitively expensive. Cottonseed oil may contain herbicides and pesticides since cotton is not considered a food and the USDA applies no rules regarding limits on levels of toxins. It behooves the consumer to read labels for the type of oil used to process the packaged food.

Oxidized oils become rancid, and thus carcinogenic. It may be that rancid oils in bags of dog and cat food could cause cancer in pets. Most pet owners purchase large bags of dry food and keep them open for weeks. Keep any food products containing oils refrigerated after opening. Unprocessed foods such as whole wheat or brown rice contain natural oils and should be refrigerated or used quickly.

Partially hydrogenated oils (transfatty oils, or "trans fats") are modified oils that have been linked to skin cancer.[41] If the label says "no cholesterol" the oil is actually artificial cholesterol. If the ingredients list contains the word "hydrogenated," the product contains trans fat. The food industry uses these fats liberally because they are flavor enhancers and have a long shelf life. Trans fats are found in most cocoas, baked goods, margarine, shortening, nondairy coffee creamer, cookies, crackers, bread, microwavable popcorn, tortillas, and nearly all so-called "junk foods." Of the items on this list, popcorn is the worst offender in terms of amount and type of fat, and 42% of the calories in the popcorn come from trans fat.[42]

Butter contains saturated fat while margarine has trans fat. The harder the margarine, the more trans fat it contains. These synthetic oils change proteins in our bodies so that they reject insulin created by the pancreas. Since the late 1970s, research has consistently linked these oils to heart disease and Type 2 diabetes. This variety of diabetes is characterized by the body's inability to use natural insulin. In October 1998, the American Heart Association finally removed their seal of approval from products containing partially hydrogenated oils and warned consumers to keep use of these to a minimum.

Salt

Public health experts estimate that we Americans consume about 9 grams of salt each day, exceeding the cautionary maximum by 3 grams. They also note that most of this sodium intake comes from processed food, including items ordered from take-out eateries and restaurants.[43] Preparing meals at home isn't always practical or possible, but limiting salt is feasible. Including more fruits, vegetables and whole grains will not only offset the effects of salt, it will help to lower cholesterol and blood pressure.

Restricting salt should be done gradually, else one's taste buds will rebel. Salt substitutes like parsley, lemon, lime, pepper, or oregano add flavor. Check food labels for sodium content; choose products and brands that lower the risk of blood pressure and hypertension. Salt aggravates hypertension but does not cause it. Salt itself is not bad, but intake of too much salt upsets the optimal balance with calcium and potassium.

Processed Sugar

Studies have shown processed sugar to be immunosuppressive.[44] Upon ingesting sugar, blood sugar levels rise. The body seeks to regain balance and signals the pancreas to produce insulin. While the pancreas is thus occupied, it is not producing enzymes to fight infection. The sugar in one 12-ounce can of soda can suppress the immune system for up to six hours. The World Health Organization in 1998 reported that Type 2 diabetes is at epidemic proportions in countries where high levels of sugar and starches.

The only sugar that does not immediately raise blood sugar levels is raw cane sugar juice that has been dehydrated and granularized. Health food stores carry this product as Sucanat™.

Stevia *(Stevia rebaudiana Bertoni)* is an herbal substitute for sugar taken from a shrub native to Paraguay. Sugar has 16 calories per teaspoon while Stevia has zero calories and is 200-300 times sweeter than sugar. It is sold in the US a dietary supplement, not as a sweetener (food product) because limited studies showed one of the glycosides to contain a component (steviol) that causes cell mutation in laboratory animals. The FDA ruling denying GRAS (generally recognized as safe) status to Stevia is puzzling when one considers that caffeine and saccharine are FDA-approved but are potentially mutagenic substances.[45]

Reducing sugar does not mean avoiding natural sugars found in fruits, vegetables, and grains. It means shunning *added* sugar, common in processed foods and beverages as high-fructose corn syrup, as well as honey, maple syrup, and white table sugar. One should consume no more than 10 teaspoons per day. Labels often list sugars in terms of grams. To convert to teaspoons, divide by 4.2. For example, one 12-ounce can of soda contains an average of 38-46 total grams of sugars, equivalent to roughly 10 teaspoons. Another way to view sugar intake is to visualize each 3 grams as one sugar packet served at restaurants. Thus a can of soda would be equivalent to about 13 sugar packets. Keep a food diary for a week. It may be a surprise to see how much added sugar is being consumed.

In the 1950s, Dr. Otto Warburg won the Nobel Prize for discovering that cancer metabolizes through a process of fermentation, which requires sugar. When a cancer patient ingests sugars, starches, and carbohydrates, the cancer cells pull the sugars from the blood stream. Oncologists know that cancer needs a sugar-rich environment to thrive. One may wonder why the American Cancer Society recommends a product like Ensure™, which contains extremely high levels of sugar (18 grams) and carbohydrates (40 grams) in the form of sucrose, corn syrup, and maltodextrin.

Using Dr. Warburg's findings, University of Minnesota researchers are now experimenting with a "smart bomb," a chemotherapeutic agent wrapped in a coating that makes it harmless until it finds an oxygen-free place in the body. Such a place is where cancer cells gather. Once settled, the "smart bomb" releases its deadly payload to kill the cancer cells. This is the way Laetrile was intended to work, using a substance called amygdalin found in the pits of apricots and other fruits. In the presence of certain enzymes, amygdalin breaks down into glucose, hydrogen cyanide coated with sugars. In theory, the cancer cells would eat away at the sugar coating, releasing the cyanide that kills it. In the 1950s and '60s, Laetrile was exploited as a miracle cure for cancer but its toxicity was not carefully controlled and it was banned for sale.[46]

Antacids and Heartburn Drugs

Acid indigestion is caused by a *lack* of stomach acid, not a surplus of it. Without enough stomach acid to break down ingested food, the undigested mass ferments in the stomach. The bubbles produced by fermentation make their way into the esophagus, bringing some stomach acid along. The result is the pain and discomfort of acid reflux. An antacid will end the painful symptoms but it will cause the partially digested food to enter the intestinal tract to wreak havoc on the already overburdened digestive system and in turn, on the immune system.

It is a simple matter to be tested for hypochlorhydria (low secretion of stomach acid). The remedy is also simple: supplement the diet with digestive enzymes or betaine HCl (a form of hydrochloric acid). Ask the nutritionist to advise on additional zinc and fish oil supplements. Zinc is the required cofactor for the enzyme that produces natural hydrochloric acid in the stomach. The essential fatty acids in fish oils produce anti-inflammatory prostaglandins.[47]

Allergies may play a role if eczema is also a problem. Try eliminating chronic offenders from the diet: eggs, soy foods, peanuts, wheat, and dairy products.

Aspirin

The claim that an aspirin per day will prevent heart attacks and stroke applies only to buffered aspirin. During a heart attack, the victim has a 25% better chance of survival if injected with magnesium, which dilates blood vessels, aids the body in potassium absorption, acts as a natural blood thinner, and keeps blood cells from clumping. Nearly all autopsies on heart attack victims reveal magnesium deficiency. The harmless buffering agent in buffered aspirin is magnesium. Plain aspirin is not as effective. For some individuals, continued use of aspirin can lead to peptic ulcers and bleeding of the stomach lining. Aspirin has also been linked to macular degeneration.

Aspirin is a known vitamin antagonist, especially toward vitamin C, destroying huge quantities in the body. If aspirin is used for anti-inflammatory purposes, vitamin C supplements become extremely important. Vitamin C is also depleted by mental stress, physical trauma, smoking, and caffeine.

Ibuprofen

This OTC drug is often suggested for rheumatoid arthritis, osteoarthritis, and flare-ups of chronic disease. Although physicians recommend that the smallest dose of ibuprofen that yields acceptable control should be used, individuals seeking pain relief routinely abuse this drug. Exceeding the suggested 50mg/kg/day maximum dose can result in gastrointestinal toxicity, liver damage, blurred vision, edema, and renal toxicity.[48]

ELIMINATION OF TOXINS

Some of the toxins resident in our bodies are inadvertently consumed along with the foods we eat. Exposure to pesticides can be by ingestion, the most common method, or by tactile contact with chemicals found in household and garden products. Another source is aerial spraying and roadside pest/weed abatement spraying. Although individual exposure may be low, the effect is cumulative over years. Certain pesticides alter the body's assimilation and use of vitamins C and A, both essential for a healthy immune system. Some pesticides alter or disrupt the way in which the thymus produces T-cells, another critical immune system element.

Buying organically grown fruits, vegetables, and meats, as well as organically produced dairy products, may minimize toxin intake. The USDA has excluded irradiated foods, crops fertilized with solid waste, and genetically manipulated foods from the "organic" category. However, use caution when buying items labeled "organic." The buyer may be protected from exposure to potential carcinogens, but bacteria in manure-based fertilizers present other risks. Wash all produce thoroughly.[49]

Toxins that are natural by-products of infection must also be flushed from the body, else they will take up residence and cause problems later. As cells take in nutrients and begin the repair process, they in turn discharge waste chemicals. The circulatory and lymphatic systems must be in tip-top working order to convey these unwanted materials to the excretory organs.

Scientists at Johns Hopkins and Tsukuba University in Japan[50] have confirmed the existence of a long-suspected natural system the body uses to block the cancer-causing effects of toxic chemicals in food and the environment. Sensing toxins, the immune system increases production of phase II enzymes to dispose of them before they can damage DNA and trigger cancer. When a specific protein called Nrf2 is in short supply because the immune system is not working properly, the phase II enzymes cannot in turn be generated, reducing one's sensitivity to carcinogens. Toxicity also plays a role in many other conditions such as atherosclerosis and neurodegenerative diseases.

The body depends on proper circulation for oxygen and nutrition as well as toxin removal. Fresh blood allows oxidation to occur in tissues. Blood leaving an area carries with it the waste products of oxidation and metabolism. As fresh blood flows to the muscles, lungs, brain and heart, healthy cells are renewed. Daily consumption of at least two quarts of pure, spring water is essential to facilitate this process. Certain herbs that aid in oxygen transport are discussed in Appendix I. Vitamins and minerals that do this are described in the following subsection.

VITAMIN AND MINERAL SUPPLEMENTS

The fewer vitamins and minerals we consume on a regular basis, the more fragile our health becomes. Although theoretically all our nutritional needs can be supplied by the foods we eat, only some of us follow a strict dietary regimen that ensures consistent intake of these elements. Also, it is doubtful that we come close to satisfying our true daily requirements because our foods are so highly processed before reaching the grocery store shelves.

In 1943 the U.S. Food and Drug Administration published the first list of Recommended Dietary Allowances (RDAs) to be used as standards for nutrition labeling of foods. The latest edition of this list was published in 1989.[51] The guide is intended to be the accepted source of nutrient allowances for "healthy people." The definition of this term is not clear.

However, the critical role of certain key nutrients in maintaining healthy body functioning is sometimes ignored in traditional medical treatment, since individual differences in the need for, and intake of, vitamins and minerals are difficult and time-consuming to determine.[52] This is where a qualified nutritionist can be of help. Also, many Internet resources allow mapping specific disorders to vitamin, mineral, and herbal supplements.[53] Nearly 24 million Americans routinely consume dietary supplements, but fewer than 40% of them discuss it with their doctors.[54]

Despite FDA rules requiring a facts panel on supplement labels, the Dietary Supplement Health and Education Act of 1994 actually requires and prohibits very little in terms of processing. Manufacturers and marketers still have considerable leeway. Although labels cannot claim to cure, treat, diagnose, mitigate, or prevent a disease, they can legally make "structure" or "function" claims.[55] For example, the phrase "reduces joint pain" is illegal but "supports healthy joints" is not. A label stating "lowers cholesterol" is not allowed but one reading "helps to maintain healthy cholesterol levels" is permitted. Under the law, skillful ad writers may use vague words and phrases to infer relief and to suggest hope for a cure, but they may not make specific claims.

The FDA mandates "good manufacturing practices" for makers of prescription drugs, over-the-counter drugs, and food products. However, these rules do not apply to supplement producers. Having no pre-market regulatory power, the FDA can act to solve a problem or recall a supplement only after the fact. Thus consumers are relying heavily on the ethics of the manufacturer to deliver a quality product.

Health food store sales personnel are no substitute for credentialed nutritionists or medical doctors. The sales clerk's job is to sell the store's products, though some come close to diagnosing and prescribing by strongly recommending a "best seller." Until recently, most pharmacists knew little or nothing about dietary supplements, as this topic was not taught to them in school. An admirable policy by Rite Aid, one of the United States' largest drugstore chains, was to train its ten thousand pharmacists on natural medications so they could in turn credibly counsel customers.[56]

The following list of vitamins and minerals are purposely unaccompanied by suggested daily amounts since specific doses should be tailored to the individual consumer. Some substances in high doses may be toxic. The reader should research the precise amount necessary for his/her biochemical profile ideally with the assistance of a nutritionist or dietitian. Individuals using an antibiotic regimen should not take supplements at the same time of day because supplements may interfere with antibiotic uptake and/or transport.[57]

Immune System Boosters

Those supplements that are especially valuable in promoting a vigorous immune system are:

- Vitamin A, a powerful antioxidant that fortifies the immune system when under the stress of viral infection. This vitamin is essential for healthy vision and skin. Along with Vitamins C and D, it is an important cofactor for calcium absorption. Vitamin A maintains epithelial tissues and mucous membranes in the respiratory, digestive, and urinary tracts, which serve as physical barriers to microorganisms;

- B-complex vitamins, needed to produce red blood cells, B-cells, T-cells, and antibodies.[58] Vitamin B_6 helps metabolize protein and amino acids, and maintains the central nervous system. Vitamin B_{12} helps build and maintain myelin—a protective sheath found around the nerves—and also synthesizes DNA;
- Bioflavonoids, which help build resistance to infection, help maintain the normal state of the walls of small blood vessels, and promote healing by facilitating the absorption of vitamin C;
- Vitamin C (ascorbic acid),[59] an antiviral agent that also helps to strengthen capillary walls, and is essential to assist the body in the production of interferon (an immune system stimulant), neutral antihistamines, and collagen. It plays a vital role in calcium absorption. Vitamin C scavenges free radicals, helps metabolize particular amino acids, stimulates adrenal function and aids in metabolizing cholesterol;
- Calcium,[60] for building and maintaining strong bones and teeth. Calcium plays a role in the transmission of nerve impulses, blood clotting, and smooth muscle contraction, which helps regulate heart rhythm. Calcium is essential for encapsulating and ensnaring harmful invaders;

- Chlorophyll, which helps to remove toxins from the bloodstream;
- Coenzyme Q_{10}, an important antioxidant that increases the activity of those immune system cells that target and destroy harmful bacteria. Several studies document extraordinary benefit to the immune system;[61]
- Copper, which aids in creating red blood cells and collagen. Copper helps in the absorption and transport of iron;
- Vitamin D, necessary to calcium and phosphorus utilization as well as promoting strong bones and teeth and protecting against muscle weakness;
- Vitamin E, an antioxidant that (a) prolongs the life of red blood cells, (b) is essential to the use of oxygen by the muscles by preventing premature reaction of oxygen, (c) has a beneficial effect on the pituitary gland, which is part of the body's antistress mechanism, (d) prevents damage to cell membranes, and (e) keeps "bad" cholesterol (i.e., LDL) from oxidizing, which is the beginning of arterial plaque;
- Folic Acid (or Folate), a B-vitamin (B_9) necessary for red blood cell production, growth, and reproduction. Folic acid metabolizes protein and converts many amino acids. It forms the nucleic acids for DNA and RNA;
- Iron, needed for hemoglobin formation and the transfer of oxygen from the lungs to every cell of the body;
- Magnesium, a key factor in the proper functioning of nerves and muscles and healthy maintenance of

bones. Magnesium helps metabolize carbohydrates and proteins, and aids in enzyme activation. It enhances the absorption and use of calcium;

- Manganese, needed to metabolize glucose, synthesize cholesterol and fatty acids, build strong bones, and produce urea for excretion;
- Niacin, which breaks down carbohydrates, fats and proteins. Niacin keeps the skin, digestive tract and nervous system functioning. It helps in the production of red blood cells and steroids;
- Pantothenic acid (calcium pantothenate), a water-soluble B-vitamin that: (a) helps in cell building (especially antibody synthesis); (b) supports the functioning of the adrenal glands and the development of the central nervous system; (c) is important for healthy skin and nerves; (d) is essential to coenzyme A production which leads in turn to the formation of components of connective tissue; and (e) is usually found to be deficient in persons with RA;[62,63]
- Phosphorus, essential for cell growth, maintenance, and repair. Excess phosphorus upsets the mineral balance and prevents calcium and other essential minerals from being assimilated;
- Potassium, which helps metabolize carbohydrates and synthesize protein, and to transmit nerve impulses. Potassium works with sodium to maintain the body's fluid balance;
- Selenium, a trace element that strengthens the immune system by stimulating lymphocytes to produce more antibodies and encouraging the

activity of phagocytes. Selenium protects cell membranes from free radicals;

- Zinc, which helps boost the immune system to fight viral infection, heal and develop new cells. Zinc helps the liver detoxify alcohol. It is needed to maintain healthy skin cells and to insure normal insulin activity. Zinc also aids in protein digestion.

A diet including daily portions of legumes, protein, green leafy vegetables, and fruit will supply many of these essential vitamins and minerals.

Table 4 shows some of these natural sources. Note that RDA amounts are not shown in the table since opinions vary widely and supplements must be tailored to an individual's needs. Those with high insulin levels, high blood pressure, high cholesterol, excess weight, and/or diabetes should avoid grains. Some extremely beneficial supplements, such as Coenzyme Q_{10}, are not yet part of the FDA's list of Recommended Daily Allowances. Biochemists and nutritionists caution against excessive supplement use.[64,65]

Some vitamins and minerals are not water-soluble and remain in the system, potentially causing harm. Exceeding selenium limits, for instance, can lead to hair loss and brittle nails. Zinc lozenges, which can mitigate the symptoms and duration of a cold, should be used in moderation. Too much zinc can drive other essential metals out of the body and cause anemia. Too high zinc levels inhibit motility of phagocytes.

Vegetables in the nightshade family (tomatoes, potatoes, bell peppers, and eggplant) contain solanine, considered a calcium inhibitor because of their binding characteristics. Fruits high in oxalates, such as cranberries, rhubarb, plums, spinach, beet greens, and chard have the same effect.

Table 4. Natural Sources of Vitamins and Minerals

Vitamin/Mineral	Natural Source (highest content in italics)
Vitamin A	Fish liver oils, eggs, dairy products, peaches, green and yellow fruits and vegetables such as *cantaloupe*, *sweet potato*, *carrots*, *squash*, tomatoes
B-Complex	Brewer's yeast, whole grains, nuts, milk, eggs, *mussels*, *liver,* kelp, *most vegetables*, avocados, *fish, crab, oysters, soybeans, tempeh, clams*
Bioflavonoids	Buckwheat and fruits (esp. citrus)
Vitamin C	Fresh fruits (especially citrus, strawberries), vegetables (especially green/red peppers, kale, potatoes, sweet potato, cauliflower, broccoli)
Calcium	*Dairy products*, salmon, soybeans, peanuts, kelp, olives, green vegetables (especially spinach and kale), *tempeh, tofu, yogurt*, *amaranth*
Coenzyme Q_{10}	Animal tissues (especially organs) of beef, pork, chicken, fish; milk, eggs, vegetables (esp. sweet potato, alfalfa, spinach, potato, soybeans), oils of rice bran, soybean, and cottonseed
Copper	*liver, oysters, crab, lobster, squid, tempeh*, nuts, lentils, soybeans, amaranth
Vitamin D	Eggs, fish, *fish liver oil, oysters*, dairy products, sunlight
Vitamin E	Vegetable oils, soybean oil, safflower oil, *wheat germ*, raw seeds and nuts (especially *sunflower seeds*), eggs, legumes, whole grains, milk, leafy vegetables, meat, liver, molasses

Table 4. Natural Sources of Vitamins and Minerals, cont'd

Folic Acid	Brewer's yeast, *liver*, deep-green leafy vegetables, egg yolk, apricots, carrots, *legumes*
Iron	*Clams, soybeans, legumes,* oysters, pine nuts, pumpkin seeds, sesame seeds, shrimp, steak, tempeh, tofu, wheat germ, mussels, *liver*
Magnesium	Nuts, whole grains, legumes, dark green vegetables, apples, soy products, figs, lemons, tofu, grapefruit, *amaranth*, corn
Manganese	*Amaranth, mussels, pineapple, tempeh, wheat germ*, berries, nuts, tofu, brown rice, soybeans
Niacin	*Swordfish*, avocados, barley, rice, corn, beef, lamb, peas, salmon, tempeh, tuna, turkey
Pantothenic Acid	Royal jelly, *liver*, whole grains, nuts, wheat germ, yogurt, green vegetables, crude molasses, *eggs, avocados, chicken, lentils, salmon*
Phosphorus	Meat, fish, poultry, eggs, whole grains, nuts, artichokes, tofu, legumes, Swiss cheese, ricotta, tempeh, yogurt
Selenium	*Fish, wheat germ*, onions, tomatoes, *couscous, liver*, broccoli, brown rice, eggs, pork, beef, tempeh, tofu, yogurt, shrimp, *Brazil nuts*
Zinc	Brewer's yeast, bone meal, wheat germ, beans, peanuts, seeds, steak, nonfat dry milk, *oysters*, crab, tempeh, turkey, wild rice, yogurt, chicken, lentils, pork, lamb

Strict vegetarians ("vegans") may require protein supplements, although many insist that the full range of requirements are satisfied through consumption of a range of fruits and vegetables rich in protein.[66] Vegans may be missing essential vitamin B_{12}, not available from plant foods. Since B_{12} deficiencies can cause anemia and nerve disorders, supplements are strongly suggested.

Lactose-intolerant individuals who are concerned about calcium deficiency should learn about the various lactase supplements that allow proper assimilation of some dairy products. Resources are readily available on the Internet.[67]

Although cell structure is standard among human beings, every individual's physiology is admittedly different. The manner in which mycoplasmas form and migrate to joints is standard among humans and similar among the other mammals. Individual metabolic profile, age, blood sugar balance, and many other factors must be considered when trying to understand why some people respond well to vitamin supplements and others do not. For example, enzymes are essential to proper digestion and metabolism of food intake. Those who do not respond to vitamin therapy may be consuming, but not assimilating, the supplements they take. The undigested material passes through the digestive system and is wasted.

Some vitamin pill formulations do not dissolve properly and are not released in time to be useful. Some supplements should be taken alone. That is, they either inhibit or enhance the action of other vitamins or minerals, so allow at least one half-hour delay before ingesting other supplements for optimum effect. A good example is MSM, which nullifies the activity of nearly all vitamins except vitamin C, which works together with MSM and acts as a booster.

Improper digestion is aggravated by consumption of caffeine in coffee, tea, and soft drinks. Alcohol and tobacco are detrimental as well. These substances dilute and may even cancel the efficacy of some vitamin supplements. A particular dilemma for arthritics is that they seek a "pick-me-up" from beverages containing caffeine to offset the fatigue and energy depression that is symptomatic of an arthritis infection and they then incur the harmful side effects of caffeine consumption. Caffeinated beverages also suppress the production of the hormone cortisol, which is essential to efficient thyroid function.[68]

Switching to decaffeinated coffee has serious drawbacks. The safety of the residue of solvents used to extract caffeine from the coffee beans is in question. One of these, methylene chloride, is suspected to cause cancer. Decaf is not completely caffeine-free. A 6-ounce cup of decaffeinated coffee could contain up to 5 mg of caffeine. The best approach is abstention or severe limitation of coffee intake.

Digestive problems are also exacerbated by stress, both internal (mental) and external (pollution). "Lunch on the run" is commonplace in busy workplaces today. It is little wonder that antacids sell well to those who make it a habit to wolf down fast food on short lunch breaks. Prolonged chewing provides necessary enzymes to aid digestion, obviating the discomfort of heartburn and the need for antacids.

Glucosamine and Chondroitin

In 1837, Johannes Müller steamed cartilage at high pressure to obtain what he called "chondrin." In the 1890s, C. S. W. Krukenberg isolated the chief component of chondrin and called it "chondroitin sulfate." In 1969, techniques used in the study of nucleic acids such as DNA allowed the extraction of proteoglycans. These macro-molecules were found to contain chondroitin sulfate intact from cartilage.[69]

Glucosamine sulfate, a component of proteoglycans, occurs naturally in the body. It is a building block of connective tissue, used to grow new cartilage, prevent enzymatic destruction of cartilage, and promote joint lubrication. It helps the body generate chondroitin, an important component of connective tissue, most highly concentrated in cartilage. Chondroitin sulfate, together with glucosamine sulfate, stimulates the growth of proteoglycans and cartilage-producing chondrocytes. Chondroitin is essential to keep cartilage strong and flexible, and also helps prevent breakdown. Vitamin C helps to stabilize collagen, a primary protein used to build cartilage.

However, for these substances to be effective, the balance of the battle at the point of infection should be tipped toward regeneration, not destruction. How to do this is unclear. Perhaps dosages should be administered in a cyclical manner to promote cycles of immune system stimulation and moderation with Glucosamine sulfate and Chondroitin sulfate taken during the moderation part of the cycle.

Glucosamine and chondroitin were tested in eight clinical trials involving 1,500 people. A daily dose of either 1,500 mg of glucosamine or 1,200 mg of chondroitin was seen to relieve arthritis pain more effectively than a placebo. These substances have long been used successfully in veterinary applications.[70]

Western, especially American, diets do not include gristle and cartilage as do many foreign recipes. One Oriental recipe calls for boiling down a whole chicken to extract the cartilage, then drinking the liquid. This practice could perhaps overcome a particular diet deficiency, proving to be as beneficial to health as purchasing processed cartilage supplements such as shark cartilage, Glucosamine sulfate, and Chondroitin sulfate.[71]

Proteoglycan structures use large volumes of water, organizing it in multiple interacting layers or shells during formation of protein chains. Additional water is trapped in the interstices of the chondrocytes' extracellular matrix. The resilience of cartilage depends on this water-structuring activity. Nourishment of cartilage in the joints does not come from blood vessels—there are no blood vessels in cartilage—but from the liquid brought there by the compressions and relaxations during bodily movement. This makes the case for daily intake of water and daily exercise.[72] Long periods of inactivity can dry out and weaken joint cartilage, making it thin and fragile.[73]

REINTRODUCING BENEFICIAL BACTERIA

Medical researchers are recognizing that much of our immune system lies along the gastrointestinal tract. The average human gut contains 400-500 different kinds of bacteria. The beneficial bacteria, such as *bifidobacteria*, stimulate the immune system and control the growth of other bacteria, while harmful bacteria, such as species of the *Clostridium* family, lead to chronic diseases like arthritis and cancer. Studies in Europe and Japan[74] have found that ingesting slow release, natural sugars found in grains, fruits, certain kinds of seaweed, and legumes encourage growth of the desired bacteria, while eating too much meat and other animal-based foods favors the bad bacteria.

Maintaining a healthy environment for natural, beneficial bacteria can be done by eating certain fermented foods such as yogurt, tempeh, cheese, sourdough bread, red grape juice, and red wine (in moderation). Freeze-dried probiotic supplements are helpful in countering *Candida* yeast infections.[75] Health food stores carry products such as dairy-free *Lactobacillus acidophilus* and caprylic acid products to maintain flora balance. It is important that the lactobacillus is properly refrigerated from manufacturer to consumer. Temperatures higher than 80 degrees can kill this beneficial bacteria and render it useless as a treatment. Most health food stores keep lactobacillus in a cold case, but it may be shipped in standard unrefrigerated delivery trucks. If in doubt, contact the supplier directly and ask about shipping methods.

Yeasty foods to avoid or drastically minimize until balance is achieved (usually for about 7-10 days) are:[76]

- wheat, barley and rye in breads, crackers, cereal and pasta;
- dairy products, especially cheese, as well as cream cheese, cheese-containing snacks, buttermilk, sour cream and sour milk products;
- alcoholic beverages and/or fermented beverages;
- cider, grape juice, and wine;
- leftovers older than 24 hours, which may be contaminated with mold;
- sugar in any form;
- dried and candied fruits;
- melons (watermelon, honeydew, and especially cantaloupe);
- all types of mushrooms, morels and truffles;
- processed and smoked meats, such as ham, hot dogs, and corned beef;
- sauces, unless homemade without peppers, sugar, vinegar or syrup;

- any foods containing vinegar, including salad dressing, pickled vegetables, sauerkraut, mustard and mayonnaise;
- peppers and horseradish;
- fried or canned foods, including vegetable juices and canned fruit;
- caffeinated beverages and products, including chocolate.

If an individual is allergic to yeast, s/he should continue to avoid yeast and mold-containing foods indefinitely. If there is no allergy, one can reintroduce these items gradually back into one's diet, but consume them in small amounts. Many individuals with yeast-connected health problems are allergic to several, often many, different foods. Specific laboratory tests can pinpoint these allergens and assist in developing a health diet that avoids them.[77]

Antifungal diet supplements sold commercially to kill yeast infections are not fully effective, since they only work in the gut. It is when the *Candida* bacteria migrates through a tear in the gut wall and moves into the systemic portion of the anatomy that an individual experiences the mental and emotional symptoms of *Candidiasis* and begins the onset of allergies that are indicative of that disease.[78] Blood Ig tests are available to confirm leaky gut syndrome.

CHOOSING A NUTRITIONIST/DIETICIAN

There are many publications, websites, and media resources offering helpful nutritional advice, but at some point the individual with chronic illness may need a personal consultation with a professional nutritionist or dietician. The usual starting point is a regimen for clearing accumulated toxins from the body. Often the cravings for allergy-producing foods will disappear along with symptoms of fatigue, low energy, depression and other signs of toxicity.

Finding a qualified dietary advisor can be problematic. Many nutritional counselors have received training through the health food industry, so their interest may be in selling certain dietary supplement firms' products. Personal trainers sometimes offer nutritional advice, but their goals are typically related to reducing body fat and building muscle tone. This focus is too narrow. Beware of nutritionists who suggest that disease is caused by faulty diet alone. Suspect those who sell vitamins in their offices or who offer a one-size-fits-all diet plan.

Registered Dietitians (R.D.'s) collectively take the view that all our nutritional needs can be obtained from the foods we eat. They tend to frown on supplements and do not accept that there are flaws in the standard American diet. A growing number of progressive R.D.'s are practicing integrative nutrition, which takes the best of modern science to detect deficiencies and uses the results to construct an individualized patient profile of dietary needs. These practitioners are Certified Clinical Nutritionists (CCNs) or Certified Nutritionists (CNs) and usually work for holistic physicians who use therapeutic nutrition as part of their treatments.

A qualified nutritionist should have an active membership in the American Society for Nutritional Sciences (ASNS) in addition to an academic degree. At the doctoral level, the American Board of Nutrition offers certification in clinical nutrition (M.D. only) and human nutritional sciences (M.D. and Ph.D.). Board certification requires the candidate to pass comprehensive examinations. Most board-certified nutritionists are affiliated with medical schools and hospitals. They may be clinical researchers as well as consultants to primary care physicians.

The American College of Nutrition offers board certification to professionals with an accredited master's or doctoral degree who have clinical experience and who pass an examination. The Certified Nutrition Specialist (CNS) credential is awarded. Professional nutritionists are listed by state at www.certifiednutritionist.com/find.html.[79]

A nutritionist will often have experience in a specific area based on their work in a particular health environment, e.g., gerontology or adult diabetes. The nutritionist's credentials are not as important as his/her clinical experience, advanced education, and success rate. Do not hesitate to interview several nutritional counselors. This can be done over the phone before making an appointment. Ask key questions such as:

- What degrees and credentials do you have?
- What sort of diets do you design?
- What diagnostic tests do you recommend?
- May I call a few of your clients for references?

Choose a practitioner with whom you feel comfortable discussing every aspect of your lifestyle. Ask for the reasons behind the nutritionist's recommendations for dietary adjustments. If you understand the explanation and agree with it, you will be more readily motivated to take an active role in reaching your health goals.

---

[1] Cox (1984) p. xxiii.

[2] A scientific and philosophic rule requiring that the simplest of competing theories be preferred to the more complex, or that explanations of unknown phenomena be sought first in terms of known quantities. Named for William of Occam, 1836.

[3] Conn, Dr. Doyt L. "Can Vitamins Cure?" *Arthritis Today*, September/October 1998.

[4] Morgan, Paul. "Ease Into Exercise." *Arthritis Today*, May/June 2001.

---

[5] Schaeffer, Rachel. "The Full-energy Workout." *Natural Health*, January/February 1999.

[6] Medical studies at Fairview General Hospital; in Keough (1986) p. 76.

[7] National Arthritis Data Workgroup statistic, cited in *Arthritis Today*, November/December 1998, page 53.

[8] Brena, Steven F. "Pain Control Facilities: Roots, Organization, and Function," in Brena and Chapman (1983) p. 19.

[9] Brena, S. F., Chapman, S.L. and Decker, R. "Chronic Pain as a Learned Experience," in Ng (1981) pp. 76-83.

[10] Crue, Jr., Benjamin L. "The Neurophysiology and Taxonomy of Pain," in Brena and Chapman (1983) pp. 25-27.

[11] Examples are Lecron (1964), Straus (1982), and Cousins (1981).

[12] Spiegel, Dr. David. "The Hypnotic Trance." Science Annual 1989. H.S. Stuttman, Inc.: Westport, CN.

[13] Kabat-Zinn, J; Wheeler, E; Light, T; Skillings, A; Scharf, MJ; Cropley, TG; Hosmer, D; and Bernhard, JD. "Influence of a mindfulness meditation-based stress reduction intervention on rates of skin-clearing in patients with moderate to severe psoriasis undergoing phototherapy (UVB) and photochemotherapy (PUVA)." *Psychosomatic Medicine* 1998 September/October;60(5):625-632.

[14] See Lidell (1984), Jarney and Tindall (1991), Namikoshi (1974) and Tappan (1988).

[15] For a list of NST practitioners in the United States and Canada see www.usbowen.com/therapist.htm.. The Bowen Research & Training Institute, North Palm Harbor, FL Institute is a nonprofit corporation. Contact: (727) 937-9077. See www.bowen.org for details.

[16] See www.tbmseminars.com, www.health-doc.com/TBM.html, www.naturaltherapies.com/base/holistic/body.htm, and www.mercola.com/article/mind_body/tbm.htm.

[17] Examples are Kauz (1974) and Chuen (1994).

[18] See www.pilatesmethodalliance.org or www.pilates-studio.com.

[19] See www.alexandertech.org or 1-800-473-0620; www.feldenkrais.com or 1-800-775-2118; www.trager.com or 1-415-388-2688. Also see Horstman, Judith. "Movement Therapies." *Arthritis Today*, March/April 1999 and Morgan, Park. "Ease Into Exercise." *Arthritis Today*, May/June 2001.

[20] Two of many examples are Blaney, Beth. "Eat Pyramid Perfect." *Arthritis Today*. May/June 2001 and Sullivan, Karin H. "Consumer Guide: Eat Healthier in 5 Weeks." *Natural Health*, November/December 1998. Also see Cousens (1999).

[21] Clark (1997) p. 24.

[22] Examples are Watt (1975) and Bricklin (1993).

[23] Toivanen (1988) p. 16 and pp. 155-7.

[24] See www.mercola.com/forms/wellness_condensed.htm. Some may find this nutritional program difficult to follow, but the benefits are extraordinarily effective. Dr. Mercola emphasizes that other factors must also be considered (spiritual, emotional, and environmental) if the regimen fails to work over time.

[25] For more information about the benefits of water, see www.wqa.org.

[26] Sobel and Klein (1989) chapter 13. Also Gorman, C. "Junk Food Takes a Hit." *TIME*, June 12, 2000.

[27] See www.mdlab.com/fees&servs/serv-athero.html.

[28] Helpful websites on this topic are www.digitalnaturopath.com and www.healthy.net.

[29] Personal communication with Dr. Mercola, July 2001.

[30] Dr. Rosenfeld, Isadore. "Are You Eating Enough Fiber?"*Parade* Magazine, 4/8/2001.

[31] Gorman, Christine. "Can the Juice!" *TIME*, May 21, 2001.

[32] See http://www.mercola.com/2000/feb/27/no_milk.htm.

[33] Vitetta-Miller, Robin. "Recipes for Relief." Natural Health, October 1999.

[34] Unattributed. "The Real Deal on Calcium." *Natural Health*, March/April 1998, p. 22.

[35] Ibid.

---

[36] Suarez, F.L., Savaiano, D.A., and Levitt, M.D., "A Comparison of Symptoms After the Consumption of Milk or Lactose-Hydrolyzed Milk by People with Self-Reported Severe Lactose Intolerance." *N Engl J Med* 1995; 333: 1-4

[37] American Dietetic Association and the U.S. Department of Agriculture. *Lactose Intolerance: A Resource Including Recipes*. Food Sensitivity Series, 1991.

[38] Enig and Fallon (1998/1999).

[39] Ibid.

[40] Smith, Dr. Ian K. "Cholesterol Alert." *TIME*, May 28, 2001.

[41] Erasmus, Udo. *Fats That Heal, Fats That Kill*. Alive Books: USA, 1999.

[42] Unattributed feature. "Health Quiz: the Big Fat Facts." *Natural Health*, May 2000.

[43] Gorman, Christine. "Don't Pass the Salt." *TIME*, January 15, 2001.

[44] Dufty (1975).

[45] Gustafson, Karen K. "Stevia." *Natural Health*, July/August 1999.

[46] The American Cancer Society and the US National Cancer Institute warn against using Laetrile. See http://www3.uicc.org/publ/uiccnews/archives/Archon0300/cn-laetrile.htm.

[47] Dr. Pizzorno Jr, Joseph E.. "Ask the Experts." *Natural Health*, November/December 1998.

[48] See www.rxlist.com/cgi/generic/ibup_ids.html.

[49] Wagner, Eliza Anne. "Dangerous Fruits and Vegetables?" *Natural Health*, May 2000 and Newsome, Melba. "What's Organic?" *Arthritis Today*, November/December 1998.

[50] See http://www.hopkinsmedicine.org/brocosystem.html.

[51] Food and Nutrition Board, Commission on Life Sciences, National Research Council, *Recommended Dietary Allowances: 10th Edition*, 1989. See also Watt, Bernice K., Merrill, Annabel L., et.al, (1975).

[52] A new online database devoted entirely to dietary supplements has been created by the National Institutes of Health. This database can be found at http://odp.od.nih.gov/ods/databases/ibids.html.

---

[53] For example, www.rxlist.com, www.healthwell.com, and www.puritan.com. A powerful search engine such as Google can be given specific keywords. E.g., "ulcers" and "willow."

[54] Estimate given in *Natural Health* magazine, May 1999, p. 20.

[55] O'Koon, Marcy with Taylor, Michele. "Shopping for a 'Cure'." *Arthritis Today*, March/April 1999.

[56] Ibid.

[57] Nicolson, G.L.; Nasralla, M.Y.; Franco, A.R.; Nicolson, N.L.; Erwin, R.; Ngwenya, R. and Berns, P.A. "Diagnosis and Integrative Treatment of Intracellular Bacterial Infections in Chronic Fatigue and Fibromyalgia Syndromes, Gulf War Illness, Rheumatoid Arthritis, and Other Chronic Illnesses." Clinical Practice of Alternative Medicine 1(2):92-102,2000.

[58] Doses of Vitamin B_{12} and Vitamin E greater than recommended daily allowance (RDA) levels are contraindicated in conditions involving infectious agents, as they interfere with immune system reactions.

[59] Aspirin is a known vitamin antagonist, especially toward vitamin C, destroying huge quantities in the body. If aspirin is used for anti-inflammatory purposes, vitamin C supplements become extremely important. Vitamin C is also depleted by mental stress, physical trauma, smoking, and caffeine.

[60] The combination calcium ascorbate helps the body to metabolize enough vitamin C to effect repairs. It also potentiates aspirin to reduce inflammation. Ordinarily, calcium ascorbate is very acidic so to be effective it must be balanced to pH-neutral by an alkaline substance, e.g., bicarbonate of soda, taken at the same time. Calcium ascorbate is often sold in buffered form to be "acid free." Calcium citrate supple-ments are usually larger and more expensive than other types, but they are well-absorbed and can be taken with or without meals. Supplements made from oyster shells, dolomite, and bone meal can contain lead and should be avoided. See Ott, Christopher. "The Surprising Benefits of Calcium." *Natural Health*, January/February 2002.

[61] Folkers, Morita, McRee (1993), Folkers, Brown, et al. (1993), Tanner (1992), and Folkers, Hanioka, et al. (1991).

[62] Mandell (1983) p. 233.

[63] Eisenstein and Scheiner (1997) offer a detailed discussion of USDA-recommended daily allowances versus actual nutritional content in the

---

American diet. The authors also explain the importance of maintaining the correct level of pantothenic acid (significantly higher than the 10 mg recommended) to enhance the immune system. Examples of common grocery item labels illustrate misleading and/or deficient nutritional values.

[64] Krinsky, Dr. Norman, Department of Biochemistry, Tufts University School of Medicine; also Coco, Donna. "The Numbers Game." *Natural Health*, May 1999; and "Vitamin Overdose." *TIME*, April 24, 2000.

[65] A comprehensive analysis of deficiency symptoms, recommended doses and possible side effects is given in Cawood (1986). See also Mead, Nathanial. "5 Plans for Vitality" in *Natural Health*'s Consumer Guide, July/August 1999.

[66] This is a matter of some controversy, but the individual on a strict vegetarian diet should be on guard for signs of protein deficiency and bring the body back to balance with supplements should that condition occur. Tempeh is an excellent source of protein. Tofu is also a good protein substitute, but is high in fat content. The fewer animal products eaten, the less vitamin D we get, so vegetarians should also be careful regarding levels of vitamin D. His assertion is also met with opposition from the vegetarian community. This author merely signals a warning and does not intend to engender debate.

[67] Many websites provide a wealth of information for the lactose intolerant. Use Google with search keywords such as: lactose, lactase, dairy, milk allergy, calcium.

[68] Ott, Chris." Underactive Thyroid." *Natural Health*, October 1999.

[69] Research was done by two graduate students at Rockefeller University: Vincent C. Hascall, Jr., and Stanley W. Sajdera.

[70] *JAMA* 3/15/00 study reported in *TIME*, April 3, 2000, p. 94.

[71] Personal conversation with the late Dr. Stefan T. Possony, Georgetown University, 1975.

[72] Two low impact exercise examples are Morgan, Park. "Your Workout: Mix It Up." *Arthritis Today*, May/June 2001 and Glentzer, Molly. "The Wake Up Workout." *Natural Health*, March/April 1998.

[73] Caplan, Arnold I. "Cartilage." *Scientific American*, 1984.

[74] Studies cited in "Better Bacteria and More of It." *Natural Health*, January/February 1996, p. 92.

---

[75] Huemer (1997) p. 48. For additional information on probiotic supplements, see the September/October 1996 issue of *Natural Health*.

[76] This short subsection is not intended to be prescriptive. There are a great many health texts which give detailed information on a balanced diet specifically for countering yeast infections. See, for example, Crook (1986, 1995). See also Jacobi, Dana. "The World's Healthiest Diet." *Natural Health*, January/February 1996.

[77] Communication in 1996 with nutritionist Dr. Victoria Arcadi, who states that 60-80% of her patients have systemic yeast overgrowth.

[78] McCabe (1988) p. 51.

[79] Also see www.holistic.com for a Practitioner Directory of Nutritionists, and www.nightingalecounseling.com/nutritionist.html for additional guidelines on choosing a nutritionist.

8. TRENDS IN INFECTION RESEARCH

The usual advice given to RA sufferers is to "just live with it." *Arthritis Today,* the publication of the Arthritis Foundation routinely carries articles on coping with symptoms. The few that feature research activities typically focus on new pain-relieving medications.

Another representative article[1], written for *AARP* magazine asserts that science is "moving closer" to an arthritis cure and describes "the latest breakthrough" but this is merely a prelude to announcing a new drug (Arava) and a new FDA-approved procedure ("viscosupplementation"). Using this procedure, synthetic hyaluronic acid is injected into the knee joint over several weeks. The product does not repair damage or stop the disease's progression. It merely reduces pain; its long-term side effects are as yet unknown.

The best science can do is augment existing drugs to lessen their side effects and introduce these as "new." An example is Arthrotec, which merely encases its predecessor Voltaren in an outer shell of misoprostol to decrease GI tract effects.[2]

Media articles usually end with a vague statement such as "In the next few years there will probably be dramatic changes in our approach to arthritis." The U.S. Pharma-copoeia and the Arthritis Foundation have at this writing only tentatively accepted tetracycline treatment for Lyme Disease and RA. The impression conveyed in the media is that these treatments are still experimental and far on the horizon, when in fact they are readily available now.

In 1988 Dr. Brown was encouraged that the medical community had at last begun to recognize the risks associated with conventional arthritis treatments. He was hopeful that researchers would revisit the neglected but successful methods of the early 1950s, before what he calls the "cortisone revolution." However, he was dismayed that fewer than a dozen of the several hundred grants awarded to pursue arthritis research were looking at the infection connection.[3]

There is still much to be done to fully understand the immune system and microbial infections. The following areas of research hold great promise to unravel long-hidden scientific mysteries related to chronic disease.

The Human Genome Project

The international Human Genome Project, launched in 1990 to perform detailed mapping of the complete set of human genes, has achieved astounding results. However, this is only the beginning of the real medical challenge: to understand the activity and complex interactions of the million or more proteins in the human body. This new scientific approach is called "proteomics." Every chemical reaction essential to life depends on proteins. They are the hormones and enzymes that direct all movement and thought in organisms from bacteria to humans.

Medications based on "genomics" and molecular biology are forecast for 2005. Treatment of disease by gene therapy is estimated to be commonplace by the year 2020.[4] The Project foresees the development of new, more effective drugs to treat arthritis symptoms in the short term, and suggests that some day gene therapy may be able to stop arthritis at the cellular level.[5]

In 1989, scientists discovered the cystic fibrosis gene. In 2000, a gene for one form of arthritis characterized by recurrent fevers was mapped. As many as six genes have been found for lupus, but it is unknown how many remain. However, there are dozens of genes linked to RA, and most forms of arthritis are caused by a combination of factors besides simply genetics.

For example, possessing the HLA-DR4 gene increases one's risk of developing adult RA, but most people with this gene do not have RA. Also, some genes may have a stronger influence than others, and this strength is likely to vary from person to person, predisposing one individual's immune system to respond differently than another's when exposed to a virus or some other antigen by attacking bones or joints. Specific genes may cause some people to be more severely stricken, and sooner, than others.

Ongoing details of the Human Genome Project are available at www.ornl.gov/hgmis/project. A monthly update in newsletter form, *Human Genome News*, is found at www.ornl.gov/hgmis/publicat/hgn/hgn.html along with the full text of all previous issues.

Biofilms

Some bacteria "hibernate"—sometimes as long as centuries—until conditions are right to awaken. Biologists are deterred from studying such microbes because of false positive results that have tainted their efforts to recover ancient DNA. Scientists have developed a database describing these elusive bacteria not only as a resource for evolutionary research but also to study the potential for using these ancient organisms in the industrial production of chemicals.[6] During their state of suspended animation, these bacteria assume different forms, often in clusters.

Mycoplasmas adapt to their environment and form colonies much as bacteria aggregate in clusters as biofilms.

More than 99 percent of all bacteria types can live in biofilm communities. Some are beneficial, such as those used in sewage treatment plants to remove contaminants. Biofilms are found wherever surfaces are in contact with water. Examples are slime on river stones, insides of household water pipes, swimming pool walls and filters, and plaque on teeth. These bacteria can adhere to clean stainless steel within 30 seconds of exposure. Biofilms have been found to cause the rejection of medical implants. They are the source of much of the free-floating bacteria found in drinking water. The common *Pseudomonas aeruginosa* biofilm bacteria can infect animals with suppressed immune systems.[7]

Although a biofilm cluster can spread by ordinary cell division, it will also release cells with the express purpose of starting new colonies. Other microorganisms within a colony act symbiotically with biofilm bacteria, sharing nutrients and providing mutual protection for community survival. Biofilms have been called "communal slime cities."

The use of water purification systems causes bacteria to alter their cell wall structure in order to increase their ability to adhere to surfaces. Biofilm resistance to biocides is remarkable according to CDC experiments.[8] The biofilm colony surrounds itself with a protective shield of polysaccharides and polymers. A disinfectant's oxidizing power is depleted before it reaches the interior cell responsible for forming the biofilm. Free-floating organisms are more vulnerable. Because biofilm bacteria anchor themselves to surfaces with exuded sticky polymers, simple flushing is inadequate to remove them. Chlorinated reverse osmosis water systems, copper piping, and water filters on all house taps can limit biofilm contamination.

The human body is about 60% water. Could it be that bacteria in our bodies' organic "pipes" exhibit the same behavior as biofilms? Is the protective coating that biofilm bacteria secrete to ward off attack from disinfectants analogous to the way antigens try to thwart the immune system's antibodies? Future research will hopefully answer these questions and lead to better understanding of these pathogenic microorganisms.

Although biofilms have been with us for eons, their behavior suddenly became a topic of intensive research in the early 1990s. Bacteriologists had persistently assumed that bacteria are simple unicellular microbes. This was because the hunt for disease-causing organisms traditionally began by isolating a single cell of the suspected pathogen. Many existing theories of bacterial behavior are based on extrapolations made from this early research. New studies have revealed that bacteria build complex communities, differentiate into various cell types, hunt prey cooperatively in groups, and secrete chemical trails to direct movement of others in the colony.[9]

Mining Microbes

Previously unknown and unstudied bacteria in ordinary soil may be the starting point for specialized metagenomic research. The proteins produced by these organisms could have beneficial properties unlike any other currently exploited substances. Most of the antibiotics used in medicine today come from soil-based microbes. Two examples are streptomycin, the first treatment for tuberculosis, and vancomycin, considered the last resort for serious infections. In the opinion of some scientists[10], the inventory of known bacteria have been "mined out" and new biological agents must be developed to combat a growing number of infectious diseases. Further, these microbes have applications in a wide variety of industrial and agricultural areas.

The DNA strings must be long enough to extract and isolate a complete set of genes for study. This is a delicate and painstaking process, complicated by the fact that most of the unknown organisms cannot be grown in the laboratory. Other research teams are experimenting with extracting DNA samples from seawater, sediment, and lichens. The microbes are found to respond to different wavelengths of light, and the proteins' light sensitivity makes them potentially useful in the construction of optical computer memory.[11]

To date, progress in the decoding of the human genome has revealed more than 200 gene sequences that come from bacteria. Microbes are part and parcel of our biochemical structure. Researchers are speculating that some diseases may be caused by a change in the body's internal microbial balance rather than invasion by a single pathogenic microorganism. It may become evident that there are other specific relationships to consider: e.g., the biochemical catalyst-to-enzyme ratio and the toxin-to-antitoxin ratio.

MICROCHIP TECHNOLOGY

Exciting applications for medical diagnosis and testing are being developed using technology borrowed from the semi-conductor industry. Numerous websites document DNA Microarray (Genome Chip) research in progress worldwide. One of the best and most comprehensive is the Massachusetts Institute of Technology's site developed by Dr. Leming Shi at www.Gene-Chips.com.[12]

Biochip Testing[13]

This technology was developed in 1987 in Germany as a testing mechanism for autoimmune and infectious diseases and as a screen for monoclonal antibodies. The biochip testing method combines three usually distinct micro-analytical techniques: indirect immunoflourescence, ELISA, and Blot techniques. Classical ELISA by itself is limited and does not include RA culture elements.

The biochip product is a mosaic that permits effective miniaturization and standardization of serological analyses. The conventional "moisture chamber" and other incubation methods are superfluous as the liquids are maintained in an enclosed area and the exact height and position of the droplets are precisely defined by the geometry of the system.

Companies are using competing methods to make state-of-the-art probes, transferring pieces of cell DNA onto half-inch glass squares (one company has more than a million squares on its chip's checkerboard) or filter paper. An assortment of masks superimposed on the pattern builds up variations of probes in the millions. This remarkable multitesting approach would seem to be the direction pathogenetic research ought to go in order to keep up with swiftly evolving microorganisms. Such a test method would give physicians a valuable tool for disease identification. It is hoped that biochip testing will some day be as common as x-rays as a diagnostic technique, yet without the risks that x-rays pose. Test results would also be available in a short period of time.

Testing for allergens is another application for biochip technology. Conventional tests require either watching for reactions after injections of suspect substances or sending blood samples to a lab for testing. Both methods are costly, cumbersome, and time-consuming. As many as

100 different allergens at once may be tested using a single drop of blood smeared on a biochip. Antibodies in the blood bind to allergens prepositioned on the chip. By amplifying the fluorescence for sensing by a chip-reading instrument, the existence and severity of particular allergens can be determined at the same time.[14]

Microarrays

DNA microarrays are about the size of a credit card. Single-stranded DNA segments called "probes" coat the surface. The microarrays help biologists define a cell's genetic makeup and determine which parts of the cell are active under particular conditions. The development of synthesized crystals called "quantum dots" may make the gene chip structure obsolete.[15] The quantum dots can analyze genes faster than gene chips, allowing researchers more flexibility in designing their experiments, and may be more economical as well. The quantum dots use the optical properties of semiconductors to measure emitted light when electrons in the crystal are excited. Combinations of the crystals are blended into tiny polystyrene capsules called "microbeads."

Each microbead is uniquely cataloged on the basis of color mix and intensity (i.e., the number of quantum dots), analogous to a bar code. The microbeads are chemically attached to the DNA probes. Fluorescent dye is attached to selected single strands of DNA and these treated strands are mixed with the microbeaded probes. The interreactions using spectroscopic analysis[16] allow researchers to discover which genes are present in an unknown DNA sample.

A quantum dot-based analysis tool developed by Indiana University researchers has the potential to identify some 40,000 genes in ten minutes, compared to 24 hours required by gene chip testing. Detection of proteins is also possible by replacing DNA probes with antibodies.

Scientists expect that within a few years detection of pathogens and disease agents may be achieved using microbeads and microscopic bar codes. The latter could be used to identify and quantify molecules in fluid samples taken as part of standard medical diagnostic tests. These "nanobarcodes" are microscopic rods striped with bold, silver, or other metal. Varying the width, number, and order of the stripes can generate hundreds of thousands of unique identifier rods. These rods could be attached to probes that bind to specific biological molecules, allowing retrieval and computer analysis of thousands of different tagged samples.

Today's biological tests use fluorescent tags, which let researchers analyze only a few types of molecules at a time. The new bar code technology will help scientists detect patterns of behavior and molecular signatures of various diseases in different stages of severity and progression. Preliminary studies are using nanobarcodes to examine molecular patterns in diabetics' blood and Alzheimer's patients' brain fluid.[17]

Protein Chips

Some scientists theorize that most of the million proteins are just variations on a few basic designs, and that there may be as few as 5,000 distinct shapes to catalog definitively. But identification is much simpler than understanding how these shapes are formed and how they behave.[18] Several high tech companies are producing biochips as two-dimensional grids of proteins as a micro-array. When this protein chip is exposed to biochemicals or protein solutions, the molecules adhering to the microarray can be identified and tagged with various markers. The binding ability of molecules is what makes pharmaceuticals effective.

The chips can be used as diagnostic tools, measuring abnormally high or low amounts of blood proteins in a given sample. Biochips could be the key to early detection of serious diseases such as heart disorders and cancer.[19] Manufacture of DNA chips is the result of innovative research done in the early 1990s, but making a protein chip is much more difficult since proteins are extremely sensitive to environmental laboratory conditions, such as temperature and humidity.

Molecular barcodes and laser scanners may be developed within a few years to be a practical code reading system.

Microchip Implants

The idea of medical implants began in the early 1990s with a polymer wafer used to treat brain cancer. This innovation, developed by Dr. Richard Langer at MIT, is an effective alternative to traditional chemotherapy.[20] After surgery has been performed to remove the tumor, the gradually dissolving wafer releases drugs directly to the site. The blood/brain barrier keeps the medications from travel-ing to other parts of the body.

A colleague of Dr. Langer, Dr. John T. Santini, Jr., is developing a variety of devices made of silicon and having circuitry. These chips have tiny etched channels, each containing a minute amount of a drug, usually a protein. The channels, sealed with a fine layer of gold, can be selectively hit with an electric charge that dissolves the gold to release the drug. A companion chip implant acts as a controller to deliver the charge on a programmed schedule or perhaps could be activated remotely on an as-needed basis. Dr. Santini's research group is experimenting with a sensor chip implant that would monitor the bloodstream to determine when drugs should be released.[21]

These targeted, specific drug applications avoid the traditional problems of long-term treatment, for example:

- injected drugs break down too quickly on their journey to the site;
- ingested drugs either can't fully survive the digestive system or react adversely to produce negative side effects;
- there is a risk of overdosing to be sure enough of the drug eventually reaches the intended site;
- scheduled lab visits for treatments are inconvenient and time-consuming for both patients and medical staff; or
- forgetful, indigent, or transient patients are not apt to maintain a regular treatment schedule.

According to Dr. Santini, in as little as five years microchips might replace injections as the preferred delivery method for cancer and hepatitis C drugs. Other chips to treat heart disease and diabetes are in the development stages.[22]

The Dark Side of Biotechnology

Researchers estimate that in just a few years it will be possible to construct synthetic viruses and perhaps even individual cells. Improved vaccines will benefit humanity, but creating deadly viruses as biological weapons is on the agenda of military planners in hostile nations. Many viral genomes have fewer than 10,000 DNA bases, i.e., letters in their genetic code. The largest molecule synthesized is approximately 3,000 bases long. HIV is a viral genome.

RESEARCH RESOURCES

For the health researcher, the amount of data and useful information to be found on the Internet is startling. A good place to start is www.medscape.com sponsored by the U.S. National Library of Medicine. One can subscribe to Medscape's free online publication *MedPulse*. At this writing, subscribers to this interactive resource number over 300,000 including physicians, nurses, naturopaths, medical students and individuals seeking information for self-help. Medscape compiles articles and medical news from a variety of sources such as those listed in Table 5.

Table 5. Medscape Sources for Internet Research

The AIDS Reader
CareNotes
Clinician Reviews
Complications in Surgery
Consumer Health USA
Drug Benefit Trends
Emerging Infectious Diseases
Hippocrates
Infections in Medicine
Infections in Urology
Medical Tribune: Family Practice
Medical Tribune: Internist & Cardiologist
Medical Tribune: Obstetrician & Gynecologist
Morbidity & Mortality Weekly Report
Respiratory Care
Electronic Journals: Mental Health, Women's Health, and *Orthopedics & Sports Medicine.*

This new information technology also brings RA sufferers from all walks of life and from around the world in touch for the first time. Nonmedical people are able to discuss their courses of treatments with physicians, naturopaths, and fellow arthritics and to compare notes about success or failure of various approaches taken by each one's health care provider. Synthesizing this knowledge enables the individual RA sufferer to benefit by exploring new methods of diagnosis and treatment that can be discussed with one's physician. A well-informed patient is also better able to seek out and evaluate skilled medical support.

Public access to medical knowledge on the Internet is akin to the revolution in literacy caused by the invention of the printing press. Ordinary people can gain easy access to the results of research heretofore unavailable to them, hidden away in obscure medical journals and dusty archives, ignored by medical school professors, accessible only through hard work or special permission or status. An individual without affiliation to the medical community as either a practicing physician or medical student can now browse journal articles and scan the medical/scientific collection catalog of a major university from one's home computer. This was never before so easy to do. Nor was it possible to find, correlate, and discuss research findings openly—across different eras and across different disciplines—globally and electronically with ease, speed, accuracy, and convenience and at low cost.

There are, unfortunately, medical information hoaxes placed on the Internet. When conducting research, it is important to seek information only from credible sources such as libraries of major universities, scientific publications by established medical journals, institutes operated by licensed physicians, and government agencies such as the CDC and the NLH. Useful websites for researching health-related information are shown in Appendix IV.

Most sites have identifiable sponsors. Those sites with unknown or hidden sponsors are suspect, especially those with a strong commercial orientation.

THE QUEST FOR A CURE

For years advertisers have conditioned us to take a pill at the first sign of discomfort, so it is no surprise that our society is looking for a single magical cure for diseases like arthritis that acts almost immediately, without altering one's lifestyle. After all, if aspirin can "cure" a headache within a few minutes, why not a similar drug to "cure" arthritis?

Unlike a physical trauma injury where tissue or bone is suddenly destroyed, arthritis is degenerative. We can hardly expect a single drug or herb to effect a complete, rapid cure for a disease that has developed over years and has so many organisms that can cause it. Yet new, marginally effective products continue to vie for market share. RA sufferers form a large and highly motivated customer base for over-the-counter drugs and natural health products. Roughly 2.5 million Americans suffer from RA and about 1.3 million seek treatment each year. Of those, some 600,000 must visit a rheumatologist because they don't respond to current treatments.[23]

The FDA has approved the drug Arava, which works by blunting DHODH, an enzyme that increases the production of cells that cause inflammation. It is intended to slow joint damage and ease pain, but will not cure RA. Enbrel, another new drug, is a genetically engineered medication that works by absorbing the tumor-killing cytokine called "tumor necrosis factor" (TNF) before it can signal immune cells to multiply unnecessarily. Enbrel should be used with great caution, as there is no data available on the long-term safety of this drug. It has caused fatal reactions as a result of aplastic anemia. It is also associated with increased risk of contracting tuberculosis.[24]

A new class of anti-inflammatory agents called COX-2 inhibitors are being designed to limit arthritis pain and inflammation by targeting prostaglandin production. None of these drugs cures the disease, but may slow its progress with fewer known side effects than medications currently prescribed. However, there are concerns about the risk of heart attacks and strokes for users of COX-2 inhibiting drugs.[25] These drugs are expected to generate $6 billion in sales and 200 million prescriptions in the United States annually.[26] The wholesale price for Arava is $3,000 for one year's treatment. Enbrel's estimated cost is $10,000 per year. Celebrex, a new anti-inflammatory that merely relieves arthritis symptoms, costs $400 per year if used daily.[27]

By comparison, a one-year supply of minocycline costs $400. Tetracycline and doxycycline are often substituted for minocycline. The cost is $30 per year. Following the anti-biotic protocol described in Appendix II not only relieves symptoms in many cases but may lead to permanent remission.

In the words of Dr. Harold Clark,[28] "A major financial consequence of a debilitating and costly disease like arthritis in a majority of senior citizens has been the serious erosion of our social security system." Costly treatments and operations sap Medicaid and Medicare funds, and increase private insurance premiums. For the patient ineligible for government assistance, financial impact can be disastrous.

Four Steps Required to Regain Health

The approach to a genuine cure for rheumatic diseases like RA involves four steps: (1) identify, understand, attack, and remove the cause of the infection; (2) neutralize toxins and destructive enzymes; (3) flush toxins from the body; and (4) restore the body's immune system to normal, healthy function.

Attempting to achieve one goal without the others is useless. Our physicians must be part of the first aim—to identify and eliminate the cause of the infection through the sophisticated testing methods at their disposal. Guessing at the cause and prescribing immunosuppressing NSAIDs or DMARDs is not the best or optimal answer.

A 1993 study[29] observed, "If the infection hypothesis proves to be correct, the treatment of RA will need to be completely revised, and the consequences for the pharmaceutical industry will be enormous. It could become unethical to use steroids or agents which block prostaglandin synthesis, as we cannot be sure they do not promote the proliferation of the organism, and so in the long term lead to more severe disease. Instead we will need to devise antibiotic regimens and immunotherapeutic protocols."

When health is undermined by improper living habits, the dysfunctional condition cannot be fixed solely by wonder drugs. The body has the potential to heal itself, but it may take time, insightful treatments, and conscientious effort to retrain all systems to work together more effectively. Rheumatoid arthritis and other degenerative diseases will occur any or all of the following factors are present:

- There is a gradual buildup of microbial parasite(s) populations and toxins in the body without sustained antibacterial prophylaxis;

- The cause(s) of the infection is/are not identified, suppressed or removed;
- The immune system is weakened by months or years of drugs, improper diet, stress, allergies, or chronic infection(s);
- Toxins and harmful enzymes are not eliminated but remain and cluster in the body;
- Cardiovascular systems have deteriorated through poor circulation, plaque, blockages, low Co-Q_{10} levels, and degraded oxygen transport;
- Muscle tone is soft because the body lacks exercise;
- Joint capsules are damaged by extreme exercise or sports injuries;
- Poor dietary habits rob cells of nourishment to grow, maintain, and repair;
- Excess weight puts strain on joints, organs, and the skeletal system; mental stress causes faster pulse, high blood pressure, anxiety, headaches;
- Lungs are weak through habitual shallow breathing or heavy smoking; or
- Environmental stresses from air, water, pollens, dust, mites, mold spores/toxins, MTBE contamination, food contamination, inorganic (chromium, nickel, lead, cadmium) residues, and pesticides affect many bodily systems, especially the immune system.

When joints, especially load-bearing joints, are surrounded by weak muscles, it does not take a significant motion out of the normal range of the joint to cause serious tissue damage to the area. Maintaining normal weight and staying physically fit is a challenging but achievable goal, one worth targeting to be free of the pain and immobility of arthritis. Avoiding the four basic kinds of stress (behavioral, spiritual, biochemical, and environmental) is a significant step forward to attaining a balanced lifestyle.

Adopting a healthy regimen requires some patience, especially if the body has been out of shape for a long time. It could take as much as one full year of proper diet and exercise to achieve effective total body functioning after the infection is removed.

Despite the claims of large U.S. pharmaceutical firms and charity organizations that they are on the trail of a cure for arthritis, particularly RA, the agenda appears to be a search for a *revenue-generating* "cure." Older drugs that have come off patent and are not profitable are not promoted in favor of new drugs that may or may not have equivalent effectiveness. For example, tetracycline is in the common domain, it is cheap to manufacture for human treatments and available in various formulations, but it is not promoted because its profit margin is low.[30] There is more money to be made in producing tetracycline antibiotics for livestock feed.

Foreign Medical Systems

Medical professionals in foreign nations have a longer history of different medical traditions, admitting a variety of approaches and philosophies of life, proven traditional plant medicines, alternative therapies, and theories of how the body works and reacts to chemical substances. Important studies have been conducted abroad, but they seem to receive little, and sometimes mocking, attention here in the United States.

Physicians in Europe, India, and Asia often prescribe herbal remedies and nutritional supplements along with standard pharmaceuticals. However, they do not have, nor do they claim to have, any magical cures for the various and complex forms of arthritis and rheumatic disease. They seem open to consideration of a wider range of treatment options than their U.S. counterparts.

There are exceptions, of course. An example is the story[31] of brilliant French microbiologist Gaston Naessens who in the 1940s developed a microscope with enlargement at 30,000X. This device used ultraviolet and light technology, and was much better than the classical optical microscope (1,800X) but certainly not as powerful as the electron microscope (400,000X).

The 714X compound he developed as a cancer treatment consists of a mixture of camphor, ammonium chloride and nitrate, sodium chloride, ethanol, and water. It must be injected daily into a lymph node in the groin. Three series of 21 daily injections are the minimum treatment. He asserted that 714X was successful in reversing the disease in over 75% of 1,000 cases of cancer and more than 30 cases of AIDS. 714X is designed to reinforce and strengthen a weakened, dysfunctional immune system by making lymph channels more efficient and directing nitrogen to the cancer cells in order to stop their toxic secretions.

His findings were publicly ridiculed and the medical bureaucracy arranged to have him deported. He continued his research in Quebec, Canada. In 1989 he was again arrested and ostracized when another physician misused his 714X formulation, resulting in the death of a patient.

Naessens hypothesized that there are microscopic, dense particles called “somatids” that energize the cells of all living beings. These somatids are living organisms distinct from bacteria and viruses, with their own life cycle observable with his high-powered “Somatoscope.” He asserted that if somatids are exposed to an assault (such as trauma, pollution, or radiation) they begin an uncontrolled growth cycle leading to cancer. 714X injections supposedly return the somatids to a normal state.

Could it be that Naessens' somatids are actually cell-wall-deficient mycoplasmas? His theories concerning the etiopathogenesis of cancer were then, and still are, not consistent with prevailing mainstream medical and scientific opinion. *M. fermentans* invades healthy cells, disrupting their ability to function. The failure of cells to auto-destruct (apoptosis) may be the root cause of cancer. Currently 714X is available in Canada, Mexico, and Western Europe but not in the United States, where it is under investigation by the FDA.[32]

The Somatoscope (UV microscope) is now finally recognized as an indispensable instrument for precise measurement of living and moving microbial life forms in some research laboratories and in industry.[33] These microscopes are available to researchers in some facilities to visualize mycoplasmas and other small microbes in the blood and synovial fluid. It is expected that a size/shape taxonomy could be developed to permit identification of specific microorganisms and immune system components charac-teristic of viral and microbial infections.

The U.S. Medical System

The needless suffering of Lyme Disease patients for the last 15 years is an indication of the failure of medical science to look beyond current limits to develop the new and more precise testing methods for alternate strains of LD-causing organisms.

It is also a failure of our government to protect the public health, yielding to pressure from lobbyists and corporations to foist new symptom-appeasing drugs on individuals desperate to assuage their pain. The collective foot-dragging is a parallel to the politicization of the search to find root causes of chronic disease as described in Dr. Clark's insightful book *Why Arthritis?*.

The problem is not that doctors are insensitive and uncaring. Access to health care has become so ineffectual and frustrating that most patients don't bother seeking help until they are in dire distress. Managed care has become a system of gatekeepers requiring authorization to perform even the most basic health care procedures. Patients pay a $10-$30 co-payment for an office visit but cannot see any doctor at any time. One cannot see a specialist without a referral from the assigned primary care physician. The wait for an appointment may take weeks. There are severe restrictions on particular tests, therapies, and medications allowed by the patient's HMO.

Denial of medical services is not always apparent. One of the more common means of withholding services is "rationing by omission." This means that patients are simply not told all of the possible options for their medical condition. They are only informed of those treatments covered by insurance.[34] The doctor receives only about 30% of the fees charged, with a large percentage of the remainder going to the insurance industry.[35]

To avoid being a victim of this sort of rationing, the patient must research his/her medical condition as deeply as possible and come prepared to discuss alternatives. When the patient or the doctor requests a particular service, and the health plan denies the request, the reason is usually that the requested service is not "medically necessary"— a subjective term based on the cost of the procedure. In some instances, doctors hamstrung by contractual commitments to perform only HMO-specified procedures will quietly send their patients to physicians who offer the required treatment but the cost of the procedure must be borne by the patient.

Admittedly, the multi-dimensional nature of etiopathogenic testing makes it difficult and expensive. However, the cost of incomplete testing is reflected in an increasing number of chronic illness patients putting a strain on government health care funds. Managed care was sold as a means to control the rising cost of health care, but it has evolved into a big business with a growing bureaucracy of its own to support.

The medical system as we know it today does not work. Existing diagnostic tests are unreliable, and unnecessary surgeries are often performed based on those tests. Patients are forced to fend for themselves, researching their own conditions using the Internet or, in some cases, self-medicating or seeking treatment or lower cost drugs outside the United States.

Those patients who are aggressive about presenting documented evidence to their doctors have a much better chance of obtaining therapy that will not only relieve their symptoms but also achieve long-term success. The primary goal of the grassroots organizations listed in Appendix IV is to educate patients in ways to approach their physicians with substantial evidence of proven treatments.

"Maverick" Doctors

Dr. Brown was not the first physician whose findings upset the medical community's status quo. As seen in the stories of Drs Matzinger, Blount, and Naessens, acceptance of new theories is glacially slow. Scientific skepticism is laudable, but when hundreds of documented experiments and studies are ignored and their authors branded as "mavericks" it calls into question the medical community's true motives.

Another example illustrates the point. Dr. Laszlo K. Csatary of the United Cancer Research Institute has been publishing clinical observations on viral oncotherapy in major medical journals for three decades. Dr. Csatary first used a viral vaccine to treat cancer patients with apathogenic (i.e., "friendly") viruses in 1968. However, this technique has only recently gained attention as a new and innovative approach.[36]

Why does it take so long for the medical establishment to recognize techniques that are proven to work? Medical journals contain countless articles on the failure of current drug therapies for RA as well as studies advancing the theory of infectious organisms as the cause. Those doctors who ignore these studies usually are convinced when they (or a member of their own family) become ill and they find that conventional therapies fail to help. U.S. doctors and dentists who seek alternative treatments that they would not prescribe for their own patients routinely visit Mexico's clinics.[37]

Rheumatologists are especially critical of Dr. Brown's work and seem to be the first to denounce any alternative to standard treatment.[38] They appear reluctant to consider any therapy that does not conform to the prevailing medical community's mindset.

WHY DR. BROWN'S REGIMEN IS IGNORED

Physicians may be reluctant to use the long-term, low-dose antibiotic regimen as advocated by Dr. Brown for any of several psychological or economic reasons, believing that:

- the Jarisch-Herxheimer reaction is mistaken for an allergy to the antibiotic and the drug use is stopped and not restarted with anti-inflammatory complement drugs;

- appropriate non-pill forms of the antibiotic are not easy to administer and pill forms are likely to result in the evolution of drug resistant microbes in the gut;
- physicians are not familiar with the appropriate administration protocols for long term treatment;
- most of their patients are not disciplined enough to stay the course of a sustained treatment lasting months;
- tetracycline-type antibiotics are not promoted by the drug companies compared to high profit NSAIDs and DMARDs;
- specific diagnostic tests for mycoplasma infection are not on approved test lists for HMOs and Insurance coverage. They are costly, and administrators have no way for patients to pay for or share the cost. Patients may be unwilling to pay for them;
- Managed care works adversely against doctors that prescribe long-term treatment. Cost controllers try to find reasons to deny any treatment that does not bring instant results;
- Only about 30% of the patients respond to treatment positively, and relapse if treatment is less than 6 months;
- tests give inconclusive results and many physicians have not had the training to interpret the test results correctly and authoritatively; or
- they cannot provide the nutritional advice required to restore the patient's immune system to proper balance in addition to the antibiotic therapy.

RESEARCH TOOLS ARE INCOMPLETE

The search for the root causes of chronic diseases and microbial infections should be among the top issues of our government's national policy. If our war against pathogenic microbes is to be given a priority on a par with national defense, we need to enlist the resources of the National Academy of Science and the NIH to develop research tools, machines, and capabilities such as:

- Complete online library of genetic codes, recipes, and shapes linked to sub-libraries of:
    - microorganism genetics and taxonomy
    - pathogenic microbe database (see Appendix 4 entry www.vm.cfsan.fda.gov/~mow/Intro.html. the FDA's "Bad Bug Book" of pathogens, diseases, tests, symptoms, etc.)
    - organic genetic specialty associations
    - DNA-PCR markers and gene associations
    - molecules' functions and shapes
- DNA sequencing tools enhancements
- Modeling and display tools based on molecular shapes
- Classification tools for microbiological taxonomy
- Classification tools for molecular recipe taxonomy
- Marker-barcode/dot chemical replication
- Antigen/molecule test marker design
- Biochip fabrication machines
- Biochip reader machines
- Molecule-shape library and recipes for molecule fabrication (either organic synthesis or via DNA-RNA templates to make useful molecules and enzymes via template-building and replication or by fermentation using gene-tailored microbes)[39]

Organizing such an enormous body of data is a huge effort requiring both a logical data framework and a professional staff with both medical training and database management skills. These essential data must not only be accurately cataloged but also organized according to retrieval and presentation standards that facilitate use.

Security of the data may become an issue based on the rights of the owner, and on the possibility of misuse. Access control will require knowing the identity, affiliation and location of each person granted access, and time and extent of access to each sensitive item in a library of sensitive data. This access record keeping is quite feasible to implement.[40]

A Suggested Testing Approach

One of the disturbing aspects of chronic illness is that it can be the result of combined infections. It is beyond the scope of this book to document and describe all chronic illnesses and so-called autoimmune disorders. However, there appear to be categories of chronic diseases clearly attributable to identified sources such as mycoplasma, insect-borne spirochetes, mycotoxins, molds, and bacteria.

The major obstacle to targeted treatment is a system of accurate testing and diagnosis. The Pareto chart in Figure 7 shows the scope of the pathogen classification problem in a hypothetical way. The chart shows a large quantity of possible causative factors for rheumatic diseases, but many of these have very low actual occurrence rates. There is also an incubation period (weeks to months or even years) from initial infection until the arthritic symptoms appear, as reported by persons who have Lyme Disease.

The numbers given in the chart are not derived from actual measurements. The chart shows what might be seen if such data could be collected in a complete manner. The values would vary by region and with time.

Figure 7. Hypothetical Pareto Chart of RA Causative Agents

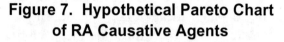

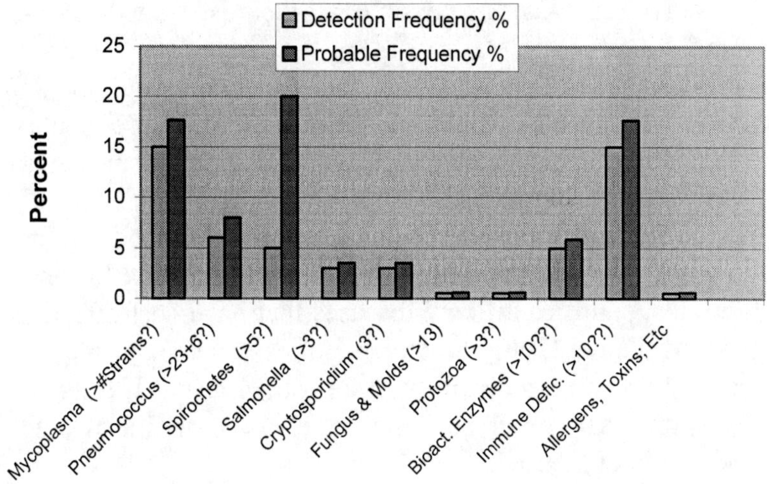

Possible Agents: Suppressor/Toxin/Enzyme/Genetic Factor

The percentage values for each pathogen-factor charted show two bars. The first (light-shaded bar) is the hypothetical measured percentage of positive test results for the factor (i.e., the detection frequency). The second (dark bar) is based on the first bar value, divided by the test effectiveness. Effectiveness depends upon the number of false negatives. No false negatives means effectiveness is 1. False positives are not considered in this simplified model.

For many of these factors' currently used test methods, a high level of false negatives exists due to unidentified factors in the category that are not tested for, so effectiveness of the test may actually be near zero.

Measured percentages also are quite possibly near zero for significant factors so the second bar reflects errors resulting from (~0)÷(~0) values. Improvements in measures of test effectiveness are needed so that such a chart will depict meaningful relationships. These improvements can only be realized by identifying as many causative organisms as possible, all their associated strains, and testing for all of them.

An added benefit of this data collection would be that blood test results would be predictive of future donors' medical problems, since the growth of the organisms is very slow, and the harm they do is slowly cumulative.

Until microchip screening tests are developed that are low cost, we will continue to be limited to testing for only the most significant likely diseases that have cost-effective tests available. HMOs, doctors, and insurance plans require some reasonable probability of a positive result. If tests are expensive and often have negative or borderline results, they will not be used.

---

[1] Eastman, Peggy. "Breaking Free of Arthritis Pain." *AARP Magazine*, November 1998.

[2] Op. cit., Eastman (1998)

[3] Brown and Scammell (1988) pg. 129.

[4] Lemonick, Michael; Cray, Dan; Park, Alice; Song, Sora, and Thompson, Dick. "The Genome is Mapped. Now What?" *TIME*, July 3, 2000.

[5] Goldfarb, Bruce. "The Human Genome: Reading the Body's Blueprint." *Arthritis Today*, March/April 2001. Also see www.genomicsnews.com.

[6] Ross, Philip E. "Ancient Sleepers." *Scientific American*, April 1993.

---

[7] The way biofilms develop, thrive, and spread are described in detail at www.edstrom.com/Lab/WaterQualityBulletins/biofilm and also at the homepage of the National Science Foundation's Center for Biofilm Engineering, Montana State University, at www.erc.montana.edu.

[8] See www.erc.montana.edu.

[9] Shapiro, James A. "Bacteria as Multicellular Organisms." *Scientific American*, June 1988.

[10] Presentation given by University of Wisconsin plant pathology professor Jo Handelsman at the annual New Horizons in Science conference in Tempe, AZ, November 2001.

[11] Raeburn, Paul. "Down in the Dirt Wonders Beckon." *BusinessWeek*, December 3, 2001.

[12] Not associated with Affymetrix, Inc. or its GeneChip® arrays.

[13] Stipp, David. "The Real Biotech Revolution" and "Gene Testing Starts to Pay Off." *Fortune*, March 31, 1997. See http://plato.tzl.de/agmt-e/ and www.chembio.t.u-tokyo.ac.jp.labs/nagamune/.

[14] Unattributed feature. "Nothing to Sneeze At." *Technology Review*. November 2001, p. 21.

[15] Morrison, Christopher. "Biotechnology Makes Quantum Dot Leap." *IEEE Spectrum*, September 2001.

[16] Weiss, Giselle. "Switzerland Builds Potent Spectroscopic Tool." *IEEE Spectrum*, September 2001.

[17] Stikeman, Alexandra. "Bar-Coding Life: Tiny tags to decode disease." *Technology Review*, January/February 2002, p. 22. SurroMed, a CA-based company, is working with the Institute for Nanotechnology at Northwestern University to perform experimental studies.

[18] Kher, Unmesh. "The Next Frontier: Proteomics." *TIME*, July 3, 2000.

[19] Voss, David. "Protein Chips." *Technology Review*, May 2001.

[20] Wood, Christina. "Implications: Medicine on a Microchip." *PC Magazine*, August 2001.

[21] This research is being done at MicroChips in Cambridge, MA. Dr. Santini is the president of MicroChips.

[22] Work is being done at iMEDD in Columbus, Ohio.

---

[23] *Investor's Business Daily*, May 20, 1997 reporting on Immunex Corporation's new drug Enbrel to relieve stiff and swollen joints.

[24] Personal communication with Dr. Joseph Mercola, November 2001.

[25] See http://jama.ama-assn.org or www.fda.gov.

[26] Tanner, Lindsey (Associated Press). "Report: Arthritis Drugs May Raise Heart Risk." In the *South Bay Daily Breeze*, August 22, 2001, p. A7.

[27] Thompson, Dick. "Arthritis Under Arrest." *TIME*, September 28, 1998. The Enbrel Support Group's website detailing patients' experiences is http://repro-med.net/guides/enbrelside.html.

[28] Clark (1997) p. 9.

[29] Rook G.A.W.; Lydyard, P.M. and Stanford J.L. (England). "A Reappraisal of the Evidence That Rheumatoid Arthritis and Several Idiopathic Diseases are Slow Bacterial Infections." *Ann. Rheum. Dis.* 1993; 52:S30-S38.

[30] At this writing, tetracycline costs about $12 per *pound*. Prescription NSAIDs cost about $1-$2 per *tablet*.

[31] Bird (1991).

[32] British Columbia Cancer Agency, Canada. "Unconventional Cancer Therapies: 714X (Gaston Naessens)." February 2000. Via the Internet.

[33] See www.cose.com and www.interlog.com.

[34] See www.YourDoctorintheFamily.com for advice on topics such as Choosing a Health Plan, Becoming a More Effective Patient, Managing Your Health Plan, Surviving Your Health Plan, and Appealing a Health Plan's Decision.

[35] Gray, Dr. Sonja. "The Managed Care Insurance Game." Internet article at www.nightingalecounseling.com.

[36] Elmer-DeWitt, Philip. "Smart Bombs for Targeting Deadly Tumors [The Future of Drugs]." *TIME*, January 15, 2001 and follow-up letter to the editor by Dr. Christine M. Csatary, May 14, 2001.

[37] Personal communication with a family friend and resident of southern Texas. She met these medical professionals (fellow patients) while obtaining her own treatments in Mexico. She interviewed them informally in the clinic's waiting room in 1999-2000.

[38] Dr. Robert A. Greenwald of the American Council on Science and Health roundly criticizes *The Road Back* on the Internet and puts Dr. Brown's regimen in the category of 'Worst of the Worst." Dr. Greenwald's website, www.drkoop.com/news/focus/june/arthritis.html has recently gone bankrupt. Rheumatologist Greenwald claims that the only effect of minocycline is to reduce the action of collagenase, and that for arthritis reduction, it has no more effect than a mild NSAID or even a placebo. The Novak and Hockhberg study Dr. Greenwald cites was done incorrectly, through no fault of Dr. Brown or his colleagues. After Dr. Brown's death, Novak offered to redo the study and publish the results. However, there was no money available to fund the work. The flawed study continues to be cited.

[39] See www.epic4health.com/whatiscoq10.html.

[40] The author has considerable experience in the design and management of large, secure databases and can attest to the feasibility of access control.

9. CONCLUSIONS

Billions of years before humans appeared on the scene, bacteria were frolicking in the primordial soup. Today, our bodies are now their "soup." We are the vehicles by which pathogenic microbes transport themselves from one place to another, to survive and reproduce. We are their world. When our bodies are invaded and colonized by these bacteria either the immune system fights them successfully, or an uneasy truce is established with the colony. Microbe-borne genetic immunosuppressive recipes generate molecules that modify various functions of the immune system. The sum of all the colonies' immunosuppressive actions degrades the immune system cumulatively.

Although knowledge of mycoplasmas has been documented since 1898, Dr. Thomas McPherson Brown and his associates worked persistently for over 40 years to understand the activity of mycoplasmas and bacterial L-forms whose sizes and genetic complexity range in-between the viruses and the cell-wall-bounded prokaryotes. An accumu-lating body of associated evidence links these microbes as factors in chronic diseases such as rheumatoid arthritis, Scleroderma and lupus. Dr. Brown observed a new lost-continent of microorganisms and encouraged others, like Dr. Harold Clark and Dr. Garth Nicolson, to join him in identifying its microscopic creatures, their biochemical offspring-molecules and their interactions with the host.

While some progress has been made to study the very complex action of these opportunistic microbial parasites, there is a great deal more research to be done. We need to fully understand the life cycle and biochemical activities of pathogenic microorganisms that have for too long been overlooked and underestimated. Microbial colonies causing arthritis-like symptoms may be responsible for all illnesses previously categorized as "autoimmune diseases."

Using new tools, numerous recent studies continue to show that mycoplasmas or other organisms can be either sole causes or cofactors of a growing number of acute and chronic diseases. Infections caused by as-yet unknown strains of insect-borne spirochetes add to the complexity of diagnosing chronic illness. Microscopic insect microbes (mites, chiggers, no-see-ums, etc) may be associated with microbial colonization similar to Lyme-disease arthritis. This area of research remains mostly a biological terra incognita and a formidable scientific challenge.

NEW PARADIGMS FOR A NEW MILLENNIUM

Chronic illness takes far more than a physical toll. It translates to billions of dollars in health care costs and lost productivity. The problems of chronic disease will not go away without deliberate action from all sectors of society.

Understanding of the *full* life cycle of every pathogenic microbe can lead to the targeting of points of vulnerability where its proliferation can be blocked. Adequate and sustained funding for basic research in this area needs to be targeted at filling in the gaps in our knowledge. This is a global information access insufficiency to detailed, catalogued scientific data that will require a sustained, multinational, cooperative effort to remedy.

Government Action

In addition to the AIDS epidemic, outbreaks of well-known diseases like tuberculosis and malaria are returning in potentially epidemic proportions. Insufficient resources have been spent in ineffective ways to control these diseases.

The events of September 11th have shifted national priorities. Top issues are now bioterrorism attacks, civilian defense, hostile nations' ongoing development of biological weapons, and disease control. Our government agencies must greatly improve their effectiveness in the interest of public health and safety as a part of national defense.

In December 2001, Congress approved an FY2002 appropriations bill (HR 3061) that increases total funding for all institutes under the NIH almost 16 percent to $26.6 Billion. However, two-thirds of the increase will be earmarked for construction to protect NIH facilities against terrorist attacks[1]—a priority of bricks and mortar over knowledge improvement. While these dollar amounts may appear large, compare NIH's net $20 Billion FY2002 budget for research with the $226.5 billion allocated to Medicare or $451.6 Billion for Social Security.[2]

Directed Funding for Chronic Illness Research

Our public health organizations (NIH, CDC, FDA, and others) are increasingly coming to terms with the hazards that pernicious pathogens represent on a global scale. They should request and receive adequate funding[3] for:

- Etiopathogenic research of organisms such as fungi and molds, mycoplasma, protozoa, worms, and spirochetes;
- Improvements in UV and multispectral microscopy;
- Development of comprehensive DNA/antibody/antigen/ antitoxin tests; and
- Development and distribution of multivalent vaccines, antitoxins, anti-enzymes, and antigens.

If these efforts are not pursued, the cost of existing chronic infections will still be paid in the form of increased costs for the health maintenance of United States Medicare participants, in decreased productivity of the workforce, and in human suffering by the millions throughout the world.

Attention to particular non-HIV organisms should be granted international project status—far more encompassing than the Human Genome Project—for a multi-disciplinary effort to find ways to render those organisms ineffective as a bioterrorism threat or as a cause of widespread medical problems approaching epidemic status.

The government should also consider humane methods to quarantine and/or treat those contagious persons who pose a public health danger to society.

With an estimated 40 million sufferers, arthritis in all its varieties is this nation's number one crippling disease.[4] It is also one of the most costly major socioeconomic problems in the United States, but arthritis takes a back seat to funding for AIDS with fewer than one million people infected.[5]

Under the 1975 National Arthritis Act, Congress approved an initial $13 Million grant, grown to over $200 Million in 1992. However, *no* funding was awarded specifically for mycoplasmal infection research.[6] As a part of the Act's strategic plan, the Arthritis Institute was founded in 1985 at the NIH. A dozen years later, the claim of the Institute was that "the causes and cures of rheumatoid disorders remain unknown."[7]

Congress should take a hard look at the outlay of tax dollars for fruitless research, and insist that NIH funds be allocated to finding the probable suspect organisms being discovered and documented in scientific publications. The 2001 NIH/ NIAMS research budget was $263 Million,[8] equivalent to $6.58 per person of the estimated 40 million stricken with arthritis, if all research dollars were actually directed to studying that particular disease.

An estimated 3 percent of the adult U.S. population[9]—approximately 8 million individuals—suffer from chronic fatigue illnesses, yet there are few federal dollars being allocated to research for the diagnosis and treatment of these chronic illnesses, even though each year Congress allocates such funds.[10, 11]

NIH National Library of Medicine

The National Institutes of Health's National Library of Medicine (NIH-NLM) has made an excellent start in providing services such as MedLine/MedScape/MedPulse (www.medline.com) for both practitioners (doctors, nurses, researchers, and medical students) and also for the public via the Internet.

The Internet is a marvelous entity operating on a global scale. It represents an electronic associative memory that permits interested and knowledgeable individuals to communicate in near real time. We need a federally funded comprehensive medical library system to provide an analogous resource—a time-spanning, information-based associative memory that will prevent the loss of knowledge from past generations of medical scientists to their successors.[12]

Many tools need to be developed to facilitate this large-scale information collection/retrieval effort. The goal is rapid and complete online access to scientific medical data for qualified persons. Some of these data must be protected in the interests of national security.

The Near Technological Horizon

Biotechnology is now producing DNA-based tools for more precise identification of pathogenic microorganisms by type and strain. In conditions like Lyme Disease where identification does not correspond with ordinarily effective treatment, more research is needed to match organisms' strains with targeted treatments or to find the right antibiotic/vaccine/antitoxin combination.

New biotechnologies will enable a better understanding of how the body's complex interrelated systems deal with resident microbes (both harmful and beneficial) as well as invading organisms. The result will be effective ways to prevent disease rather than merely deal with symptoms.

The next goal will be a giant step toward reducing the permanent damage and debilitating effects of powerful chemotherapeutic drugs. Vaccines against each of the pathogenic slow-growing parasitic organisms found in epidemic proportions in humans and livestock will help achieve this goal.

To the extent that mycoplasmas, malaria-like microbes, and viruses invade the body's cells, ways to identify the invaded cells and kill all of them must be found. This calls for more research on the mechanisms of apoptosis; for example, how radiation and toxic medicines potentiate apoptosis, and why apoptosis genes fail to make an invaded cell destroy itself.

Microscopy Improvements

Improvements in microscopy including ultraviolet (UV) microscopes with multi-spectral sensors connected to color TV displays can provide an extension of our viewing capability, from the size range of viruses through the range of the mycoplasmas, a size range where we have lacked widely available multi-spectral visibility.

Researchers must thoughtfully explore and catalog the shapes of objects found in blood samples in this newly visible size range. Additional efforts need to be provided to collect associated patient data—symptoms, test results (ELISA, Ig, antibody, antigen, etc.), DNA markers, and so forth—and to correlate any newly found remarkable shapes with these recorded patient blood attributes.

Abnormal molecular forms and organism shapes can now be cataloged in electronic databases and related to specific nutrients, expressed enzymes, syndromes, diseases, and organisms. Interpreting the interrelationships will be one of the primary challenges, and one of the most productive effects, of 21st century medical research. The NIH-NLM should take a very proactive and aggressive approach to establishing these databases and overseeing data collection, correlation and dissemination. DARPA can administer hardware research and development while the National Academy of Science and the American Association for the Advancement of Science can assist in an advisory capacity.

Effective Food Sanitation and Sterilization

It is time for our government to stop indulging the meat and dairy industries at the expense of public health. More effective enforcement of existing regulations is needed. Faster, better, and cheaper tests for contamination need to be developed, applied, and the noncompliant processing plants and procedures either cleaned up or shut down.

Meat irradiation and milk pasteurization are effective in preserving sealed, uncontaminated food, but the bacterial toxins produced by unsanitary food handling prior to sterilization create a health issue.[13] The current high levels of food poisoning could be significantly reduced by meat irradiation in the packaging process. Bagging, dating, and chilling are not effective enough measures to insure that meat free of the salmonella toxin and live microbial parasites will always reach the consumer's table. Bacteria growth during packing is very short. Toxin generation is greater on food displayed or stored for a long time since bacteria have a chance to grow after packing.

Medical Community Participation

The presence of *Mycoplasma* (and other co-infecting microbes) in Rheumatoid Arthritis, Lupus, Scleroderma, and other chronic diseases are currently not fully or effectively testable, recognized, nor are they correctly treated. Tests for *Mycoplasma*, Lyme parasites, and other pathogens are not routinely done as part of a physician's typical diagnosis procedure. Some tests give undependable, marginal, or false-negative results. The more specific tests may not be authorized by the patient's insurance-managed HMO because statistics show the chance of a positive result is low versus the cost of the test. The physician may only trust those tests s/he is familiar with interpreting.

Since testing today is often missing or inconclusive, the proper antibiotic combination to kill the specific strain of microbe is not considered. Therefore, critical treatment steps are missing to obtain a rapid, conclusive diagnosis and an effective, targeted treatment. It is up to the government and industry to fund research programs to fill in these gaps.

The conventional RA treatment with powerful steroids, antibiotics, antihistamines, interferon- and TNF-disablers, T-cell killers, and immunosuppressive drugs upset the immune system, sometimes facilitating the gradual proliferation of the invading colonies. It is countered by use of poisons (such as gold salts, methotrexate, and arsenic-based drugs used if patient is allergic to penicillin) or DMARDs to suppress the microparasites.

The use of antibiotics upsets the symbiotic microbial ecology of, and in, the body, resulting in an immune system imbalance that is not yet well understood. NSAID drugs also work to suppress pain and inflammation at the expense of disabling the body's natural defenses against infection.

Effective anti-mycoplasmal antibiotics intensify an inflammation reaction. Therefore a combination of an anti-microbe antibiotic and an effective anti-inflammatory should be used together.[14]

Tetracycline family (minocycline), quinine-based, and fluoroquinolone antibiotics such as Ciprofloxacin have strong effectiveness against the various strains of mycoplasma and bacterial L-forms.[15] Longer term, lower dosage use of certain tetracyclines, sometimes with short periods of on/off administration, often starts to become effective after 4-6 months. Treatments spanning eighteen months or more are frequently needed to avoid relapses.

Administration of pills passing through the gut provides opportunities for intestinal flora to develop antibiotic resistance. Serum infusions (approximately $2,000 per series) or injected forms can avoid this but are not as convenient to administer, especially over a long period of months.[16] Appropriate antibiotic delivery methods need to be developed, made affordable, used at the right stage of the disease, and administered for a period of time necessary to be effective.

As long as some influential scientists still think of mycoplasmas as having only bacterial or viral properties and force-fit outdated criteria on the research, diagnostic testing and treatment relating to these elusive microorganisms, no progress will be made. More realistic standards than Koch's postulates must be developed to account for infections caused by today's drug-resistant, evolving microbes that are slow-growing and difficult to culture *in vitro*. In the words of Dr. Clark, "Looking for causative agent(s) in test tubes in a lab may be the most scientifically controlled research but is the least significant and relevant to the complex human host."[17]

New, effective methods of identifying the infectious agents must be used in place of the ineffective isolation, culture, viewing, and identification methods applicable to the bacteria having cell walls. Much more timely tests must be developed, and tests must be sensitive to all strains that can be possibly considered in the diagnosis. Tests now becoming available are based on detecting pathogenic enzymes, toxins/antitoxins, antigens, DNA-PCR markers, and other molecules uniquely manufactured by the pathogenic organ-isms being identified.

Diagnosis of Multiple Infections

The traditional search for a single cause of GWI and other chronic diseases is indicative of a flawed mindset—oversimplification based on Occam's razor. Just as new testing methods and diagnostic tools have demonstrated that individuals can be afflicted with *both* osteoarthritis and rheumatoid arthritis, it is only logical to believe that in a lifetime a person will become colonized with a multitude of microorganisms. The entrenched practice of seeking a single common pathological process to explain a given disease is outmoded and ripe for revision. Substantial research has now shown that co-infections are present in patients with chronic illness.

A new approach to the understanding of chronic rheumatic diseases like arthritis and Lyme Disease must be developed. To do so will involve knowledge from medical disciplines such as virology, microbiology, lymphology, bacteriology, immunology, epidemiology, and parasitology. These are currently considered separate fields with their own goals and methodologies. Perhaps the new field of microbial ecology will unite rather than divide scientists, emphasizing links rather than differences.

One goal of research is to understand and to map the genetic complexity of these microorganisms and then to relate this genetic map to harmful/beneficial effects on the host. The traditional two-dimensional matrix that maps antibiotic drug to microorganism has become 5-dimensional as we add strains, the various pathogens' toxin/enzymes and the effects of the drugs on bioactive molecules/cells' physiology/organs/systems of the body. These data need to be online for all to reference. Some data are beginning to appear on the Internet at NIH/NLM, but persistent searching must be done.

Obstacles to Antibiotic Treatment

Anti-mycoplasma antibiotic treatment has long been labeled as "not adequately tested in humans" by the "authorities" controlling research, who themselves have worked to deny funding for such testing or have established test criteria based on short-term tests when long-term tests are indicated. Thus, mycoplasma research has been steadfastly ignored by certain segments of the medical research community. Dr. Clark calls this "one of the greatest failures in medical history."[18]

Arthritis sufferers are faced with the problem of finding physicians who will not only agree to test for mycoplasmal infection but also monitor their progress through a course of antibiotic treatment over a long period of time. A starting point is the Arthritis Center of Riverside, Dr. Mercola's website, and Dr. Nicolson's Institute for Molecular Medicine and the resources they offer to bring doctor and patient together.[19] The Internet has enabled sharing of data and experiences among victims of chronic disease. Discussion groups offer increased odds of finding a physician who will be receptive to the idea of trying Dr. Brown's protocol.[20]

Advantages of a Holistic Approach

Bolstering the patient's immune system while working to suppress a relentless infection requires a holistic view of the individual.

We are each unique in terms of nutritional needs, physiological factors, emotional outlook, environmental factors, stressors, genetic inheritance, and allergies. It is encouraging to note that a growing number of physicians are using "integrative medicine" (also called "functional medicine" or "complementary medicine") to better treat their RA patients. This holistic approach combines the best of conventional diagnosis and clinically proven treatments with documented, effective alternative therapies.

Once the pathogenic microorganisms have been correctly identified, their destructive features suppressed or the organisms eliminated, naturopathic methods can be very effective in revitalizing the body's collective system of systems—especially the immune system—to ward off future infections and to reduce the pain and spread of chronic disease.

Health Care Industry's Role

Large private or non-profit organizations such as the Arthritis Foundation are part of the Health Care Industry. They use collected funds to cover the costs of managing a sizable bureaucracy, promoting the Foundation operating classes teaching arthritis sufferers how to cope with symptoms, publishing an informative magazine, and lobbying for research. The Arthritis Foundation accepts funds not only from charitable contributions but also from major pharmaceutical companies who advertise in their monthly magazine.

The Arthritis Foundation's aggressive appeals for federally funded research have paid off, but not to the extent where it might make a significant difference. E.g., the Foundation was able to lobby for increased funding for the FY2001 National Arthritis Action Plan to $13.3 Million, but in the annual duel for scarce federal funds, the CDC lost $27 Million for its Chronic Disease program. The Foundation is seeking to obtain $460 Million for the FY2002 National Institute of Arthritis and Musculoskeletal and Skin Diseases (NIAMS) research budget.

Such advocacy efforts are laudable, but they seek narrow applications. For each specific rheumatic illness there is at least one private foundation appealing for donations to find a cure, but because their research funding is uncoor-dinated and sometimes misdirected, their efforts have little payoff. Meanwhile, the pharmaceutical industry continues to develop "improved, new" drugs to relieve symptoms but with associated serious side effects.

The question arises: "Will there ever be a cure for arthritis?" High profits are needed to support developmental research leading towards a cure, but if a cure were found, the drug companies would suffer a huge loss of business. The answer is clear: as long as arthritis is a billion-dollar per year industry—why work to find a cure and kill the golden goose?

Because of the latent harmful nature of some of these drugs the FDA must carefully review their safety and effectiveness. Continuation of high drug company profits is needed to pay the high cost of the cumbersome FDA drug approval process imposed by government bureaucracy.

Fixing a Broken Health Care System

The U.S. health care system is broken. Six major areas need to be fixed:

1. timely access to effective medical care;
2. treatment authorization process;
3. overcharging for drugs;
4. targeted tests for infectious agents not widely available;
5. cautious, selective use of antibiotics; and
6. development and availability of vaccines.

1. Access to care. Insurance companies and HMOs have come to terms with the financial realities of chronic illness. They are finding new ways to deny coverage for the high cost chronically ill patient. By refusing to authorize crucial diagnostic tests in the short term they only delay later claims for disabilities brought about by chronic disease.

2. Treatment authorization. Insisting that doctors prescribe only from a mandated list of treatments limits the physician's ability to treat the patient's condition properly and in a timely manner. It makes it difficult if not impossible for new treatments to be authorized and applied. Doctors should not be censured for prescribing more effective long-term (and perhaps higher cost) drug treatments.

3. Drug costs. The double cost of a physician visit and a high profit drug could both be eliminated in many cases by making more drugs subject to pharmacist-controlled dispensing without a prescription. Low-cost drugs for arthritis such as quinine sulfate, doxycycline, and aureomycin are candidates for this category. In many other countries, the professional pharmacist has a much greater role in drug selection and customer assistance without a physician intermediary. The very low cost of anti-allergy drugs in these foreign counties makes one suspect that the American drug companies are grossly overcharging on a massive scale.[21]

Federal efforts to make more OTC medications available would shift costs from insurance to the patients.

4. Lack of effective tests. A wider variety of comprehensive tests for infectious agents must be made available to doctors so that diseases can be detected and suppressed in the early stages. However, those tests have not yet been fully developed. Until databases matching organism strains to symptoms and to targeted treatments (drugs, antitoxins, vaccines, etc) become routinely available to the physician, access to crucial diagnostic indicators will not be possible. Doctors will continue to depend on a minimal set of tests and guesswork.

5. Cautious use of antibiotics. Dr. Brown's low-dose, long-term antibiotic regimen trains the RA patient's immune system to fight resident pathogens gradually, over several months, or in some cases, years. It does not introduce the harmful side effects usually associated with indiscriminately prescribed broad-spectrum antibiotics that suddenly suppress the immune system and leave the patient open to new assaults. The protocol is described in Appendix II.

6. Availability of vaccines. Many more vaccines that are now proven to be effective on animal subjects need to be developed for human use. Prevention of chronic illnesses caused by microbial parasites should be a priority. Without vaccines, pathogenic organisms have ample opportunity to establish colonies before symptoms become evident. By that time, these pathogens are difficult to eradicate.

Patient's Responsibility

The more we understand about our body's cellular makeup, its functions, and its nutritional needs, the better we know how to keep our body's systems in balance. This understanding is an essential first step. The next step is to seek out a health care provider who can do more than prescribe pills to relieve symptoms. The doctor-patient relationship is a team effort to identify the cause(s) of the infection(s) and remove it/them. Diligence and commitment are necessary for a long-term course of treatment.

In parallel, the patient must make lifestyle adjustments to strengthen the immune system. These adjustments include improving one's eating habits, avoiding allergens, quitting harmful addictions to cigarettes, alcohol, antidepressants, etc., and adding vitamins and supplements to counter deficiencies. Specific tests may be required to identify allergens. A nutritionist can help develop a personalized dietary profile. Counseling may be required to help conquer addictions, reduce stress, and deal with negative emotions.

Each chronically ill patient must take an active role in regaining his/her own health. This means learning more about one's condition and the resources available to find the root cause. Using the Google search engine on the Internet with appropriate key words is one way. Appendix IV lists some of the best references now available. Regional medical libraries are federally funded and are available for public use in most major cities. The payoff is a decrease in RA symptoms and possibly full remission.

The Road to Remission

There have been many books written about arthritis. Typically these books either describe coping techniques or they advocate a particular substance that will act as a magic bullet to relieve and stop pain. This substance could be yucca root or olive leaf extract or some unique combination of herbs. The truth is, there is no magic bullet because each of us has a unique biochemical makeup.

We also eat a typical American diet high in fats, sugar, and salts and deficient in fiber and essential nutrients. So many influential factors contribute to our physiology—diet, metabolism, allergens, environmental conditions, immune system genetics, level of exercise, the way we handle stress, past exposure to chemicals (especially insecticides), and interactions with other medications—that the idea of a single cure is preposterous.

Various strains of infectious organisms have different sensitivities to the substances that may be able to suppress their activities. They can also send a "stop doing that" signal to the host via allergic flare-ups such as the Jarisch-Herxheimer reaction when they are adversely threatened by an effective treatment.

The anti-mycoplasma antibiotic protocol, if diligently followed and coupled with good nutrition, will train the body to combat the microbial infection that is the root cause of many chronic diseases. For those who do not respond to long-term antibiotic treatment, other options may be available based on results of specific tests for co-infections and/or allergies as described in Chapter 5.

The Road Back Foundation estimates that over 40 million people currently suffer from some form of rheumatic disease. For many of these individuals, the 30-40 percent probability of remission or significant reduction in symptoms using antibiotic protocols is significant.

This means that approximately 15 million individuals in the United States are eligible for new hope and restored health.

---

[1] Source: American Association for the Advancement of Science analyses of R&D in AAAS Reports VIII-XXCI.

[2] Source: www.whitehouse.gov/omb/budget/fy2002.

[3] See www.niaid.nih.gov/ncn/ for details on the "New Bioterrorism-Related Funding Opportunities." *NIAID Council News*.

[4] See www.med.umich.edu/opm/newspage/art.htm.

[5] See www.niaid.nih.gov/factsheets/aidsstat.htm.

[6] See American College of Rheumatology's Action Plan Agenda and Recommendations site: www.rheumatology.org/gov/alert.html.

[7] For a disheartening history of misdirected arthritis research in the United States, see Clark (1997) Ch. 5.

[8] See http://www.niams.nih.gov/an/budget/FY2001/fy01actmechpie.htm.

[9] The April 2000 Census reports a total of 281,421,906 people.

[10] Written testimony of Dr. Garth L. Nicolson to the Congressional Committee on Government Reform (Subcommittee on National Security, Veterans' Affairs and International Relations), January 24, 2002.

[11] Dr. William Reeves of the CDC in Atlanta sought protection under the "Federal Whistle Blower's Act" after he exposed misappropriation of funds allocated for Chronic Fatigue Syndrome research at the CDC.

[12] This assertion is based on the late Alfred Korzbyski's argument for improving upon general semantics and the concept of time binding. See www.kcmetro.cc.mo.us/pennvalley/biology/lewis/akbio.htm.

[13] See http://arborcom.com/frame/food_chem.htm#Food irradiation.

[14] Brown and Scammel (1988), p. 202.

[15] See www.intmed.mcw.edu/drug/InfectionRx.html.

[16] See www.thearthritiscenter.com for protocols.

[17] Clark (1997) p. 21.

[18] Clark (1997) p. 40.

[19] The Institute for Molecular Medicine in Huntington Beach, CA (www.immed.org) is a nonprofit organization with a certified laboratory which can perform a variety of tests that are covered by private insurance as well as Medicare, Medicaid, and other government-funded medical

---

assistance programs. The laboratory's website is www.imd-lab.com. See also www.mercola.com, www.rheumatic.org, and www.shasta.com.

[20]E.g., www.uams.edu/physician_directory is useful. See also www.miningco.org, which provides links to over 700 arthritis-related websites.

[21] A package of 30 tablets of 30 mg Claritin costs approximately $67 in the U.S. but about $2.25 for the same chemical formulation in Chile. Source: personal experience of the author.

BIBLIOGRAPHY

Actor, Paul, et al., eds. *Antibiotic Inhibition of Bacterial Cell Surface Assembly and Function*. American Society for Microbiology, Washington, DC, 1988.

Atkins, Dr. Robert C., M.D. *Dr. Atkins' Vita-Nutrient Solution*. Simon & Schuster: New York, 1998.

Aladjem, Henrietta. *Understanding Lupus*. Macmillan: New York, 1985.

Alexander, Dan D. *Arthritis and Common Sense*. Witkower Press, Inc.: West Hartford, CT, 1954.

Baker, S.M., McDonnell, M., and Truss, C.V. "Double Blind Placebo-Controlled Crossover Study Proves Effectiveness of IgG Food ELISA Testing." Seminar Presentation to the American Academy of Environmental Medicine, Virginia Beach, VA, October 1994.

Barnes, Broda O., M.D. and Galton, Lawrence. *Hypothyroidism: the Unsuspected Illness*. Thomas Y. Crowell Company: New York, 1976.

Baseman, J.B. and Tulley, J.G. "Mycoplasmas: Sophis-ticated, Reemerging, and Burdened by Their Notoriety." *Emerging Infectious Diseases*. 1997;3(3): 21-32.

Benenson, Abram S., ed. *Control of Communicable Diseases in Man*.12th edition, American Public Health Association, 1979.

Berger, Stuart M., M.D. *Dr. Berger's Immune Power Diet*. New American Library: New York, 1985.

________. *How to be Your Own Nutritionist*. Avon Books: New York, 1987.

Bingham, Robert, M.D. *Fight Back Against Arthritis*, Desert Arthritis Medical Clinic: Desert Hot Springs, CA, 1984.

Bird, Christopher. *The Persecution and Trial of Gaston Naessens*. H.J. Kramer, Inc.: Tiburon, CA, 1991.

Bliznakov, Emile G., M.D., and Hunt, Gerald L. *The Miracle Nutrient: Coenzyme Q_{10}*. Bantam Books: New York, 1989.

Bottone, Edward J., ed. *Unusual Microorganisms: Gram-Negative Fastidious Species*. Marcel Dekker, Inc.: New York, 1983.

Brena, Steven F. and Chapman, Stanley L., eds. *Management of Patients with Chronic Pain.* Spectrum Publications, Inc.: NY, 1983.

Bremness, Lesley. *Herbs*. Dorling Kindersley: New York, 1994.

Bricklin, Mark, ed. *The Natural Healing and Nutrition Annual 1989*. Rodale Press: Emmaus, PA, 1989.

_________. *Prevention Magazine's Nutrition Advisor*. Rodale Press: Emmaus, PA. 1993

Brown, Thomas McPherson, M.D., and Scammell, Henry. *The Road Back: Rheumatoid Arthritis—Its Cause and Its Treatment.* M Evans and Company, Inc.: New York, 1988.

Cambier, John C., ed. *Ligands, Receptors and Signal Transduction in Regulation of Lymphocyte Function*. American Society for Microbiology, Washington, DC, 1990.

Canby, Thomas Y. "Bacteria: Teaching Old Bugs New Tricks." *National Geographic*, August 1993.

Cawood, Frank. *Vitamin Side Effects Revealed*. FC&A Publishing: Peachtree City, GA, 1986.

Chopra, Deepak, M.D. *Perfect Health: The Complete Mind/Body Guide*. Crown Publishers, Inc.: New York, 1994.

Chuen, Lam Kam. *Tai Chi: The Natural Way to Strength and Health*. Simon & Schuster: New York, 1994.

Clark, Harold W. *Why Arthritis? Searching for the Cause and the Cure of Rheumatoid Disease*. Axelrod Publishing: Tampa Bay, FL, 1997. Available through the Mycoplasma Research Institute. See www.digitalusa.net/~hwcmri.

Corrigan, A.B., M.D. *Living With Arthritis*. Grosset & Dunlap: New York, 1971.

Cousens, Dr. Gabriel. *Conscious Eating*. North Atlantic Books: Berkeley, CA, 1999.

Cousins, Norman. *Anatomy of an Illness as Perceived by the Patient*. Bantam Books: New York, 1981.

Cox, Michael A. *Oxycal® Vs. Arthritis*. Ralph Tanner Associates: Prescott, AZ, 1984.

Crook, William G., M.D. *The Yeast Connection*. Random House: New York, 1986.

________. *The Yeast Connection and The Woman*. Professional Books, Inc.: Jackson, TN, 1995.

Cummings, Stephen, M.D. and Ullman, Dana. *Everybody's Guide to Homeopathic Medicines*. G.P. Putnam's Sons: New York, 1991.

Dewey, Laurel. *The Humorous Herbalist*. Safe Goods: Glenwood Springs, CO, 1996.

Diamond, Harvey and Diamond, Marilyn. *Fit For Life*. Warner Books: New York, 1985.

Dixon, Dr. Bernard, ed. *Health, Medicine and the Human Body*. MacMillan Publishing Company: New York, 1986.

Dufty, William. *Sugar Blues*. Chilton Book Co.: PA 1975.

Dworkin, Martin, ed. *Microbial Cell-Cell Interactions*. American Society for Microbiology, Washington, DC, 1991.

Eisenstein, Phyllis and Scheiner, Samuel M., M.D. *Overcoming the Pain of Inflammatory Arthritis: The Pain-Free Promise of Pantothenic Acid.* Avery: Garden City Park, New York, 1997.

Enig, Mary G., and Fallon, Sally. "The Oiling of America (The Cholesterol Myth)." Published in two installments of *Nexus*, November/December 1998 and February/March 1999.

Feltelius, N. and Hällgren, R.. "Sulphasalazine in Anky-losing Spondylitis." *An Rheum Dis*. 1986; 45:396.

Folkers, K.; Brown, R.,; Judy, W.V. and Morita, M. "Survival of Cancer Patients on Therapy with Coenzyme Q_{10}." *Biochem-Biophys-Res-Commun.* 1993; 192(1):241-5.

Folkers, K., Hanioka, T., Xia, L.J., and McRee, Jr., J.T. "Coenzyme Q_{10} Increases T4/T8 Ratios of Lymphocytes in Ordinary Subjects and Relevance to Patients Having the AIDS Related Complex." *Biochem-Biophys-Res-Commun.* 1991; 176(2):786-91.

Folkers, K.; Morita, M. and McRee, Jr., J.T. "The Activities of Coenzyme Q_{10} and Vitamin B_6 for Immune Responses." *Biochem-Biophys-Res-Commun.* 1993; 193(1): 88-92.

Foster, Steven. *Herbs for Your Health*. Interweave Press: Loveland, CO, 1996.

Fox, Nicols. Spoiled: The Dangerous Truth About a Food Chain Gone Haywire. BasicBooks: New York, 1997

Fredericks, Carlton. *Arthritis: Don't Learn to Live With It.* Grosset & Dunlap: New York, 1981.

Garrett, Laurie. *The Coming Plague*. Penguin Books: New York, 1995.

Hilborne, Lee H. and Golomb, Beatrice A. *A Review of the Scientific Literature as it Pertains to Gulf War Illnesses,* Vol I: *Infectious Diseases*. RAND, MR-1018/1-OSD, 2001.

Hoffman, R.W.; O'Sullivan, F.X.; Schafermeyer, K. R.; Moore, T.L.; Roussell, D.; Watson-McKown, R.; Kim M. F. and Wise, K.S. "Mycoplasma Infection and Rheumatoid Arthritis: Analysis of Their Relationship using Immuno-blotting and an Ultrasensitive Polymerase Chain Reaction Detection Method." *Arthritis Rheum*. 1997;40(3): 1219-1228.

Huemer, Richard, M.D. and Challem, Jack. "Outsmart the Supergerms." *Natural Health*, May/June 1997.

Isada, Carlos M., M.D.; Kasten, Jr., Bernard, L., M.D.; Goldman, Morton P.; Pharm.D.; Gray, Larry D., PH.D and Aberg, Judith A., M.D. *Infectious Diseases Handbook 1995-96, Including Antimicrobial Therapy and Laboratory Diagnosis*. American Pharmaceutical Association and Lexi-Comp, Inc.: Hudson, OH, 1995.

Ishida, K.; Kaku, M.; Irifune, K.; Mizukane R.; et al. "*In-vitro* and *In-vivo* Activity of a New Quinolone AM-1155 Against Mycoplasma pneumoniae." *J Antimicrob Chemo*. 1994; 34:875-83.

Jarney, Chris and Tindall, John. *Acupressure for Common Ailments.* Simon & Schuster: New York, 1991.

Jarvis, D. C, M.D. *Arthritis and Folk Medicine.* Fawcett Publications: Greenwich, CN, 1960.

Johnson, Hillary. *Osler's Web: Inside the Labyrinth of the Chronic Fatigue Syndrome Epidemic*. Crown Publishers, Inc.: New York, 1996.

Kauz, Herman. *Tai Chi Handbook: Exercise, Meditation, and Self-defense*. Doubleday & Co., Inc.: Garden City, NY, 1974.

Keough, Carol and the editors of *Prevention* magazine. *Natural Relief for Arthritis*. Simon & Schuster: New York, 1986.

Kremer, J.M.; Lawrence, D.A.; Jubix W.; et al. "Dietary Fish Oil and Olive Oil Supplementation in Patients With Rheumatoid

Arthritis: Clinical and Immunological Effects." *Arth Rheum* 1990; 33:810-20.

Kushner, Irvin; Volanakis, John E. and Gewurz, Henry. *C-Reactive Protein and the Plasma Protein Response to Tissue Injury*. New York Academy of Sciences, New York, 1982.

Lamba, Surendar S. and Walker, Charles A.. *Antibiotics and Microbial Transformations*. CRC Press, Inc.: Boca Raton, FL, 1987.

Lappe, Marc. *When Antibiotics Fail*. North Atlantic Books: Berkeley, CA, 1986.

Lecron, L. M. *Self Hypnotism: The Technique and its Use in Daily Living*. Prentice-Hall: Englewood Cliffs, N.J., 1964.

Lessof, Maurice H., ed. *Immunology of Cardiovascular Disease*. Marcel Dekker, Inc.: New York, 1981.

Lidell, Linda. *The Book of Massage: The Complete Step-by-Step Guide to Eastern and Western Techniques*. Simon & Schuster: New York, 1984.

Lorig, Kate, R.N., and Fries, James F., M.D. *The Arthritis Helpbook*. 3rd edition, Addison-Wesley: New York, 1990.

Lucas, Richard M. *Herbal Health Secrets From Europe and Around the World*. Parker Publishing Co.: West Nyack, New York, 1983.

Maduro, Rogelio A. and Schauerhammer, Ralf. *The Holes in the Ozone Scare: The Scientific Evidence That the Sky Isn't Falling*. 21st Century Science Associates: Washington, D.C. 1992.

Mandell, G.L.; Bennett, J.E. and Dolin, R., eds. *Principles and Practice of Infectious Diseases*. Vol. 2, 5th ed. Churchill Livingstone, Inc.: New York, 2000.

Mandell, Marshall, M.D. *Dr. Mandell's Lifetime Arthritis Relief System*. Berkley Books: New York, 1983.

Maniloff, Jack, ed. *Mycoplasmas: Molecular Biology and Pathogenesis*. American Society for Microbiology, Washing-ton, DC, 1992.

Martin, David W., M.D.; Mayes, Peter A.; Rodwell, Victor W. and Granner, Daryl K., M.D. *Harper's Review of Biochemistry*. 20th ed., Lange Medical Publications: Los Altos, CA, 1985.

Mattman, Lida H. *Cell Wall Deficient Forms—Stealth Pathogen*. 2nd ed., CRC Press: Boca Raton, FL, 2000.

Mazza, J.G., and Ooma, G.D., eds. Functional Foods: Herbs, Botanicals and Teas. Publ: location, 2000.

McCabe, Edward. *O2Xygen Therapies: A New Way of Approaching Disease*. Energy Publications: Morrisville, NY, 1988.

McGrady, Sr., Pat. *The Persecuted Drug: The Story of DMSO*. Charter Books: New York, 1981.

Michaud, Ellen and Feinstein, Alice, and the editors of *Prevention* magazine. *Fighting Disease: The Complete Guide to Natural Immune Power*. Rodale Press: Emmaus, PA, 1989.

Mindell, Earl. *Vitamin Bible*. Warner Books: New York, 1979.

Mizel, Steven B. and Jaret, Peter. *In Self Defense: The Human Immune System—The New Frontier in Medicine*. Harcourt Brace: Jovanovich, NY, 1985.

Mowrey, Daniel B. *The Scientific Validation of Herbal Medicine*. Keats Publishing: New Canaan, CT, 1986.

Nagler, Willibald, M.D., and von Estorff, Irene, M.D. *Dr. Nagler's Body Maintenance and Repair Book*. Simon & Schuster: New York, 1987.

Namikoshi, Toru. *Shiatsu Therapy: Theory and Practice*. Japan Publications: Tokyo, 1974.

Ng, L.K.Y., ed. *New Approaches to Treatment of Chronic Pain.* Washington: U.S. Department of Health and Human Services, 1981.

Nicolson, G.L.; Nasralla, M.Y.; Haier, J.; Erwin, R.; Nicolson, N.L. and Ngwenya, R. "Mycoplasmal Infections in Chronic Illnesses: Fibromyalgia and Chronic Fatigue Syndromes, Gulf War Illness, HIV-AIDS and Rheumatoid Arthritis." *Medical Sentinel* 1999; 4:172-176.

Nicolson, Garth L. and Rosenberg-Nicolson, Nancy L. *Doxycycline Treatment and Desert Storm.* University of Texas M.D. Anderson Cancer Center, Houston, Texas, December 1995.

Olszewski, Waldemar L. *Peripheral Lymph: Formation and Immune Function.* CRC Press, Inc.: Boca Raton, FL, 1987.

Palmer, D. G. "Total Leukocyte Enumeration in Pathologic Synovial Fluids." *Am J Clin Path.* 1968; volume 49.

Pascoe, Elaine. "The 1987 Nobel Prize in Physiology or Medicine." *Science Annual 1989.* H.S. Stuttman, Inc.: Westport, CN, 1989.

Physician's Drug Handbook. 5th ed., Springhouse Corp.: Springhouse, PA, 1993.

Qu, Zhuqing; Lu, Dinghuo and Wang, Yirun. "Effect of Acupuncture on Ion Distribution in Cells of Normal and Injured Skeletal Muscles." *Journal of Beijing Institute of Physical Education.* 1993; Vol. 16, no. 4.

Roberts, Elizabeth H. *On Your Feet.* Rodale Press: Emmaus, PA, 1975.

Roitt, I.; Brostoff, J. and Male, D. *Immunology.* 2nd ed., J.B. Lippincott Co.: New York, 1989.

Rose, Noel R.; Friedman, Herman and Fahey, John L. *Manual of Clinical Laboratory Immunology*. 3rd ed., American Society for Microbiology, Washington, DC, 1986.

Rosenberg, Steven A., M.D., and Barry, John M. *The Transformed Cell*. G.P.Putnam's Sons: New York, 1992.

Samuels, Mike, M.D. and Samuels, Nancy. *Arthritis: How to Work with Your Doctor and Take Charge of Your Health*. Summit Books: New York, 1991.

Sherris, David; Kern, Eugene and Jens, Ponikau. "Mayo Clinic Study Implicates Fungus as Cause of Chronic Sinusitis." *Mayo Clinic Proceedings*, September 1999.

Shoemaker, Dr. Ritchie C. *Desperation Medicine: The Inside Story of How an American Doctor Discovered a Threatening New Family of Environmental Diseases…and How to Stop Them*. Gateway Press: Baltimore MD, 2001.

Shou-Jiang, G. and Moore, P.S. "Molecular Approaches to the Identification of Unculturable Infectious Agents." *Emerg Infec Dis* 1996; 2(3): 159-167.

Sinatra, Dr. Stephen T. *The Coenzyme Q10 Phenomenon*. Keats, a division of NTC/Contemporary Publishing Group, Lincolnwood (Chicago), IL, 1998.

Sittig, Marshall, ed. *Handbook of Toxic and Hazardous Chemicals and Carcinogens*. 2nd ed., Noyes Publications: Park Ridge, NJ, 1985.

Smyth, Angele. *The Complete Home Healer*. Harper-Collins: New York, 1994.

Sobel, Dave and Klein, Arthur C. *Arthritis: What Works*. St. Martin's Press: New York, 1989.

Solomon, Neil, M.D. and Lipton, Marc. *Sick & Tired of Being Sick & Tired*. Wynwood Press: New York, 1989.

Spiegel, Dr. David. "The Hypnotic Trance." *Science Annual 1989*. H.S. Stuttman, Inc.: Westport, CN, 1989.

Stanway, Andrew. *Alternative Medicine: A Guide to Natural Therapies*. Bloomsbury Books: London, 1979.

Stollerman, G.H. "Trends in Bacterial Virulence and Antibiotic Susceptibility: *Streptococci*, *pneumococci*, and *gonococci*." *Annals of Internal Medicine*. 1978:89 (Part 2): 746-48.

Straus, R. A. *Strategic Self-Hypnosis*. Prentice-Hall: Engle-wood Cliffs, N.J., 1982.

Tanner, H.A. "Energy Transformations in the Biosynthesis of the Immune System: Their Relevance to the Progression and Treatment of AIDS." *Med-Hypotheses*. 1992; 38(4):315-21.

Tappan, Frances M. *Healing Massage Techniques*. 2nd ed., Appleton & Lange: Norwalk, CN, 1988.

Tarshis, Barry. *DMSO: The True Story of a Remarkable Pain-Killing Drug*. William Morrow and Company: New York, 1981.

Tilly, B.C.; Alarcon, G.S.; Heyse, S.P.; et al. "Minocycline in Rheumatoid Arthritis: a 48-week, Double-Blind, Placebo-Controlled Trial." *Ann Int Med* 1995; 122:147-148.

Toivanen, Auli and Toivanen, Paavo. *Reactive Arthritis*. CRC Press, Inc.: Boca Raton, FL, 1988.

Toppo, Frank R., M.D. and Schramm, Alan T., Ph.D. *The ToppFast™ Diet Plan*. TOPPFAST, Newport Beach, CA, 1986.

Tyler, Varro. *The Honest Herbal*. Lubrecht & Cramer Ltd.: Port Jervis, NY, 1993.

Ullman, Dana. *Discovering Homeopathy*. North Atlantic Books: Berkeley, CA, 1991.

Vierck, Elizabeth. *Osteoporosis: How to Stop It; How to Prevent It; How to Reverse It*. Parker Publishing Company: West Nyack, NY, 1993.

Volker, D.; Fitzgerald, P.; Major, G.; et al. "Efficacy of Fish Oil Concentrate in the Treatment of Rheumatoid Arthritis." *J Rheum* 2000; 27:2343-2346.

Wallace, Dr. Daniel. *The Lupus Book.* Oxford University Press: New York, 1995.

Wallace, Jean. *Arthritis Relief.* Rodale Press: Emmaus, PA, 1989.

Watt, Bernice K.; Merrill, Annabel L.; et.al., prepared for the United States Department of Agriculture. *Handbook of the Nutritional Contents of Foods*. Dover, Inc.: New York, 1975.

Wyburn-Mason, Dr. Roger. *The Causation of Rheumatoid Disease and Many Human Cancers: A New Concept in Medicine.* Arthritis Trust of America: Fairview, TN, 1983.

Weil, Andrew, M.D. *Eight Weeks to Optimum Health*. Alfred A. Knopf: New York, 1997.

________. *Health and Healing*. Houghton Mifflin: Boston, 1988.

Williams, Dr. Roger J. *Nutrition Against Disease*. Pitman Publishing Corporation: New York, 1971.

Wilson, J., Braunwald; E., Iselbacher, K.; et al., eds. *Principles of Internal Medicine*. 12th ed. McGraw-Hill: New York, 1991.

Wistreich, George A. and Lechtman, Max D. *Microbiology*. 5th ed., MacMillan: New York, 1988.

Witkin, Steven S. "Defective Immune Responses in Patients with Recurrent Candidiasis." *Infections in Medicine*, May/ June 1985.

Yates, George and Shermer, Michael B. *Meeting the Challenge of Arthritis*. Lowell House: Los Angeles CA, 1990.

Yoshikawa, Thomas T., M.D.; Chow, Anthony W., M.D. and Guze, Lucien B., M.D., eds. *Infectious Diseases: Diagnosis and Management*. Houghton Mifflin: Boston, 1980.

Zimmerman, Barry E. and Zimmerman, David J. *Killer Germs: Microbes and Diseases That Threaten Humanity.* Contemporary Books, Inc.: Chicago, IL, 1996.

APPENDIX I:

COMMON HERBAL TREATMENTS

The substances described in this appendix are well-known, well-documented, and popular remedies—an indication of the wealth of available natural substances that have been used in place of drugs whose side effects can be as harmful as the disease itself.[1] Because there are many herbs that strengthen the immune system, many others that improve circulation, and still others that relieve symptoms of inflammation, pain, and swelling, a comprehensive list is beyond the scope of this book.

The herbal substances listed below are among those referenced consistently in texts dealing with naturopathic treatment for arthritis, rheumatism, and related ailments[2]. The focus here is on those substances that remove toxins, are natural antibacterial and antibiotic agents, and offer relief from common rheumatoid arthritis symptoms of fatigue, pain, and inflammation. Providing this list is by no means intended to be prescriptive, merely informative.

Despite the fact that these substances are "natural," they are by no means completely risk-free. They should not be applied internally or externally before one has consulted with a qualified and knowledgeable health care practitioner who is well versed in their use. Some substances are contraindicated when the individual has specific health problems and/or is taking prescription medication.[3] Reputable Internet sites can be explored to identify specific interreactions[4] before consulting with one's physician.

Manufacturers and suppliers of herbal products may adulterate these substances, adding fillers or preservatives or they may blend the herbs with a related herb of lower quality. These additions, although identified as "inactive," may cause allergic reactions. Herbs and vitamins lose potency and effectiveness after one to two years. Herbal products bought at clearance sales are likely to be past their prime. Products in gelatin capsules should be refrigerated.

The "herbal remedy" industry is at this writing unregulated by the FDA to a great extent. Fortunately, labels are legally required to list the percentage of herbal substance included in each package. Let the buyer beware. A qualified health care professional should know which brands are reputable and which substances may interfere with prescribed medications.[5]

Standardization ensures that herbal products contain the same amount of a plant's biologically active substance(s) found to have therapeutic effect. This is important because many factors contribute to a varying level of potency—soil quality, plant genetics, time of harvest, part of the plant used, etc. Some herbs contain so little active substance that it must be extracted from many plants and concentrated to have any therapeutic effect.[6] Ginkgo is one example. The glycosides must be carefully extracted and other undesirable compounds like tannins removed before marketing. Herbal products are standardized in three ways[7]:

1. Extract the principal ingredient(s) by dissolving in a solvent such as alcohol or hexane to make a tincture;

2. Blend various batches of extracts to achieve some degree of consistent potency; or

3. Introduce an active compound (this is called "spiking").

Spiking may create a chemical imbalance and/or diminish the intended effect of the herbal substance. In Germany, many herbal products are sold by prescription and thus must meet pharmaceutical criteria. Standardization is difficult because the chemical constituents of any given therapeutic herb act together in synergy. Extracts represent only one or a few of these active constituents. Generally, fresh processed herbs are most highly potent. The longer a harvested herb is left to the air, the more active molecules will escape. An herb in powdered form, including those in capsules, has been subjected to oxidation and has lost much of its potency. However, some herbs, like cascara sagrada bark, must be dried and aged, else its laxative effects will be too powerful.

One should choose those brands of herbal products whose constituent phytochemicals have been proven in scientific studies to have therapeutic effects. These may cost more compared to other similar standardized but untested products, however, the buyer has the assurance that the brand name product's efficacy is supported by clinical studies.[8]

Alfalfa (*Medicago sativa*)

This herb has been a traditional folk treatment for rheumatoid arthritis, diabetes, indigestion, anemia, and atherosclerotic plaque. It is high in protein and contains vitamins A, B_1, B_6, B_{12}, C, E, and K as well as the minerals calcium, potassium, phosphorus, iron, and zinc. Eating alfalfa seeds or sprouts has been said to be beneficial to those with Lupus, a chronic illness characterized by the inflammation of connective tissue, which also is a symptom of rheumatoid arthritis. However, this assertion is controversial. Alfalfa seeds contain a substance called L-canavanine, present in all legumes, and may cause lupus flares in some individuals.[9] These flares may indicate the temporary destruction of a colony of infectious organisms.

Astragalus (*Astragalus membranaceaous*)

This member of the pea family is one of the most important stamina tonics in Chinese medicine and was mentioned as *huang-qi* in a 2,000-year-old Chinese medical text. Numerous recent studies confirm its immunostimulant, antibacterial, antiviral, adaptogenic, anti-inflammatory, and diuretic effects. It is often combined with ginseng for the commercial market.

Barberry (*Berberis vulgaris*)

Besides its powerful antibiotic properties, barberry is believed to stimulate the immune system, reduce high blood pressure, and shrink tumors. Studies have shown significant infection-fighting properties against germs responsible for wound infections, diarrhea, dysentery, cholera, urinary tract infections, and yeast infections. The herb may be able to stimulate macrophages, the germ-destroying white blood cells of the immune system.

Blackstrap Molasses

A mixture of one teaspoonful in 6 ounces of hot water, drunk before each meal, is a centuries-old folk remedy for arthritis. Molasses is high in vitamins E and

B_5, substances that fight infection by building natural anti-bodies. Molasses is the residue of sugar cane refining. It contains all the organic molecules removed from processed sugar.

Boneset (*Eupatorium perfoliatum*)

Related to marigolds and dandelions, this herb stimulates the immune system. Native Americans used it to treat fevers, ward off colds and influenza, and to relieve arthritis symptoms. Studies have shown it to mobilize white blood cells to destroy infection-causing bacteria and viruses.

Boswellia (*Boswellia serrata)*

Boswellia serrata is a shrub indigenous to India and related to *Boswellia carteri* (frankincense or olibanum). The plant produces a resin called salai guggal, used for millenia in India by Ayurvedic medical practitioners to treat arthritis. The active ingredient is boswellic acid, which has an anti-inflammatory effect. A 1996 issue of *Phytomedicine* was devoted to studies of boswellia.

Bromelain

An extract of pineapple, this herb has significant anti-inflammatory effects, as well as being able to assist proper digestion. However, individuals with ulcers should avoid this herb.

Burdock Root (*Arctium lappa*)

Usually brewed as tea, this herb helps to purify the blood and detoxify poisons.

Capsaicin

This herb is the fruit of a number of plant species, including paprika and chili peppers, and has been used for many years as a topical treatment for aches and pains, especially those associated with arthritis and shingles. Capsaicinoids are presumed to relieve pain because they inhibit neuro-transmitter release from afferent pain receptors. They may also stimulate endorphin production in those brain areas related to joint sensations.

Capsaicinoids block the release of neuropeptides to mediate pain and neurogenic inflammation. The chemical action initially stimulates the nerve endings, evoking the sensation of warmth and mild stinging. Recently some very expensive compounds whose only active ingredient is capsaicin have appeared on the market. Capsaicin powder can be obtained fresh, in bulk, for a fraction of the cost of these compounds heavily advertised as providing "miraculous relief." A poultice is simple to make and apply.

If there is any skin irritation over the affected joint, topical creams containing capsaicin should be avoided. Never use an analgesic ointment, particularly those containing capsaicin, in conjunction with a heating pad because of the potential for deep burns.

Cider Vinegar

References to mixtures of apple cider vinegar with honey as a tonic appear frequently in folk medicine literature. An organism that survives after the yeast fermentation cycle produces cider vinegar. Natural cider vinegar may contain chemicals that suppress the growth of yeasts. Honey is a natural antibiotic.

Cod Liver Oil

A perennial favorite for centuries in Europe and America, cod liver oil is a rich source of the omega-3 class fatty acids EPA (Eicosapentaenoic Acid) and DHA (Docosahexaenoic Acid) as well as vitamin D. This vitamin assures that calcium is available to be deposited in the bones by allowing the intestine to absorb it more efficiently. If there is enough vitamin D in the diet, the amount of calcium absorbed by the intestine can triple.

With the advent of prescription steroids, cod liver oil was all but forgotten as a natural, safe, and inexpensive way to ensure adequate vitamin D intake, despite credible clinical studies that showed that fish oil brought blood sedimentation rates down dramatically in arthritic individuals.[10] Results of thirteen double-blind placebo-controlled studies involving a total of over 500 participants indicate that supplementation with omega-3 fatty acids can significantly reduce RA symptoms.[11]

A daily tablespoon of fish oil is a traditional folk remedy to keep arthritic joints lubricated. This is based on the misconception that our joints work like a mechanical ball and socket, and that the ingested oil is somehow squirted into the assembly for smoother functioning. In reality it is the EPA, DHA, and vitamin D that nourishes the cells forming the synovial fluid that surrounds all joints. Those who take fish oil supplements should take care not to exceed the safe maximum intake of vitamins A and D. Fish oil has a mild blood thinning effect, so it should not be combined with any anticoagulant drugs unless approved by a physician.

Curcumin

See Turmeric.

Devil's Claw (*Harpagophytum procumbens*)

This herb has been used for centuries to help reduce pain and swelling. Scientific research done in Germany[12] shows that Devil's Claw has produced good results in certain disorders of the liver and kidneys, stimulating the detoxifying and protective mechanisms of the body. Devil's Claw must be taken for a course of eight or nine weeks to see results, and then should be discontinued. Diabetics should not use the herb except under medical supervision.

Echinacea (*Echinacea purpurea*)

Native Americans used this herb for more medicinal purposes than any other plant, treating everything from colds to cancer. It is valued in China for its antibiotic and immune system-stimulating properties, applicable even to severe immune disorders such as cancer and AIDS. American doctors adopted it in 1895 to treat malaria, measles, mumps, chicken pox, arthritis, scarlet fever, yeast infections, and chronic nasal congestion. The natural antibiotic (echinacoside) in the plant works in a way comparable to penicillin to kill viruses, bacteria, fungi, and other germs. Several studies show echinacea extract as being able to increase the production of infection-fighting T-cells by 30 percent.

Echinacea was later replaced by synthetic antibiotics in the United States, but still enjoys widespread popularity in Europe. It is used for relief from the symptoms of seasonal allergies. Herbalists consider *Echinacea purpurea* root to be a blood purifier and an aid to fighting infections. Persons allergic to pollens such as ragweed may be also allergic to echinacea. This herb should not be used in cases of seriously impaired immune response illnesses such as tuberculosis, multiple sclerosis, and HIV infection. Stimulating badly infected T-cells is unwise. Caution: too much of this herb over a long period of time can actually have immunosuppressive effects in otherwise healthy individuals. It should be used at the onset and during a cold or allergy attack, but not as a daily supplement.

Eleuthero (*Eleutherococcus senticosus*)

Also known as Siberian ginseng, Eleuthero has been used in China as an invigorating tonic for more than two thousand years. It strongly stimulates the immune system and counters symptoms of fatigue. It is used to treat a variety of illnesses ranging from the common cold to severe respiratory and inflammatory conditions.

The active eleutherosides in this herb have been studied, revealing an ability to support immune function and adrenal gland function, especially under stressful conditions.[13] In Russia, inhabitants of the Taiga region of Siberia originally used eleuthero to decrease infections and increase vitality. Russian Olympic athletes use this herb for stamina and endurance. The Soviet government distributed eleuthero to its citizens to counter the effects of radiation after the Chernobyl nuclear accident. The herb has been shown to alleviate the side effects of chemotherapy and radiation therapy and to help bone marrow recover more quickly.[14]

Research reveals that eleuthero assists in maintaining aerobic activity for longer periods and in recovery from strenuous workouts more quickly.[15] Increase in blood oxygen transport to inflamed areas is especially beneficial to arthritis sufferers. Some microorganisms in the body are very sensitive to oxygen levels in the blood. If this level is impaired, the organisms are not controllable.

Studies have shown a potential value of this herb in the long-term management of various diseases of the immune system by a measurable increase in the number of T-cells (lymphocytes).[16]

Garlic (*Allium sativum*)

Cultivated as food and medicine for over five thousand years, garlic's antibacterial activity was first recognized in 1858 by Louis Pasteur. The following are among the well-documented properties of garlic: anti-inflammatory, antibacterial, antifungal, antiparasitic, antioxidant, and immunostimulant. At this writing, nine epidemiological studies show that garlic significantly decreases the incidence of cancer, especially cancer of the gastrointestinal tract, among those who consume it regularly.[17] Its action is believed to be similar to that of sulfa drugs. Its potency is so strong that it is typically used in sausage recipes to prevent spoilage. The European livestock industry is currently considering adding garlic to animal feed rather than chemical antibiotics, which are seen to cause consumer health problems.

Whole cloves of garlic are less expensive and far more potent than commercially prepared garlic capsules. It is necessary to crush the clove before consuming it to obtain maximum benefit. Cooking the garlic decreases its beneficial action.

Ginger (*Zingiber officinalis*)

The anti-inflammatory actions of ginger help relieve the pain of arthritis, menstrual cramps, and headache. An easy way to obtain this herb's benefits is to use it liberally in cooking. Add the fresh root to soups, stir-fry recipes, and sauces. Scrub the root but do not peel it, since active properties are primarily contained in the skin. Three to four cups of ginger tea daily can be beneficial. Use two teaspoons of chopped fresh root in one cup of water simmered in a covered pot for ten minutes.

Ginkgo (*Ginkgo Biloba)*

This herb has been found to improve both blood circulation and oxygen metabolism in the brain. Unique compounds called ginkgolides are potent inhibitors of a platelet-activating factor involved in the development of inflammatory, cardiovascular, and respiratory disorders. The action of ginkgolides helps explain the herb's broad spectrum of biological effects, such as antioxidant activity.

Olive Leaf Extract

This phytochemical substance has antiviral, antibacterial, antifungal and antiparasitic activity. The elenolic acid contained in the extract (oleuropein) is the active biological agent that combats infectious diseases. Oleuropein stimulates phagocytosis and increases T-call counts. It is used in China to suppress cancer and rebuild the immune system. Oleuropein acts as a free radical scavenger in a manner similar to vitamin E. It also inhibits the oxidation of LDL cholesterol. Individuals suffering from a viral or bacterial infection or from Chronic Fatigue Syndrome may experience a Jarisch-Herxheimer effect during the detoxification process.

Pectin

This substance is found in the cell walls of plants. Because of its ability to gel and hold water molecules together, pectin is valuable in ridding the body of toxins. Fruit (usually apple) pectin is sold commercially where canning supplies are available. It has been used for decades as a folk remedy for bursitis or "tennis elbow." It may assist in lubricating joint-tendon synovial interfaces. A tablespoon of fruit pectin may be stirred in a small glass of water or fruit juice and taken daily. An alkaline juice such as apricot or apple works best. Pectin is also sold in capsule form at health food stores.

Propolis

This unusual remedy is a sticky resinous substance collected by bees from the bark or leaf buds of trees, especially poplars. Its medicinal value has been known since the first century A.D. Propolis contains resin, balsam, wax, fragrant essential oils, pollen, and amino acids. It is rich in minerals, antibiotics and vitamins, especially the B vitamins. It has an unusually high concentration of pantothenic acid, which is required by and stimulates the function of the adrenal glands. Propolis also contains tannins, which cause proteins in the blood to coagulate. Propolis compounds are used extensively in Europe and in Russia.

Reishi

This herb is the fruiting body of a mushroom native to the Orient. Although related species occur in North America, they are not grown commercially nor have their medicinal properties been seriously studied. Reishi has been a prized folk remedy in China for thousands of years, once available only to emperors as an important tonic to increase longevity. Its Chinese name *ling zhi* means "spirit plant." It was traditionally used to treat hepatitis, nervous conditions, hypertension, arthritis, insomnia, and lung disorders. Recent studies confirm Chinese reishi's antiallergenic, antioxidant, antiviral, anti-inflammatory, and immunostimulant properties. It is also a calmative and reduces blood pressure. It may be cultivated from spores if a dried reishi is placed in a bed of moist sawdust or wood chips. Non-Chinese varieties may not possess true reishi properties.

Saint John's Wort (*Hypericum perforatum*)

Known in Europe as a healing agent since the 16th century, the herb's wound-healing ability and its capability to stimulate the immune system make it a valuable traditional remedy. Studies have shown that it contains a family of chemicals known as flavonoids, which strengthen the immune system for antibacterial, anti-inflammatory, and antiviral effects. There is no evidence to support the contention that this herb is an effective treatment for chronic depression, although it has mild antidepressant properties. Mild depression often accompanies systemic mycoplasmal/bacterial infections.

Stinging Nettle (*Urtica dioica*)

Nettle tea has been used in folk medicine to stimulate blood circulation and as a tonic for chronic skin ailments. It is a traditional folk treatment for arthritis, probably because it increases oxygen transport to inflamed areas, providing relief. Research has shown that the leaf tea aids coagulation and formation of hemoglobin in red blood cells, while the leaf extract depresses the central nervous system and inhibits bacteria and adrenaline.[18] In Germany the herb is used extensively for rheumatic complaints and kidney infections.

Thyme (*Thymus vulgaris*)

Thyme is a medicinal herb indigenous to the Mediterranean area and is a member of the mint family. Although used extensively in cooking, its medicinal properties have been known in Europe since the time of Charlemagne in the eighth century. Thyme is said to relieve muscle pains and spasms, inhibit the growth of harmful microorganisms such as strep and candida, relieve or prevent coughs, act as an expectorant and settle upset stomachs.[19]

The more than 60 active compounds called phenols in thyme, especially thymol and carvacrol, are known to have muscle-relaxant and antiseptic properties. Research must still be done to identify the exact source of thyme's other healing properties.

Thyme should not be used without first consulting a health care professional if one suspects a dysfunctional thyroid condition or if pregnant or nursing. While powdered thyme is usually used for tea or in recipes, a drop or two of essential oil can be gently inhaled using a vaporizer. It can also be added sparingly to massage oil or bath water for topical treatment. Thyme essential oil should never be ingested, applied directly to the skin, or used in other than very small quantities.

Tiger Balm

Although this topical compound was developed in China only about 60 years ago, its ingredients (oils of camphor, menthol, mint, clove, cajuput, wintergreen, and cassia) have been used for centuries in various liniments to afford relief of minor aches and pains due to strain, fatigue, exposure, or cold. There are many other external herbal poultices one could make from scratch using the Tiger Balm ingredients or a blend of comfrey, willow, thyme oil, tumeric, or capsaicin. A good herbal healing text should provide useful recipes and procedures.

Turmeric (*Curcuma longa*)

According to Ayurvedic medicine, turmeric can relieve inflammatory joint pain and ligament problems associated with arthritis, bursitis, and tendinitis. Turmeric's main ingredient is curcumin, a natural anti-inflammatory agent as helpful as cortisone but without the immunosuppressive side effects. Ayurvedic practitioners advise taking one ounce of powdered turmeric (obtainable in bulk) stirred into water or juice daily until the inflammation subsides. As a preventive measure, the recommended dose is one-half to one ounce daily.[20] This herb is a flavorful seasoning for rice and chicken soup.

White Willow Bark (*Salix alba*)

This herb contains salicylin, the same active ingredient found in aspirin (acetylsalicylic acid), used to reduce pain and inflammation. Hippocrates advised women of 400 B.C. Greece to chew willow bark to relieve the pains of childbirth. Native people of the North America have used Willow bark for over two thousand years as a blood thinner, to reduce fevers, to treat respiratory problems, headaches, and to relieve the inflammation, aches, and pains of rheumatism and arthritis. Willow bark has been called a "natural aspirin" but without aspirin's potency or side effects. It does not cause stomach upset as aspirin often does. Willow bark is high in tannins, which could damage the liver if taken in extraordinary quantities. However, it would take about a gallon of willow bark tea to provide a single dose of salicin equivalent to one dose of aspirin. Salicin produced by the bark does not metabolize in the same way as aspirin, so the same contraindications may not apply for stomach ulcers.

Yucca (*Yucca schidigera*)

All parts of the *Yucca schidigera* were used for centuries by the native people of the southwestern United States and Baja California deserts to combat the pain and inflammation caused by arthritis and rheumatism. The extract of this plant is still used commercially as a foaming agent in alcoholic beer, root beer, shampoos, and detergents. It is also used as a food supplement for livestock. The yucca root is rich in steroid-like saponins that elevate the body's production of cortisone to reduce and eliminate the pain, swelling, and joint stiffness associated with arthritis. Saponins also reduce cholesterol by binding with bile acids, making them unavailable for reabsorption. These acids pass into the colon for excretion. The process forces the liver to produce more bile, which it does by removing cholesterol from the blood and leaving less to accrue in the arteries.

The late Dr. Robert Bingham, director of the Desert Hot Springs Medical Clinic in Palm Springs, CA supervised thousands of successful case studies using yucca extract supplements. According to Dr. Bingham, toxic substances or harmful bacteria provoke allergic responses taking a variety of forms—migraines, skin rashes, joint pain—so an antistress agent such as yucca saponin may have the same beneficial effect as direct action on the invader by simply improving and protecting the intestinal flora. Yucca seems to inhibit harmful intestinal bacteria while helping maintain the natural balance of normal resident bacteria.[21]

---

[1] See Rosenberg (1992) for scientific case studies of cancer treatment-related death, especially pp. 228-232, 236-238, 251 and 300-301 and also for accounts of spontaneous remission.

[2] One of many articles dealing with naturopathic approaches to pain relief is Horn, Clare. "13 Ways to Wipe Out Pain." *Natural Health*, January/ February 1999.

[3] Rosenfeld, Dr. Isadore. "A Doctor's Guide to Herbs." *Parade Magazine*, May 31, 1998.

[4] For example, www.healthwell.com , and www.puritan.com . A powerful search engine such as Google can be given specific keywords. E.g., "athritis" and "yucca."

[5] Horstman, Judith. "Label-Smart." *Arthritis Today*. May/June 2001.

[6] Challem, Jack. "The Problem With Herbs." *Natural Health*, January/ February 1999.

[7] Ibid.

[8] For specifics of problems and drawbacks, see *The Complete German Commission E Monographs* published in *Integrative Medicine Communications*, 1998. Also see Tyler (1993) and publications like *Nutrition Action Healthletter, Environmental Nutrition, Tufts University Health and Nutrition Letter*. Useful websites are www.herbalgram.org and www.healthy.net/clinic/therapy/herbal/index.html.

[9] Wallace (1995) p. 44.

[10] Among these, a study at the Brusch Medical Center in Cambridge, MA, referenced in Keough (1986) p. 163. See also Kremer (1990).

[11] James, M.S. and Cleland, L.G. "Dietary n-3 Fatty Acids and Therapy for Rheumatoid Arthritis." *Semin Arthritis Rheum*. 1997; 27:85-97. See also Volker, et al. (2000).

[12] Lucas (1983) pp. 186-7.

[13] H. Wagner, H. Nörr and H. Winterhoff. "Plant Adaptogens." *Phytomed* 1994;1: 63-76.

[14] Kupin, V.I. and Polevaia, E.B. "Stimulation of the Immunological Reactivity of Cancer Patients by *Eleutherococcus* Extract." *Vopr Onkol* 1986;32: 21-26 [in Russian]

[15] Asano, K.;Takahashi, T.; Miyashita, M.; et al. "Effect of *Eleutherococcus senticosus* Extract On Human Working Capacity." *Planta Medica* 1986;37: 175-77.

[16] Bohn, B.; Nebe, C.T.; Birr, C. and Flow, C. "Cytometric Studies With *Eleutherococcus senticosus* Extract as an Immunomodulating Agent." *Arzneim-Forsch Drug Res* 1987;37: 1193-96.

[17] Foster (1996) p. 42.

[18] Ibid. p. 92.

[19] Block, Betsy. "Thyme." *Natural Health*. July/August 1999 and Duke, James. *The Green Pharmacy*. St. Martin's Press: New York, 1997.

[20] Vukovic, Laurel, "Home Remedies," *Natural Health*, July/August 1999.

[21] Results of a placebo-controlled study on the effects of yucca in the *Journal of Applied Nutrition*, 1978; Vol 27: Nos. 2 and 3. See also Pike, Dr. Arnold. "The Healing Properties of Yucca." *Let's Live*, August 1990.

APPENDIX II:

Physicians' Protocol for Using Antibiotics in Rheumatic Disease

by Dr. Joseph M. Mercola, D. O.

Introduction

Rheumatoid arthritis affects about 1 percent of our population and at least two million Americans have definite or classical rheumatoid arthritis. It is a much more devastating illness than previously appreciated. Most patients with rheumatoid arthritis have a progressive disability. More than 50% of patients who were working at the start of their disease are disabled after five years of rheumatoid arthritis. The annual cost of this disease in the U.S. is estimated to be over $1 billion.

There is also an increased mortality rate. The five-year survival rate of patients with more than thirty joints involved is approximately 50%. This is similar to severe coronary artery disease or stage IV Hodgkin's disease. Thirty years ago, one researcher concluded that there was an average loss of eighteen years of life in patients who developed rheumatoid arthritis before the age of 50.

Most authorities believe that remissions rarely occur. Some experts feel that the term "remission-inducing" should not be used to describe ANY current rheumatoid arthritis treatment. A review of contemporary treatment methods shows that medical science has not been able to significantly improve the long-term outcome of this disease.

My Experience with Dr. Brown's Protocol

I first became aware of Doctor Brown's protocol in 1989 when I saw him on 20/20 on ABC. This was shortly after the introduction of his first edition of *The Road Back*. The newest version is *The New Arthritis Breakthrough* that is written by Henry Scammel. Unfortunately, Dr. Brown died from prostate cancer shortly after the 20/20 program so I never had a chance to meet him. By the year 2000, I treated over 1,500 patients with rheumatic illnesses, including SLE, scleroderma, polymyositis and dermatomyositis.

My application of Dr. Brown's protocol has changed significantly since I first started implementing it. Initially, I followed Dr. Brown's work rigidly with very little modification other than shifting the tetracycline choice to Minocin. I believe I was one of the first people who recommended the shift to Minocin, which seems to have been widely adopted at this time.

In the early 90s, I started to integrate the nutritional model into the program and noticed a significant improvement in the treatment response. I cannot emphasize strongly enough the importance of this aspect of the program. It is absolutely an essential component of the revised Dr. Brown protocol. One may achieve remission without it, but the chances are much improved with its implementation. The additional benefit of the dietary changes is that they severely reduce the risk of the two to six month worsening of symptoms that Dr. Brown described in his book.

In the late 80s, the common retort from other physicians was that there was "no scientific proof" that this treatment works. Well, that is certainly not true today. If one peeks ahead at the bibliography, one will find over 200 references in the peer-reviewed medical literature that supports the application of Minocin in the use of rheumatic illnesses. The definitive scientific support for minocycline in the treatment of rheumatoid arthritis came with the MIRA trial in the United States.

This was a double blind randomized placebo controlled trial done at six university centers involving 200 patients for nearly one year. The dosage they used (100 mg twice daily) was much higher and likely less effective than what most clinicians currently use. They also did not employ any additional antibiotics or nutritional regimens, yet 55% of the patients improved. This study finally provided the "proof" that many traditional clinicians demanded before seriously considering this treatment as an alternative regimen for rheumatoid arthritis.

Dr. Thomas Brown's effort to treat the chronic mycoplasma infections believed to cause rheumatoid arthritis is the basis for this therapy. Dr. Brown believed that most rheumatic illnesses respond to this treatment. He and others used this therapy for SLE, Ankylosing spondylitis, scleroderma, polymyositis, and dermato-myositis.

Dr. William Osler was also a preeminent figure of his time (1849-1919). Many regard him as the consummate physician of modern times. An excerpt from a commentary on Dr. Osler provides a useful perspective on application of alternative medical paradigms:

Osler would be receptive to the cautious exploration of nontraditional methods of treatment, particularly in situations in which our present science has little to offer. From his reading of medical history, he would know that many pharmacological agents were originally derived from folk medicine. He would also remember that in the 19th century physicians no less intelligent than those in our own day initially ridiculed the unconventional practices of Semmelweis and Lister.

Osler would caution us against the arrogance of believing that only our current medical practices can benefit the patient. He would realize that new scientific insights might emerge from as yet unproved beliefs. Although he would fight vigorously to protect the public against frauds and charlatans, he would encourage critical study of whatever therapeutic approaches were reliably reported to be beneficial to patients.

Nutritional Considerations

Limiting sugar is a critical element of the treatment program. Sugar has multiple significant negative influences on a person's biochemistry. Its major mode of action is through elevation of insulin levels. However, it has a similarly severe impairment of intestinal microflora. Patients who are unable to decrease their sugar intake are far less likely to improve.

One of the major benefits of implementing the dietary changes is that one does not seem to develop worsening of symptoms the first three to six months that is described in Dr. Brown's book. Most of my patients tend not to worsen once they start the antibiotics. I believe this is due to the beneficial effects that the diet has on the immune response. I ask all new patients to read my 6-page handout on the dietary changes on my web site at www.mercola.com under the tab heading on the left side of the page entitled “Read This First.”

Antibiotic Therapy with Minocin

There are three different tetracyclines available: simple tetracycline, doxycycline, or Minocin (minocycline). Minocin has a distinct and clear advantage over tetracycline and doxycycline in three important areas:

1. Extended spectrum of activity
2. Greater tissue penetrability
3. Higher and more sustained serum levels

Bacterial cell membranes contain a lipid layer. One mechanism of building up a resistance to an antibiotic is to produce a thicker lipid layer. This layer makes it difficult for an antibiotic to penetrate. Minocin's chemical structure makes it the most lipid-soluble of all the tetracyclines.

This difference can clearly be demonstrated when one compares the drugs in the treatment of two common clinical conditions. Minocin gives consistently superior clinical results in the treatment of chronic prostatitis. In other studies, Minocin was used to improve between 75-85% of patients whose acne had become resistant to tetracycline. Strep is also believed to be a contributing cause to many patients with rheumatoid arthritis. Minocin has shown significant activity against treatment of this organism.

There are several important factors to consider when using Minocin. Unlike the other tetracyclines, it tends not to cause yeast infections. Some infectious disease experts even believe that it even has a mild anti-yeast activity. Women can be on this medication for several years and not have any vaginal yeast infections. Nevertheless, it would be prudent to have patients on prophylactic oral Lactobacillus acidophilus and bifidus preparations. This will help to replace the normal intestinal flora that is killed with the Minocin.

Another advantage of Minocin is that it tends not to sensitize patients to the sun. This minimizes the risk of sunburn and increased risk of skin cancer. However, one must incorporate several precautions with the use of Minocin. As with other tetracyclines, food impairs its absorption. However, the absorption is much less impaired than with other tetracyclines.

This is fortunate because some patients cannot tolerate Minocin on an empty stomach. They must take it with a meal to avoid gastrointestinal (GI) side effects. If they need to take it with a meal, they will still absorb 85% of the medication, whereas tetracycline is only 50% absorbed. In June of 1990, a pelletized version of Minocin became available. This improved absorption when taken with meals. This form is only available in the non-generic Lederle brand and is a more than reasonable justification not to substitute for the generic version. Clinical experience has shown that many patients will relapse when they switch from the brand name to the generic.

Clinically it has been documented that it is important to take Lederle brand Minocin. Most all generic minocycline is clearly not as effective. A large percentage of patients will not respond at all or not do as well with generic non-Lederle minocycline.

Traditionally it was recommended to only receive the brand name Lederle Minocin. However, there is one generic brand that is acceptable-- the brand made by Lederle. The only difference between Lederle generic Minocin and brand name Minocin is the label and the price.

The problem is finding the Lederle brand generic. Some of my patients have been able to find it at WalMart. Since WalMart is one of the largest drug chains in the US, this should make the treatment more widely available for a reduced charge.

Many patients are on NSAIDs, which contribute to microulcerations of the stomach that in turn cause chronic blood loss. It is certainly possible they can develop a peptic ulceration contributing to their blood loss. In either event, patients frequently receive iron supplements to correct their blood counts. IT IS IMPERATIVE THAT MINOCIN NOT BE GIVEN WITH IRON. Over 85% of the dose will bind to the iron and pass through the colon unabsorbed. If iron is taken, it should be at least one hour before the Minocin or two hours after. One recent uncommon complication of Minocin is a cell-mediated hypersensitivity pneumonitis.

Most patients can start on Minocin 100 mg. every Monday, Wednesday, and Friday evening. Doxycycline can be substituted for patients who cannot afford the more expensive Minocin. It is important to not give either medication daily, as this does not seem to provide as great a clinical benefit.

Tetracycline type drugs can cause a permanent yellow-grayish brown discoloration of the teeth. This can occur in the last half of pregnancy and in children up to eight years old. One should not routinely use tetracycline in children. If patients have severe disease, one can consider increasing the dose to as high as 200 mg three times a week. Aside from the cost of this approach, several problems result may result from the higher doses. Minocin can cause quite severe nausea and vertigo. Taking the dose at night does tend to decrease this problem considerably.

However, if one takes the dose at bedtime, one must tell the patient to swallow the medication with TWO glasses of water. This is to insure that the capsule doesn't get stuck in the throat. If that occurs, a severe chemical esophagitis can result which can send the patient to the emergency room.

For those physicians who elect to use tetracycline or doxycycline for cost or sensitivity reasons, several methods may help lessen the inevitable secondary yeast overgrowth. Lactobacillus acidophilus will help maintain normal bowel flora and decrease the risk of fungal overgrowth. Aggressive avoidance of all sugars, especially those found in non-diet sodas will also decrease the substrate for the yeast's growth. Macrolide antibiotics like Biaxin or Zithromax may be used if tetracyclines are contraindicated. They would also be used in the three pills a week regimen.

Clindamycin

The other drug used to treat rheumatoid arthritis is clindamycin. Dr. Brown's book discusses the uses of intravenous clindamycin. It is important to use the IV form of treatment if the disease is severe. Nearly all scleroderma patients should take an aggressive stance and use IV treatment. Scleroderma is a particularly dangerous form of rheumatic illness that should receive aggressive intervention.

A major problem with the IV form is the cost. The price ranges from $100 to $300 per dose if administered by a home health care agency. However, if purchased directly from Upjohn, significant savings will be appreciated. A case of two-dozen 900-mg pre-filled IV bags can be purchased directly from Upjohn for about $200.

For patients with milder illness, the oral form is preferable. If the patient has a mild rheumatic illness (the minority of cases), it is even possible to exclude this from their regimen. Initial starting doses for an adult would be a 1200-mg dose once a week. Patients do not seem to tolerate this medication as well as Minocin. The major complaint seems to be a bitter metallic type taste, which lasts about 24 hours after the dose. Taking the dose after dinner does seem to help modify this complaint somewhat. If this is a problem, one can lower the dose and gradually increase the dose over a few weeks.

Concern about the development of *C. difficile pseudo-membranous enterocolitis* as a result of the Clindamycin is appropriate. This complication is quite rare at this dosage regimen, but it certainly can occur. It is important to warn all patients about the possibility of developing a severe uncontrollable diarrhea. Administration of the acidophilus seems to limit this complication by promoting the growth of the healthy gut flora.

If one encounters a resistant form of rheumatic illness, intravenous administration should be considered. Generally, weekly doses of 900 mg are administered until clinical improvement is observed. This generally occurs within the first ten doses. At that time, the regimen can be decreased to every two weeks with the oral form substituted on the weeks where the IV is not taken.

What to Do if Severe Patients Fail to Respond

The most frequent reason for failure to respond to the protocol is lack of adherence to the dietary guidelines. Most patients will be eating too many grains and sugars, which disturb insulin physiology. It is important that patients adhere as strictly as possible to the guidelines. A small minority, generally fewer than 15%, of patients will fail to respond to the protocol described above despite rigid adherence to the diet. These individuals should already be on the IV Clindamycin.

It appears that the hyaluronic acid, a potentiating agent commonly used in the treatment of cancer, may be quite useful. It seems that hyaluronic acid has very little to no direct toxicity but works in a highly synergistic fashion when administered directly in the IV bag with the Clindamycin. Hyaluronic acid is also used in orthopedic procedures. The dose is generally from 2 to 10 cc into the IV bag. Hyaluronic acid is not inexpensive as the cost may range up to $10 per cc. One does need to exert some caution with its use as it may precipitate a significant Herxheimer flare reaction.

Patients will frequently have emotional traumas that worsen their illness. Severe emotional traumas can seriously impair the immune response to this treatment. A particularly useful and rapid technique called Emotional Freedom Technique (EFT) can be used to resolve this problem. Practitioners using this technique can be found by calling the One Foundation at 800-638-1411.

Anti-Inflammatories

The first non-aspirin NSAID, Indomethacin, was introduced in 1963. Now more than 30 are available. Relafen is one of the better alternatives, as it seems to cause less of an intestinal dysbiosis. If cost is a concern, generic ibuprofen can be used. Unfortunately, recent studies suggest this drug is more damaging to the kidneys. One must be especially careful to monitor renal function studies periodically. It is important for the patient to understand and accept the risks associated with these more toxic drugs.

Unfortunately, these drugs are not benign. Every year, they do enough damage to the GI tract to kill 2,000 to 4,000 patients with rheumatoid arthritis alone. That is ten patients EVERY DAY. At any given time patients receiving NSAID therapy have gastric ulcers in the range of 10-20%. Duodenal ulcers are lower at 2-5%. Patients on NSAIDs are at approximately three times greater relative risk for developing serious GI side effects than are non-users.

Approximately 1.2% of patients taking NSAIDs are hospitalized for upper GI problems per year of exposure. One study of patients taking NSAIDs showed that a life-threatening complication was the first sign of ulcer in more than half of the subjects.

Celebrex has received much recent press due to its decreased toxicity to the gut. That is certainly a step in the right direction. Celebrex inhibits a specific type of prostaglandin and is called a COX-2 inhibitor. A similar new drug introduced in 1999 is Vioxx. There was a report in early 1999 in the Proceedings of the National Academy of Science, which showed that these drugs might increase the risk of heart attack, stroke and blood clotting disorders.

Researchers found that the drugs suppress production of prostacyclin, which is needed to dilate blood vessels and inhibit clotting. Earlier studies had found that mice genetically engineered to be unable to use prostacyclin properly were prone to clotting disorders. Anyone who is at increased risk of cardiovascular disease should steer clear of these two new medications. Ulcer complications are certainly potentially life threatening, but heart attacks are a much more common and likely risk, especially in older individuals.

Risk factor analysis helps to identify those that are at increased danger of developing these complications. Those factors associated with a higher frequency of adverse events are:

1. Old age
2. Peptic ulcer history
3. Alcohol dependency
4. Cigarette smoking
5. Concurrent Prednisone or corticosteroid use
6. Disability
7. High dose of the NSAID
8. NSAID known to be more toxic

Studies clearly show that the non-acetylated salicylates are the safest NSAIDs. Celebrex and Vioxx likely cause the least risk for peptic ulcer. But as mentioned, they pose an increased risk for heart disease. Factoring these newer medications out would leave the following less toxic NSAIDs: Relafen, Daypro, Voltaren, Motrin, and Naprosyn. Meclomen, Indocin, Orudis, and Tolectin are among the most toxic or likely to cause complications. They are much more dangerous than the antibiotics or non-acetylated salicylates. One should run an SMA at least once a year on patients who are on these medications. One must monitor the serum potassium levels if the patient is on an ACE inhibitor as these medications can cause hyperkalemia. One should also monitor their kidney function. The SMA will also show any liver impairment that the drugs might cause.

These medications can also impair prostaglandin metabolism and cause papillary necrosis and chronic interstitial nephritis. The kidney needs vasodilatory prostaglandins (PGE2 and prostacycline) to counterbalance the effects of potent vasoconstrictor hormones such as angiotensin II and catecholamines. NSAIDs decrease prostaglandin synthesis by inhibiting cyclooxygenase, leading to unopposed constriction of the renal arterioles supplying the kidney.

One might consider the use of non-acetylated salicylates such as salsalate, sodium salicylate and magnesium salicylate (i.e., Salflex, Disalcid, or Trilisate). They are the drugs of choice if there is renal insufficiency. They have minimal interference with anticyclooxygenase and other prostaglandins.

Additionally, they will not impair platelet inhibition of those patients who are on every other day aspirin to decrease their risk for stroke or heart disease. Unlike aspirin, they do not increase the formation of products of lipoxygenase-mediated metabolism of arachidonic acid. For this reason, they may be less likely to precipitate hypersensitivity reactions. These drugs have been safely used for patients with reversible obstructive airway disease and a history of aspirin sensitivity.

They also are much gentler on the stomach than the other NSAIDs and are the drug of choice if the patient has problems with peptic ulcer disease. Unfortunately, all these benefits are balanced by the fact they may not be as effective as the other agents and are less convenient to take. One needs to push them to 1.5-2 grams bid and tinnitus is a frequent complication.

One should warn patients of this complication and explain that if tinnitus does develop they need to stop the drugs for a day and restart with a dose that is half a pill per day lower. They repeat this until they find a dose that relieves their pain and doesn't give them any ringing in the ears.

Prednisone

One can give patients with severe disease a prescription for Prednisone 5 mg. They can take one of them a day if they develop a severe flare-up as a result of going on the antibiotics. They can use an additional tablet at night if they are in really severe flare. Explain to all patients that the Prednisone is very dangerous and every dose they take decreases their bone density. However, it is a trade-off. Since they will only be on it for a matter of months, its use may be justifiable. This is the first medicine they should try to stop as soon as their symptoms permit.

Blood levels of cortisol peak between 3 a.m. and 9 a.m. It would, therefore, be safest to administer the Prednisone in the morning. This will minimize the suppression on the hypothalamic-pituitary-adrenal axis. Patients often ask the dangers of these medications. The most significant one is osteoporosis. Other side effects that usually occur at higher doses include adrenal insufficiency, atherosclerosis acceleration, cataract formation, Cushing's syndrome, diabetes, ulcers, herpes simplex and tuberculosis reactivation, insomnia, hypertension, myopathy, and renal stones.

One also needs to be concerned about the increased risk of peptic ulcer disease when using this medicine with conventional non-steroidal anti-inflammatories. Persons receiving both of these medicines may have a 15 times greater risk of developing an ulcer.

If a patient is already on Prednisone, it is helpful to give him a prescription for 1 mg tablets so he can wean himself off the Prednisone as soon as possible. Usually one lowers the dose by about 1 mg per week. If a relapse of the symptoms occurs, than further reduction of the Prednisone is not indicated.

Remission

The following criteria can help establish remission:

- A decrease in duration of morning stiffness to no more than 15 minutes
- No pain at rest
- Little or no pain or tenderness on motion
- Absence of joint swelling
- A normal energy level
- A decrease in the ESR to no more than 30
- A normalization of the patient's CBC. Generally the HGB, HCT, & MCV will increase to normal and his "pseudo"-iron deficiency will disappear
- ANA, RF, & ASO titers returning to normal

The natural course of rheumatoid arthritis is quite remarkable. Less than 1% of patients who are rheumatoid factor seropositive have a spontaneous remission. Some disability occurs in 50-70% of patients within five years after onset of the disease. Half of the patients will stop working within 10 years. This devastating natural prognosis is what makes the antibiotic therapy so exciting.

Approximately one third of patients have been lost to follow-up for whatever reason and have not continued with treatment. The remaining patients seem to have a 60-90% likelihood of improvement on this treatment regimen. That is quite a stark contrast to the numbers quoted above.

There are many variables associated with an increased chance of remission or improvement. The younger the patient is the better they seem to do. The more closely they follow the diet, the less likely they are to have a severe flare-up and the more likely they are to improve. Smoking seems to be negatively associated with improvement. The longer the patient has had the illness and the more severe the illness the more difficult it seems to treat.

If patients discontinue their medications before all of the above criteria are met, there is a greater risk that the disease will recur. If the patient meets the above criteria, one can have them to try to stop their anti-inflammatory medication once they start to experience these improvements. If the improvements are stable for six months, then discontinue the Clindamycin. If the improvements are maintained for the next six months, one can then discontinue their Minocin and monitor for recurrences. If symptoms should recur, it would be wise to restart the previous antibiotic regimen.

Overall, nearly 80% of the patients do remarkably better with this program. Approximately 5% of the patients continued to worsen and required conventional agents, like Methotrexate, to relieve their symptoms. Approximately 15% of the patients who started the treatment dropped out of the program and were lost to follow-up. The longer and more severe the illness, the longer it takes to cure. Smokers tend not to do as well with this program. Age and competency of the person's immune system are also likely important factors.

Dr. Brown successfully treated over 10,000 patients with this protocol. He found that significant benefits from the treatment require on the average one to two years. I have treated nearly over 2,000 patients and find that the dietary modification I advocate accelerates the response rate for several months. Most patients who follow the program actually notice improvement in their symptoms in a few weeks. The length of therapy can vary widely. In severe cases, it may take up to thirty months for the patients to gain sustained improvement. One requires patience because remissions may take up to 3 to 5 years. Dr. Brown's pioneering approach represents a safer less toxic alternative to many conventional regimens and results of the NIH trial have finally scientifically validated this treatment.

Preliminary Laboratory Evaluation for Non-Rheumatologists

It is important to evaluate patients to determine if indeed they have rheumatoid arthritis. Most patients will have received evaluations and treatment by one or more board certified rheumatologists. If this is the case, the diagnosis is rarely in question and one only needs to establish some baseline laboratory data.

However, patients will frequently come in without having any appropriate workup done by a physician. Arthritic pain can be an early manifestation of 20-30 different clinical problems. These include not only rheumatic disease, but also metabolic, infectious and malignant disorders. These patients will require a more extensive laboratory analysis.

Rheumatoid arthritis is a clinical diagnosis for which there is not a single test or group of laboratory tests which can be considered confirmatory. When a patient hasn't been properly diagnosed, one needs to establish the diagnosis with the standard Rheumatism Association's criteria found at the end of this Appendix.

One must also make certain that the first four symptoms listed in the table are present for six or more weeks. These criteria have a 91-94% sensitivity and 89% specificity for the diagnosis of rheumatoid arthritis. However, these criteria were designed for classification and not for diagnosis. One must make the diagnosis on clinical grounds. It is important to note that many patients with negative serologic tests can have a strong clinical picture for rheumatoid arthritis.

The metacarpophalangeal joints, proximal inter-phalangeal and wrists joints are the first joints to become symptomatic. In a way, the hands are the calling card of rheumatoid arthritis. If the patient completely lacks hand and wrist involvement, even by history, the diagnosis of rheumatoid arthritis is doubtful. Rheumatoid arthritis rarely affects the hips and ankles early in its course.

Fatigue may be present before the joint symptoms begin. Morning stiffness is a sensitive indicator of rheumatoid arthritis. An increase in fluid in and around the joint probably causes the stiffness. The joints are warm, but the skin is rarely red.

When the joints develop effusions, the patients holds them flexed at 5 to 20 degrees, as it is too painful to extend them fully.

The general initial laboratory evaluation should include a baseline ESR, CBC, SMA, U/A, and an ASO titer. One can also draw RF and ANA titers to further objectively document improvement with the therapy. However, they seldom add much to the assessment.

Follow-up visits can be every two months for patients who live within 50 miles, and every three to four months for those who live farther away. An ESR at every visit is an inexpensive and reliable objective parameter of the extent of the disease. However, one should run this test within several hours of the blood draw. Otherwise, one cannot obtain reliable and reproducible results. This is nearly impossible with most clinical labs that pick up your specimen at the office.

Inexpensive disposable ESR kits are a practical alternative to the commercial or hospital labs. One can then run them in the office, usually within one hour of the blood draw. One must be careful to not run the test on the same countertop as your centrifuge. This may cause a falsely elevated ESR due to the agitation of the ESR measuring tube.

Many patients with rheumatoid arthritis have a hypochromic, microcytic CBC. This is probably due to the inflammation in the rheumatoid arthritis impairing optimal bone marrow utilization of iron. This type of anemia does NOT respond to iron.

Patients who take iron can actually worsen if they don't need it as the iron serves as a potent oxidant stress. Ferritin levels are generally the most reliable indicator of total iron body stores. Unfortunately it is also an acute phase reactant protein and will be elevated anytime the ESR is elevated. This makes ferritin an unreliable test for patients with rheumatoid arthritis.

Fibromyalgia

One needs to be very sensitive to this clinical problem when treating patients with rheumatoid arthritis. It is frequently a complicating condition. Many times, patients will confuse the pain from it with a flare-up of their arthritis. One needs to aggressively treat this problem. If this problem is ignored, the likelihood of successfully treating the arthritis is significantly diminished.

Fibromyalgia is a very common problem. Some experts believe that 5% of people are affected with it. Over 12% of the patients at the Mayo Clinic's Department of Physical Medicine and Rehabilitation have this problem. It is the third most common diagnosis by rheumatologists in the outpatient setting. Fibromyalgia affects women five times as frequently as men.

Signs and Symptoms of Fibromyalgia

One of the main features of Fibromyalgia is the morning stiffness, fatigue, and multiple areas of tenderness in typical locations. Most patients with Fibromyalgia complain of pain over many areas of the body, with an average of six to nine locations. Although the pain is frequently described as being all over, it is most prominent in the neck, shoulders, elbows, hips, knees, and back.

Tender points are generally symmetrical and on both sides of the body. The areas of tenderness are usually small (less than an inch in diameter) and deep within the muscle. They are often located in sites that are slightly tender in normal people. Patients with Fibromyalgia, however, differ in having increased tenderness at these sites than normal persons. Firm palpation with the thumb (just past the point where the nail turns white) over the outside elbow will typically cause a vague sensation of discomfort. Patients with Fibromyalgia will experience much more pain and will often withdraw the arm involuntarily.

More than 70% of patients describe their pain as profound aching and stiffness of the muscles. Often it is relatively constant from moment to moment, but certain positions or movements may momentarily worsen the pain. Other terms used to describe the pain are dull and numb. Sharp or intermittent pain is relatively uncommon. Patients with Fibromyalgia often complain that sudden loud noises worsen their pain. The generalized stiffness of Fibromyalgia does not diminish with activity, unlike the stiffness of rheumatoid arthritis, which lessens as the day progresses.

Despite the lack of abnormal lab tests, patients can suffer considerable discomfort. The fatigue is often severe enough to impair activities of work and recreation. Patients commonly experience fatigue on arising and complain of being more fatigued when they wake up then when they went to bed. Over 90% of patients believe that pain, stiffness, and fatigue are made worse by cold, damp weather. Overexertion, anxiety and stress are also factors. Many people find that localized heat, such as hot baths, showers, or heating pads, give them some relief. There is also a tendency for pain to improve in the summer with mild activity or with rest.

Some patients will date the onset of their symptoms to some initiating event. This is often an injury, such as a fall, a motor vehicle accident, or a vocational or sports injury. Others find that their symptoms began with a stressful or emotional event, such as a death in the family, a divorce, a job loss, or similar occurrence.

Pain Location

Patients with Fibromyalgia have pain in at least 11 of the following 18 tender point sites (one on each side of the body):

1. Base of the skull where the suboccipital muscle inserts.
2. Back of the low neck (anterior intertransverse spaces of C5-C7).
3. Midpoint of the upper shoulders (trapezius).
4. On the back in the middle of the scapula.
5. On the chest where the second rib attaches to the breastbone (sternum).
6. One inch below the outside of each elbow (lateral epicondyle).
7. Upper outer quadrant of buttocks.
8. Just behind the swelling on the upper leg bone below the hip (trochanteric prominence).

9. The inside of both knees (medial fat pads proximal to the joint line).

Treatment of Fibromyalgia

There is a persuasive body of emerging evidence that indicates that patients with Fibromyalgia are physically unfit in terms of sustained endurance. Some studies show that cardiovascular fitness training programs can decrease Fibromyalgia pain by 75%. Sleep is critical to the improvement. Many times, improved fitness will correct the sleep disturbance.

Allergies, especially to mold, seem to be another common cause of Fibromyalgia. There are some simple interventions using approaches called Emotional Freedom Technique (EFT) and Neurostructural Therapy (NST) described in Chapter 7 of this book. These methods have proved be helpful in rapidly resolving the problem.

Exercise For Rheumatoid Arthritis

It is very important to exercise or increase muscle tone of the non-weight bearing joints. Experts tell us that disuse results in muscle atrophy and weakness. Additionally, immobility may result in joint contractures and loss of range of motion (ROM). Active ROM exercises are preferred to passive. There is some evidence that passive ROM exercises increase the number of WBCs in the joint. If the joints are stiff, one should stretch and apply heat before exercising. If the joints are swollen, application of ice for ten minutes before exercise would be helpful.

The inflamed joint is very vulnerable to damage from improper exercise, so one must be cautious. People with arthritis must strike a delicate balance between rest and activity. They must avoid activities that aggravate joint pain. Patients should avoid any exercise that strains a significantly unstable joint.

A good rule of thumb is that if the pain lasts longer than one hour after stopping exercise, the patient should slow down or choose another form of exercise. Assistive devices are also helpful to decrease the pressure on affected joints. Many patients need to be urged to take advantage of these. The Arthritis Foundation has a book, *Guide to Independent Living*, which instructs patients about how to obtain them.

Of course, it is important to maintain good cardiovascular fitness. Walking with appropriate supportive shoes is also another important consideration.

The Infectious Cause of Rheumatoid Arthritis

It is quite clear that autoimmunity plays a major role in the progression of rheumatoid arthritis. Most rheumatology investigators believe that an infectious agent causes rheumatoid arthritis. There is little agreement as to the involved organism. Investigators have proposed the following infectious agents: Human T-cell lymphotropic virus Type I, rubella virus, cytomegalovirus, herpes virus, and mycoplasma. This review will focus on the evidence supporting the hypothesis that mycoplasma is a common etiologic agent of rheumatoid arthritis.

Mycoplasmas are the smallest self-replicating prokaryotes. They differ from classical bacteria by lacking rigid cell wall structures and are the smallest known organisms capable of extracellular existence. They are considered to be parasites of humans, animals, and plants.

In 1939, Dr. Sabin, the discoverer of the polio vaccine, first reported a chronic arthritis in mice caused by a mycoplasma. He suggested this agent might cause that human rheumatoid arthritis. Dr. Thomas Brown was a rheumatologist who worked with Dr. Sabin at the Rockefeller Institute. Dr. Brown trained at John Hopkins Hospital and then served as chief of medicine at George Washington Medical School before serving as chairman of the Arthritis Institute in Arlington, Virginia. He was a strong advocate of the mycoplasma infectious theory for over fifty years of his life.

Culturing Mycoplasmas from Joints

Mycoplasmas have limited biosynthetic capabilities and are very difficult to culture and grow from synovial tissues. They require complex growth media or a close parasitic relation with animal cells. This contributed to many investigators failure to isolate them from arthritic tissue. In reactive arthritis immune complexes rather than viable organisms localize in the joints. The infectious agent is actually present at another site. Some investigators believe that the organism binding in the immune complex contributes to the difficulty in obtaining positive mycoplasma cultures.

Despite this difficulty some researchers have successfully isolated mycoplasma from synovial tissues of patients with rheumatoid arthritis. A British group used a leukocyte-migration inhibition test and found two-thirds of their rheumatoid arthritis patients to be infected with *Mycoplasma fermentans*. These results are impressive since they did not include more prevalent Mycoplasma strains like *M salivarium, M ovale, M hominis, and M pneumonia*.

One Finnish investigator reported a 100% incidence of isolation of mycoplasma from 27 rheumatoid synovia using a modified culture technique. None of the non- rheumatoid tissue yielded any mycoplasmas. The same investigator used an indirect hemagglutination technique and reported mycoplasma antibodies in 53% of patients with definite rheumatoid arthritis. Using similar techniques other investigators have cultured mycoplasma in 80-100% of their rheumatoid arthritis test population.

Rheumatoid arthritis follows some mycoplasma respiratory infections. One study of over 1000 patients was able to identify arthritis in nearly 1% of the patients. These infections can be associated with a positive rheumatoid factor. This provides additional support for mycoplasma as an etiologic agent for rheumatoid arthritis. Human genital mycoplasma infections have also caused septic arthritis.

Harvard investigators were able to culture mycoplasma or a similar organism, *Ureaplasma urealyticum*, from 63% of female patients with SLE and only 4% of patients with CFS. The researchers chose CFS as these patients shared similar symptoms as those with SLE, such as fatigue, arthralgias, and myalgias.

Animal Evidence for the Protocol

The full spectrum of human rheumatoid arthritis immune responses (lymphokine production, altered lymphocyte reactivity, immune complex deposition, cell-mediated immunity and devel-opment of autoimmune reactions) occurs in mycoplasma induced animal arthritis. Investigators have implicated at least 31 different mycoplasma species. Myco-plasma can produce experimental arthritis in animals from three days to months later. The time seems to depend on the dose given and the virulence of the organism.

There is a close degree of similarity between these infections and those of human rheumatoid arthritis. Mycoplasmas cause arthritis in animals by several mechanisms. They either directly multiply within the joint or initiate an intense local immune response. Mycoplasma produces a chronic arthritis in animals that is remarkably similar to rheumatoid arthritis in humans. Arthritogenic mycoplasmas cause joint inflammation in animals by many mechanisms. They induce nonspecific lymphocyte cytotoxicity and antilymphocyte antibodies as well as rheumatoid factor. Mycoplasma clearly causes chronic arthritis in mice, rats, fowl, swine, sheep, goats, cattle and rabbits. The arthritis appears to be the direct result of joint infection with culturable mycoplasma organisms.

Gorillas have tissue reactions closer to man than any other animal. Investigators have shown that mycoplasma can precipitate a rheumatic illness in gorillas. One study demonstrated mycoplasma antigens occur in immune complexes in great apes. The human and gorilla IgG are very similar and express nearly identical rheumatoid factors (IgM anti-IgG antibodies). The study showed that when mycoplasma binds to

IgG it can cause a conformational change. This conformational change results in an anti-IgG antibody, which can then stimulate an autoimmune response.

The Science of Why Minocycline Is Used

If mycoplasma were a causative factor in rheumatoid arthritis, one would expect tetracycline-type drugs to provide some sort of improvement in the disease. Collagenase activity increases in rheumatoid arthritis and probably has a role in its cause. Investigators demonstrated that tetracycline and minocycline inhibit leukocyte, macrophage, and synovial collagenase.

There are several other aspects of tetracyclines that may play a role in rheumatoid arthritis. Investigators have shown minocycline and tetracycline to retard excessive connective tissue breakdown and bone resorption (dissolution) while doxycycline inhibits digestion of human cartilage. It is also possible that tetracycline treatment improves rheumatic illness by reducing delayed-type hypersensitivity response. Both Minocycline and doxycycline inhibit phosolipases, which are considered proin-flammatory and capable of inducing synovitis.

Minocycline is a more potent antibiotic than tetracycline and penetrates tissues better. These characteristics shifted the treatment of rheumatic illness away from tetracycline to minocycline. Minocycline may benefit rheumatoid arthritis patients through its immunomodulating and immunosuppressive properties. *In vitro* studies demonstrated a decreased neutrophil production of reactive oxygen intermediates along with diminished neutrophil chemotaxis and phagocytosis.

Investigators showed that minocycline reduced the incidence of severity of synovitis in animal models of arthritis. The improvement was independent of minocycline's effect on collagenase. Minocycline has also been shown to increase intracellular calcium concentrations that inhibit T-cells.

Individuals with the Class II major histocompatibility complex (MHC) DR4 allele seem to be predisposed to developing rheumatoid arthritis. The infectious agent probably interacts with this specific antigen in some way to precipitate rheumatoid arthritis. There is strong support for the role of T-cells in this interaction. Minocycline may suppress rheumatoid arthritis by altering T-cell calcium flux and the expression of T-cell derived from collagen binding protein.

Minocycline produced a suppression of the delayed hypersensitivity in patients with Reiter's syndrome. Investigators also successfully used minocycline to treat the arthritis and early morning stiffness of Reiter's syndrome.

Clinical Studies

In 1970 investigators at Boston University conducted a small, randomized placebo-controlled trial to determine if tetracycline would treat rheumatoid arthritis. They used 250 mg of tetracycline a day. Their study showed no improvement after one year of tetracycline treatment. Several factors could explain their inability to demonstrate any benefits. Their study used only 27 patients for a one-year trial, and only 12 received tetracycline. Noncompliance could have been a factor. Additionally, none of the patients had severe arthritis. Patients were excluded from the trial if they were on any anti-remittive therapy.

Finnish investigators used lymecycline to treat the reactive arthritis in *Chlamydia trachomatous* infections. The study compared the effect of the medication in patients with two other reactive arthritis infections Yersinia and Campylobacter. Lymecyline produced a shorter course of illness in the Chlamydia-induced arthritis patients, but did not affect the other enteric infections-associated reactive arthritis. The investigators later published findings that suggested lymecycline achieved its effect through non-antimicrobial actions. They speculated it worked by preventing the oxidative activation of collagenase.

Breedveld published the first trial of minocycline for the treatment of animal and human rheumatoid arthritis. In the first published human trial, Breedveld treated ten patients in an open study for 16 weeks. He used a very high dose of 400 mg per day.

Most patients had vestibular side effects resulting from this dose.

However, all patients showed benefit from the treatment. All variables of efficacy were significantly improved at the end of the trial. Breedveld concluded an expansion of his initial study and observed similar impressive results. This was a 26-week double-blind placebo-controlled randomized trial with minocycline for 80 patients. They were given 200 mg twice a day. The Ritchie articular index and the number of swollen joints significantly improved ($p < 0.05$) more in the minocycline group than in the placebo group.

Investigators in Israel studied 18 patients with severe rheumatoid arthritis for 48 weeks. These patients had failed two other DMARDs. They were taken off all DMARD agents and given minocycline 100 mg twice a day. Six patients did not complete the study, three withdrew because of lack of improvement, and three had side effects of vertigo or leuko-penia.

All patients completing the study improved. Three had complete remission, three had substantial improvement of greater than 50% and six had moderate improvement of 25% in the number of active joints and morning stiffness.

Criteria for Classification of Rheumatoid Arthritis

- Morning Stiffness: Morning stiffness in and around joints lasting at least one hour before maximal improvement is noted.
- Arthritis of three or more joint areas: At least three joint areas have simultaneously had soft-tissue swelling or fluid (not bony overgrowth) observed by a physician. There are 14 possible joints: right or left PIP, MCP, wrist, elbow, knee, ankle, and MTP joints.
- Arthritis of hand joints: At least one joint area swollen as above in a wrist, MCP, or PIP joint

- Symmetric arthritis: Simultaneous involvement of the same joint areas (as in criterion 2) on both sides of the body (bilateral involvement of PIPs, MCPs, or MTPs) is acceptable without absolute symmetry. Lack of symmetry is not sufficient to rule out the diagnosis of rheumatoid arthritis.
- Rheumatoid Nodules: Subcutaneous nodules over bony prominences, or extensor surfaces, or in juxta-articular regions, observed by a physician. Only about 25% of patients with rheumatoid arthritis develop nodules, and usually as a later manifestation.
- Serum Rheumatoid Factor: Demonstration of abnormal amounts of serum rheumatoid factor by any method that has been positive in less than 5% of normal control subjects. This test is positive only 30-40% of the time in the early months of rheumatoid arthritis.

Radiological Changes

Radiological changes typical of rheumatoid arthritis on PA hand and wrist X-rays, which must include erosions or unequivocal bony decalcification localized to or most marked adjacent to the involved joints (osteoarthritic changes alone do not count).

Note: Patients must satisfy at least four of the seven criteria listed. Any of criteria 1-4 must have been present for at least 6 weeks. Patients with two clinical diagnoses are not excluded. Designations as classic, definite, or probable rheumatoid arthritis is not to be made.

An extensive bibliography of over 200 references supporting this appendix may be found at www.mercola.com.

Appendix III:

DIETARY CONSIDERATIONS FOR PATIENTS WITH CHRONIC ILLNESSES AND MULTIPLE CHRONIC INFECTIONS

A Brief Outline of Eighteen Dietary Steps to Better Health

(Version current as of 8/2001)

by Prof. Garth L. Nicolson and Dr. Richard Ngwenya

The Institute for Molecular Medicine (Website www.immed.org)
15162 Triton Lane, Huntington Beach, CA 92649-1401

James Mobb Immune Enhancement
132 Josiah Chinamano Ave., Harare, Zimbabwe

There are a number of considerations when undergoing therapy for chronic illnesses, including whether to use allopathic or traditional Western medical approaches as well as integrative nutraceutical supplements and an appropriate diet. Paramount in these considerations is a patient's diet, irrespective of the type of therapy that is being used to control chronic illness. We have found that most chronic illness patients, including those with Chronic Fatigue Syndrome, Fibromyalgia Syndrome, Gulf War Illness, Rheumatoid Arthritis, Hepatitis, Diabetes, Coronary Diseases, Inflammatory Bowel Diseases, Autoimmune Diseases, HIV/AIDS, among other chronic illnesses, usually have poor diets that contribute significantly to their illnesses. Furthermore, we have found that patients that refuse to change their dietary habits usually do not recover from their illnesses. Thus diet is extremely important, and chronic illness patients must follow some simple procedures to correct their dysfunctional gastrointestinal tracts and restore proper nutrition to their bodies.

General Nutritional Considerations for Chronic Illness Patients

Chronic illness patients are often immunosuppressed or have dysfunctional immune systems and are susceptible to opportunistic infections, so proper nutrition is extremely important. Patients should not smoke or drink alcohol or caffeinated products, and should drink as much fresh fluids as possible, such as vegetable juices and pure water. High sugar and high fat foods, such as Military Ready to Eat (MRE) or other fast foods and acid-forming, allergen-prone and system-stressing foods and especially high sugar/fat junk foods should be avoided. Increased intake of fresh vegetables, some low-sugar fruits and grains, and decrease intake of saturated fats are useful. Note that *simple or refined sugars can suppress the immune system.* To build the immune system cruciferous vegetables, soluble fiber foods, such as prunes and bran, wheat germ, fish and whole grains are useful. Meat and fish can be consumed for protein, but it should be lean and well cooked. In some patients exclusive use of 'organic' foods has been beneficial, as these do not contain the levels of pesticides and chemicals as the usual commercial sources of foods.

The important points for chronic illness patients to remember are:

1. Do not eat sugar or high-sugar-containing foods. This is the number one problem in the diets of most chronic illness patients. Simple processed sugars can stimulate disease-causing microorganisms that require sugars for their growth. Pathogenic or disease-causing micro-organisms usually require simple sugars for their growth and are found in the overwhelming majority of chronic illness patients, so high sugar diets can actually stimulate their proliferation. For example, high sugar diets stimulate bacteria, yeast and fungal forms and even parasites, and patients eating processed sugars often show signs of thrush or yeast and bacteria on their tongue and at other places in and on their bodies, in their blood and in body secretions.

Since most untreated chronic illness patients have excessive levels of yeasts and other fungi, these can overwhelm the immune system and produce fatigue and other signs and symptoms. In addition to stimulating the overgrowth of yeasts and other fungi, simple sugars can also directly suppress the immune system. Examples of foods that are particularly stressing to chronic illness patients are carbonated drinks, cookies, biscuits, dried fruits, and any food that contains added sugar. Certain sugar substitutes can be used, but we recommend natural sugar substitutes, such as Stevia made from *Stevia rebaudiana* (for infor-mation call: 1-800-4STEVIA).

2. Do not consume caffeine. Caffeine can stimulate the growth of certain microorganisms and can change blood properties and stimulate certain biochemical pathways that are not helpful for chronic illness patients. In addition, excess caffeine can modify a patient's immune system and its ability to fight disease.

3. Reduce or eliminate milk products. Milk and milk products stimulate the growth of yeast and fungi. Milk also contains high amounts of sugar and fat, two dietary components that should be reduced in the diet of chronic illness patients. Sour milk or its products, such as yogurt, can be troublesome for some patients. We usually suggest that patients use supplementation with *Lactobacillus acidophilus* and other friendly bacteria (from 3-6 billion live organisms twice per day) to restore gastrointestinal balance. The gut contains approximately 2 kilograms of bacteria, and these bacteria are important in digestion and maintenance of a healthy gastrointestinal system. The use of friendly bacteria sup-plements is discussed in more detail below.

4. Reduce starch intake. Starches are broken down to simple sugars, and simple sugars as discussed above are not useful for chronic illness patients. Since starches are complex carbohydrates, they are broken down gradually to simple sugars, so some starch is not bad for chronic illness patients, but an attempt should be made to limit the amount of starches in any diet. Diets rich in pastas and breads should be avoided.

5. Increase intake of vegetables. Vegetables, especially green vegetables, are especially useful in helping to restore the food balance in chronic illness patients, because they contain important vitamins, minerals and fiber. They also tend to decrease the amounts of pathogenic bacteria and fungi in the gut because these mainly use simple sugars and lipids to grow. Vegetables also help cleanse the bowel by moving pathogenic bacteria and fungi through the gut. Eating lots of vegetables also increases bowel movements, and this can be beneficial to restoring the gut and removing toxins from the body.

6. Reduce intake of yeast-containing foods. High yeast breads, cheeses, and other milk products that contain yeast are not particularly useful for chronic illness patients because they add to the overall burden of yeast and fungi in the gut. Although the types of yeast in such food products are not pathogenic or disease causing, they can under certain circumstances overburden a fully taxed immune system and must be limited in any diet for chronic illness patients.

7. Increase intake of dietary fiber. Dietary fiber increases bowel movements and helps to remove harmful bacteria from the gastrointestinal system. Increasing the number of bowel movements per day is important in helping to remove partially digested food and bacteria from the gut. Most chronic illness patients have problems with constipation (producing small, hard stools). Increasing the number of bowel movements and their volumes are important. To help remove pathogenic bacteria from the bowel and bladder some recommend a non-dietary sugar, D-mannose (Biotech Co., 800-345-1199). This natural sugar inhibits binding of bacteria to biological membranes and does not contribute to bacterial sugar fermentation in the gut.

8. Eat small amounts every one and one-half to two-hours. Eating small amounts of food often, as much as every 1-1/2 hours is necessary to keep the stomach partially full so that stomach acid and bile will not be overproduced and irritate the gastrointestinal system. Eating small amounts of natural foods also aids in digestion and movement of digested food. The strategy is to never be hungry and have lots of fresh vegetables and other foods available all of the time.

9. Reduce the intake of cured or over-refined canned foods. These foods contain preservatives, nitrites and high levels of salt and curing substances. These can cause problems by irritating the gastro-intestinal lining, and nitrites can contribute to carcinogenesis. High salt levels are detrimental to maintaining normal blood pressure and homeostasis.

10. Eliminate alcohol and tobacco. Alcohol is converted to sugars and most alcoholic beverages contain high levels of sugar, such as beer, wine and other spirits. In addition to the problems with sugar discussed above, alcohol damages the nervous tissue (brain and peripheral nerves) and irritates the gastrointestinal lining. Some have recommended small amounts of alcohol, but we are against the use of alcohol in any form by chronic illness patients. Overuse of tobacco can result in emphysema, lung and thoracic cancers, high blood pressure, heart disease and other problems; so chronic illness patients should not use tobacco products in any form.

11. Increase water and juice intake. Purified water is a natural cleanser, and chronic illness patients usually do not drink enough water. They should be drinking the equivalent of 8 full glasses of water each day. Juices, especially vegetable juices are especially good sources of vitamins and minerals and other phytonutrients. Increased water intake is also good for bladder and urinary tract infections. Some have used dried cranberry (without the usual high levels of sugars) powder dissolved in water with natural sweeteners to cleanse the urinary tract of pathogenic bacteria.

We suggest the following approximate ratios of basic foods for chronic illness patients:

2/3 vegetables, such as fresh, uncooked (in moderation) or cooked (mostly) in-season green, orange and yellow vegetables, such as salads, squash, beans, etc. in vegetable oils (olive or sunflower are best), and juices made from vegetables. A wide variety of juices can be made with mixtures of various vegetables, and we recommend that these be taken as often as possible. Some fruit can be added, but most fruit contains sugars and acids, and so they must be used in moderation.

1/6 starch, such as whole grains, rice, non-yeast or low-yeast breads, oats, and other natural sources. Some intake of complex carbohydrates is not bad, because these will be broken down slowly to sugars in your body but they should not be a large part of any diet for chronic illness patients.

1/6 protein, such as chicken, fish and well-cooked lean meat. Beans are also a good source of protein. High protein foods are good, but they must be balanced with vegetables so that they do not remain for excessive times in the gut and cause constipation.

Of course, it is not always possible to follow completely the above suggestions, so moderation should be the rule. Since vegetables do not contain the calories that are present in most diets, most patients will gradually lose weight unless the quantities eaten are increased. This is why we recommend eating every 1-1/2 or 2 hours per day. Many professionals have recommended fruit juices for chronic illness patients, but these are often high in simple sugars so they must be used in moderation. For patients who are under-weight, we recommend that they eat substantial meals as often as possible and increase the amounts of protein. Teas (especially herbal), vegetable juices, water and soups should not be counted as substantial sources of any of the foods listed above and can be eaten at any time.

Vitamins and Minerals for Chronic Illness Patients

Chronic illness patients are often depleted in vitamins (especially B-complex, C, E, Co-Q_{10}) and certain minerals. The reason for this is that chronic illnesses often result in poor absorption. Therefore, high oral doses of some vitamins are useful; others, such as vitamin B-complex, cannot be easily absorbed by the gut (in oral dose form). Sublingual (under the tongue) natural B-complex vitamins in capsules or liquids (also injectable) should be used instead of swallowed capsules. B-complex vitamins are especially important in Chlamydia and Mycoplasma infected patients.

Patients should take a daily General Vitamin capsule, but they may have to supplement with extra vitamin B-complex and vitamins C and E, Co-Q_{10}, beta-carotene, folic acid and bioflavonoids. Some amino acids, such as L-cysteine, L-tyrosine and L-glutamine have been recommended for chronic illness patients, and L-carnitine and malic acid are reported to be useful. Also, it is useful to supplement with oils that contain high amounts of 'omega' fatty acids, such as fish oils and flaxseed oils.

Certain minerals are depleted in chronic illness patients, such as zinc, magnesium, chromium and selenium. Some recommend up to 200 mcg/day sodium selenite, followed by lower doses. The best multivitamins come with extra antioxidants. If patients are on antibiotics for treatment of chronic infections, vitamins and minerals should not be taken at the same time of day as antibiotics. Vitamins and minerals should be taken 3 hours after antibiotics, because they can affect antibiotic absorption. Some recommend that antioxidant vitamins be taken at least 4 hours before or after oxygen therapy.

The suggested doses of vitamins can vary dramatically among patients; consult with your physician or nutritionist for appropriate dosage. Many chronic illness patients have excess heavy metals in their system, such as mercury, lead, cadmium and other heavy metals. For heavy metal removal, chelation therapy or certain oral products, such garlic supplements and oral chelation products have been shown to useful in many patients.

12. Add at least a multi-vitamin, sublingual vitamin B complex and Co-Q_{10} to the diet. As described above, most chronic illness patients are depleted in certain vitamins, and a multi-vitamin and B-complex vitamins and Co-Q_{10} will help restore this imbalance. Other supplements should be considered as well, such as certain amino acids, fish oils, etc. These are often low in chronic illness patients and must be increased by supplementation.

13. Add a mineral supplement if certain minerals are not present in a multi-vitamin. Zinc, magnesium, calcium, and especially selenium are often present in multivitamins, but the amounts may be too low for chronic illness patients. Some patients live in areas with especially low mineral content in the drinking water and soil, such as selenium, and they should always supplement these depleted minerals in the diet. Physicians or nutritionists need to make sure that patients are receiving the most optimal amounts of minerals.

14. Make sure that enough helpful lipids are being eaten, such as the lipids in fish or fish oils. Fish contain useful oils, such as omega-3 and omega-6 fatty acids, among others, and these have been shown to be beneficial for the heart and other organs. Flaxseed oils and some other oils can substitute for fish oils. These oils are healthy and should not be considered harmful or useless fats.

Replacement of Gut Flora and Digestive Enzymes

Patients undergoing treatment with antibiotics and other substances risk destruction of normal gut flora or friendly bacteria that provide important digestive enzymes for processing food in the gut. Antibiotic use depletes normal gut bacteria and can result in overgrowth of less desirable bacteria. To supplement bacteria in the gastrointestinal system, yogurt and especially live cultures of *Lactobacillus acidophilus* in capsules or powder are strongly recommended (at least 3-6 billion live organisms at least two or three times per day). Mixtures of *Lactobacillus acidophilus, L. bifidus, B. bifidus, L. bulgaricus* and FOS (fructoologo-saccharides) to promote growth of these probiotics in the gut are important. *L. acidophilus* mixtures (above 3 billion live organisms) should be taken three times per day.

For irritable bowel, certain mixtures of Chinese herbs have proven to be very effective in clinical trials. Another problem in chronic illness patients is the lack of digestive enzymes that can process foods to useful metabolites in the gut. We recommend a combination of natural digestive enzymes (usually from plant sources) plus antioxidants.

15. Take a probiotic supplement containing at least 3 billion live *Lactobacillus acidophilus* plus other 'friendly' bacteria at least twice per day. These supplements are available at most drug and food stores, but the best products are available in health food stores. Most recommend the mixtures of at least three different types of friendly bacteria, and these products are especially good for the gut.

16. Take a supplement of natural digestive enzymes that aid in digestion. These natural sources of digestive enzymes help digest food and make it available in a form that can be readily absorbed. These should be taken at least twice per day with meals to aid digestion, food uptake and help to minimize leaky gut problems that can introduce pathogenic bacteria into the blood.

Natural Immune Modulators and Natural Remedies

A number of natural remedies, such as ginseng root, herbal teas, lemon/olive drink, olive leaf extract with antioxidants are sometimes useful, especially during or after antibiotic therapy. More important examples are immune modulators, such as bioactive whey protein, oral transfer factors and plant glycans. Some additional remedies are olive leaf extract, lactoferrin, and some natural plant products or herbal mixtures. Good immune boosters have been isolated from certain mushroom extracts. These products have been used to enhance immune systems. Although they appear to help many patients, their clinical effectiveness in chronic illness patients has not been carefully evaluated, and in our experience patients show individual differences in responses to these nutraceutical supplements. They appear to be useful during therapy to stimulate the immune system or after antibiotic/antiviral therapy in a maintenance program to prevent relapse and opportunistic secondary infections.

17. Add an immune modulator and a natural remedy. Several types of immune modulators are listed above. Unfortunately, each patient is different and may respond differently to the many products that are on the market, so patients will have to decide with the advice of a health care provider what is best. Similarly, there are many natural remedies on the market, and although these are generally good for chronic illness patients, each patient is different and may respond disparately to different products. In some cases, foods can substitute for a portion of the natural remedies. For example, fresh garlic, olive leaf extract, oregano oil (in enteric-coated capsules), among others have been shown to be useful. Purified milk products, such as bioactive whey and transfer factors made from colostrum (mother's milk) are also useful for many patients and contain natural substances that suppress pathogenic organisms and stimulate the immune system. Mixtures of herbal formulations are especially useful and very popular as a method to boost immune responses.

Yeast/Fungal Overgrowth while on Antibiotics

Yeast overgrowth occurs often in chronic illness patients, especially in females (usually first seen as vaginal infections or thrush [white coating] on the tongue). Gynecologists recommend Nizoral, Diflucan, Sporanox, Mycelex, or anti-yeast creams. Metronidazole [Flagyl, Prostat] has been used to prevent fungal or parasite overgrowth or other antifungals [Nystatin, Amphotericin B, Fluconazole, Diflucan, Sporanox or Pau d' arco] have been administered for fungal infections that can occur while on antibiotics. Some patients have as their principal problem systemic fungal infections that can be seen using dark field microscopy of blood smears. For superficial fungal infections, such as fungal nail, topical antifungals are effective.

As mentioned above, *L. acidophilus* mixtures are used to restore gut flora. Bacterial overgrowth can also occur, for example, in between cycles of antibiotics or after antibiotics/antivirals have been stopped. Natural or nutraceutical approaches to controlling yeast infections include supplementation with the following formulations: Pau d' arco, grapefruit extract, olive leaf extract (most of these require at least 2 capsules 3X per day), caprylic acid, garlic extract and enteric-coated oregano oil. These can be found in health food stores, along with instructions on how they are used to control yeast and fungal infections. Diet is especially important in controlling yeast overgrowth, and the dietary instructions in this section should be followed, such as the elimination of most simple or refined sugars from the diet.

18. When necessary, take an anti-fungal medication or a natural yeast and fungal controlling remedy. Most chronic illness patients have trouble with yeast/fungal infections, and these must be controlled to permit recovery of the immune system. If the yeast or fungi are not excessive, the natural anti-fungal food supplements (Pau d' arco, grapefruit extract, olive leaf extract, caprylic acid, garlic extract or enteric-coated oregano oil) should be used first because they may be less stressing on the body, and they are certainly less expensive.

If the instructions above are followed, patients will start to notice a change in health within a short period of time. However, recovery from chronic illnesses is long, slow process, and patients should not be discouraged if cyclic periods of more and less severity of illness (morbidity) persist. Patients must decide to make diet an important part of their recovery, and the recommendations above are only a part of the program of recovery. We consider it unlikely that patients will recover from their chronic illnesses unless they change their diet and eating habits, so diet is as important as other factors in recovery.

For Further Information:
Professor Garth L. Nicolson, Ph.D.
The Institute for Molecular Medicine
15162 Triton Lane
Huntington Beach, CA 92649
Tel: (714) 903-2900

Note: this dietary protocol has been published in the online Townsend Letter. See www.tldp.com.

Selected References

Nicolson GL. "Considerations when undergoing treatment for chronic infections found in Chronic Fatigue Syndrome, Fibromyalgia Syndrome and Gulf War Illnesses (Part 1)." *International Journal of Medicine* 1998; 1:115-117.

Nicolson GL; Nasralla M; Franco AR; Erwin R; Nicolson NL; Ngwenya R and Berns, P. "Diagnosis and Integrative Treatment of Intracellular Bacterial Infections in Chronic Fatigue and Fibromyalgia Syndromes, Gulf War Illness, Rheumatoid Arthritis and other Chronic Illnesses." *Clinical Practice of Alternative Medicine* 2000;1(2): 92-102.

Tietelbaum, J. "Fighting those persistent infections in Chronic Fatigue Syndrome." *From Fatigued to Fantastic Newsletter* 2000 and 2001; 3(3) and 4(1).

Appendix IV:

WEBSITES FOR HEALTH-RELATED RESEARCH

The following pages contain pointers to useful resources on the Internet.

HOW TO USE THIS APPENDIX

Tables 6 and 7 represent Research attributes and Practical Resources of these sites, respectively. The first column in each table shows the website's top-level Home Page.

An "X" in a box for a given Home Page means that the information in that category is well worth reading. For example, the site www.stanford.edu has an "X" in the Arthritis and Lupus categories. Of course, much more than this specific information on a few illnesses is available on this Stanford University medical library site. It is just that for research pertinent to topics covered in this book, that set of data is judged to be authoritative and outstanding.

Note that this website also has an "X" in the box for "Autoimmune Diseases" and "Rheumatic Diseases." This means that the site is comprehensive, providing information on many other illnesses in those categories, too many to list individually.

Any site with an "X" in the "Topic Search" category has a local keyword search feature leading to subcategories of useful information within the site. The lack of an "X" does not mean to imply that the site has minimal data on a particular topic. It only means that the topic area was not fully explored as part of the research done for this book. The reader is encouraged to visit these websites and type in topic keywords of personal interest.

Certain websites, like that of Dr. Gabe Mirkin, are so stellar that an "X" appears in nearly every category.

[*continued on page 375*]

Table 6.

Research-related Websites: Home Pages

Site Name URL Address	Topic Search (TS)	Links to Other Great Sites (Lnks)	Studies, Journal Articles, Abstracts (S,J,A)	Pharmaceuticals, Prescription Drug Info (PPDI)	Case Histories (CH)	Alternative Medicine (AM)	Infectious Diseases (ID)	Mold, biofilms (M,B)	AIDS/HIV (HIV)	Multiple Sclerosis (MS)	Lyme Disease (LD)	Chronic Fatigue Syndrome (CFS)	Fibromyalgia (FM)	Autoimmune Diseases (AID)	Rheumatic Diseases (RD)	Arthritis (Arth)	Scleroderma (SD)	Lupus (Lup)	Allergy (Alrg)	Blood, Drug Research (BDR)	Mycoplasma Research (MR)	Treatment Protocols (TP)
www.albany.net/~tjc/hhv-6.html (HHV-6 linked to Multiple Sclerosis)			X				X		X	HHV-6											X	
www.aarda.org (RH Disease Ass'n)	X	X												X	X							
www.AllOneSearch.com (Multiple Search Engines)	X		Search FAQ																			
www.alternativemedicine.com	X		X			X																
www.altvetmed.com (Veterinary)	X	X	X	X		X													X			
www.arthritis.about.com (Extensive)	X	X	X	X		X								X	X	X						X
www.arthritis.org (ArthritisFoundat'n)	X	X		X												X						
www.arthritistrust.org	X	X	X		X		X								X	X						
www.biomedcentral.com	X		Many	X											X	X						
www.bloodbook.com (Great Online Blood Textbook)		X	All About Blood				X		X					X		X				X		
www.bowen.org (Pain/Stress)			X		X						X		X									

Site Name URL Address	TS	Lnks	S,J,A	PPDI	CH	AM	ID	M,B	HIV	MS	LD	CFS	FM	AID	RD	Arth	SD	Lup	Alrg	BDR	MR	TP
www.bulkmsm.com			X	MSM		X																
www.cbshealthwatch.com	X		Nutr'n			X	X		X					X	X	X			X			
www.cdc.gov (Disease Stats)	X	X	Vaccine		X		X		X		X									X		
www.chronicneurotoxins.com					X	X					X	X										X
www.clinicaltrials.gov	X		X				X	X	X	X	X	X	X	X	X	X	X	X	X		X	X
www.consumerlab.com (SafetyTests)	X		Warn'gs																			
www.drmirkin.com (Radio Host)	X	X	Archive	X		X	X		X	X	X	X	X	X	X	X	X	X	X	X	X	X
www.drweil.com (Author's Site)	X	X	Archive	X		X				X	X	X	X			X						
www.edstrom.com (WaterQual,biofilm)	X							X														
www.erc.montana.edu (biofilms)	X	X	Library					X														
www.fda.gov (Food/Drug Admin)	X		NewDvl.	Vaccine			X													X		X
www.gene.com (Genentech)	X		NewDvl.	X										X					X			
www.gene-chips.com (Multi-Tests)	X	X	X	X															X	X		
www.genomicsnews.com	X	X	X	X															X	X		
www.google.com (Best web-s'rch Site)	X	X	Images	X	X	X	X	X	X	X	X	X	X	X	X	X	X	X	X	X	X	X
www.healingwell.com (HealthBooks)	X	X	X			X			X	X	X	X	X		X	X		X	X			
www.healingwithnutrition.com	X			Vitamins		X	X				X	X		X	X	X		X				
www.healthfinder.gov (Resources, Dr's, Organizations)	X	X	X			X																
www.healthgrades.com (Resource)	X		X	Finder		X																
www.healthmall.com	X	X	Archive	Herbs		X																
www.healthwell.com (Drug-Nutrient Interactions)	X		Archive	Herbs		X			X	X	X		X	X	X	X		X	X	Chem		X
www.hemex.com (Blood Testing)	X		FAQ								X	X	X							X		X
www.herbalgram.org (American. Botanical Council)	X		Herbals			X								X	X							

Site Name URL Address	TS	Lnks	S,J,A	PPDI	CH	AM	ID	M,B	HIV	MS	LD	CFS	FM	AID	RD	Arth	SD	Lup	Alrg	BDR	MR	TP
www.herbmed.org (Herbal DataBase)	X	X	Archive	Herbals		X																
www.hopkins-arthritis.org (Clinic)	X	X	X		X				X	X	X		X	X	X	X	X	X	X			X
www.igenex.com (LD Testing)		X	X				X						X	X	X		X	X				
www.ilads.org (Intern'l LymeDis.Soc.)	X		Lyme	Tests	X		X				X	X		X						X		X
www.immed.org (Molecular Med.)	X		Multi-	Tests			X		X	X		X	X	X	X	X	X		X	X	X	X
www.immuno-sci-lab.com (Multi-PCR Tests via Site-map)	X	X	X	Tests			X					X		X					X	X	Tst	
www.intelihealth.com (Harvard M.Sch)	X		Archive	Refrnc.		X			X	X			X			X		X	X			X
http://jama.ama-assn.org	X		X				X		X	X	X	X	X	X	X	X	X	X	X	X		
www.lib.uiowa.edu/hardin/md (Links to Meta Directory)	X	X	X	X			X		X		X		X	X	X	X			X	X	X	
www.lymealliance.org (Support)	X	X	FAQ		X	X	X				X											X
www.lymenet.org (Libr.Abstracts)	X	X	Archive				X				X											
www.mayoclinic.com (Authoritative)	X		X	x			X	Fng	X	X	X	X	X	X	X	X	X	X	X		X	
www.mdlab.com (Multi-PCR Tests)	X	X	X	Tests							X	X							X	X	X	X
www.medscape.com (Medline+)	X	X	X	Vaccines	X	X	X	X	X	X	X	X	X	X	X	X	X	X	X	X	X	X
www.mentalhealthandillness.com	X	X	X				X				X					X						X
www.merckhomeedition.com	X		X	X		X	X	X	X		X			X	X	X			X	X	X	
www.mercola.com (Great Med Site)	X	X	X	X	X	X	X	X	X	X	X	X	X	X	X	X	X	X	X	X	X	X
www.miningco.com/health	X	X	Nutr'n	Herbs		X			X			X	X			X			X			
www.molecularstaging.com (PCR)			X	Tests															X	X	X	
www.muhealth.org (Univ.Med.Library)	X	X	D.Base	X		X			X													
www.naet.com (Allergic Therapy)			FAQ		X											X			X			X
www.navigator.tufts.edu (Links DB)	X	X	Nutr'n	Diet												X						
www.ncf.carleton.ca (Arthritis)	X	X	D.Base													X						

Site Name URL Address	TS	Lnks	S,J,A	PPDI	CH	AM	ID	M,B	HIV	MS	LD	CFS	FM	AID	RD	Arth	SD	Lup	Alrg	BDR	MR	TP
www.niaid.nih.gov (Infect. Diseases)	X	X	X	Vaccines			X	X	X		X			X					X	X	X	
www.ncbi .nlm.nih.gov/Entrez (Links NLM Genetic & Taxonomy Dbases)		Db	Multi-				X													X		
www.ncbi.nlm.nih.gov/ltbin-post/Taxonomy.... (NLM Taxonomy/ Genetic-sequence Dbase)		Db	Multi-				X													X		
www.nccam.nih.gov (FAQ, Dbase, Drug Trials)	X	X	FAQ F,D,T			X	X							X	X							
www.nih.gov (Natnl. Inst'ts Health)	X	X	FAQ											X	X							
www.nih.gov/icd/od (Directorate)	X	X	X																			
www.nlm.nih.gov PubMed, Medscape /Dbases, etc (National Library of Medicine)	X	X	Archive	D.Bases	X	X	X	X	X	X	X	X	X	X	X	X	X	X	X	X	X	X
www.nutriteam.com (Parasites, Mold)	X		Nutr'n	Vitamins			X	X											X		X	
www.nutritionreporter.com (Archive)	X	X	Lnks	Vitamins		X	X			X						X						
www.pdr.net (Physician'sDeskReference)	X	X	FAQ	Rerence												X			X			
www.pilates-studio.com DanceTherapy, mind-body training; like Tai Chi			FAQ Theory	Brain Chems		X										X						
www.pitsburgh.com (D.Base: Lookup-Terms = "Arthritis","infection", "Allergy", etc,)	X		D.Base	X			X									X			X			
www.puritan.com (Nutrit'n: Interact'n)	X		DrugsVs	Vitamins		X										X			X			
http://repro-med.net (Fertility)	X		X	X										X								
www.rheumatic.org (AntibioticTreatm't)		X	FAQ		X	X	X				X			X	X	X	X	X				X
www.rheumatology.org (Links)		X	Rheum.												X	X	X	X	X			
www.roadback.org (Dr Brown's Heritage)		X	FAQs	Anti-Biotic	X		X						X	X	X	X	X	X	X	X	X	X
www.scleroderma.org (Support)		X	X											X	X		X					

Site Name URL Address	TS	Lnks	S,J,A	PPDI	CH	AM	ID	M,B	HIV	MS	LD	CFS	FM	AID	RD	Arth	SD	Lup	Alrg	BDR	MR	TP
www.seniors.gov (Social Security Admin Links)	X	X	X													X						
www.shasta.com/cybermom (CFS/GWI)		X	FAQ		X		X		X			X	X	X	X				X	X	X	
www.stanford.edu (MedCenter Libr.)		X	Libr.	Health			X							X	X	X	X	X	X	X		
http://store.springnet.com (Drug Ref)			X	X																		
www.thearthritiscenter.com (In Riverside California)	X		Infect'n X	Anti-biotic	X	X	X	X	X	X	X	X	X	X	X	X	X	X	X	X	X	X
www.thecanadiandrugstore.com	X		FAQ	Drugs																		
www.the-thyroid-society.org		FAQs	X	X										X								
http://thyroid.about.com (Extensive)	X	X	X	X									X			X						
www.tldp.com (Townsend Letter)	X	X	X	X	X	X								X	X			X				
www.toxnet.nlm.nih.gov (Toxics Database)	X	X	X																	X		
www.uams.edu (U Ark Med Library)		X	Hlth.Lnk			X	X		X					X						X		
www.usda.gov (Dept of Agriculture)	X		X				X													X		
www.vm.cfsan.fda.gov/~mow/Intro.html (Bad Bug Book = Pathogenic Entities List)																						
www.webmd.com (Drugs & Herbs)	X	X	Library	D.base		X			X	X			X		X	X		X	X			
www.yahoo.com (Search Engine)	X	X	Search	X	X	X	X	X	X	X	X	X	X	X	X	X	X	X	X	X	X	X

[*continued from page 369*]

An overwhelming amount of information is available on the web, but not all of it is accurate or founded on solid scientific investigation. Some data is intentionally bogus, placed there by mean-spirited individuals to deceive or by others who crave attention.

Every effort has been made to distill the wheat from the chaff and to provide the reader with the cream of the Internet crop of credible health-related websites. This book is written for those who wish to take an active role in achieving good health. The more informed the patient, the better s/he is able to enter into a partnership with a health care provider. Dealing with illness then becomes a stronger, more focused team approach and the probability is increased for a positive, rewarding outcome.

Caution: Websites and information on sites are subject to change. Site names and URLs (Universal Resource Locator) listed here are sometimes case-sensitive. First look up the website directly to get the current, exact URL spelling. For categories of health interests, use a powerful search engine such as Google or Yahoo using well-chosen, definitive keywords. One simple keyword like "arthritis" or "lupus" will result in thousands of hits (i.e., websites located). Google will often prompt you about misspellings. Try to refine your search as much as possible with additional specific keywords.

Apologies are extended to the reader for any pointers that may have changed since this book went to print. The Internet is a dynamic and evolving resource. What appears in the following tables is a snapshot in time. Some websites, like Dr. Joseph Mercola's, are well established and continue to provide a wealth of information while other sites may be ephemeral.

However, the most important site an individual can visit is probably the office of a caring, physician who takes a holistic approach to treating patients.

Table 7. **Resource-related Websites: Home Pages**	Toxic Substances Data	Diseases \ Condition	Lab(s), Testing Info	Medicines / Treatments	Search by Query-term(s)	Doctor Query (email)	Frequently Asked Questions (FAQs)	Newsletter, Magazine	Health Books	Support / Interest Group(s)	Practitioner List	Alternative Medicine Site	Nutrition, Diet	Vitamins, Herbs	General Health, Fitness	University Site	Medical Site	U.S. Government Site	Non-profit, Foundation	Commercial Site
Web-site URL Address / (Comment)	Txx	Dis	LT	Med	Qry	DrQ	FAQ	NL	HB	Sprt	PL	Alt	ND	VH	HF	U.S	Med	Gov	NFP	Com
www.albany.net/~tjc/hhv-6.html		MS			X		HHV -6												X	
www.aarda.org (Rheumatic Disease Ass'n)		X	X		X		x	X	X										X	
www.AllOneSearch.com (Multiple-Qrys)		X			X															
www.alternativemedicine.com		X		X	X		x	X	X			X	X	X	X					X
www.altvetmed.com Veterinary Alt med		X		X	X		X			X		X	X		X					
www.amazon.com (Books Sales)		X		X	X		Lnk		X						X					
www.arthritis.about.com	X	X		X	X		Mult						X	X	X		X			
www.arthritis.org (Arthritis Foundation)		X			X		X	X	X	X				X					X	X
www.arthritistrust.org		X			X		X	X			X								X	
www.biomedcentral.com	X	X		X	X		X					X	X	X	X		X			X

Web-site URL Address / (Comment)	Txx	Dis	LT	Med	Qry	DrQ	FAQ	NL	HB	Sprt	PL	Alt	ND	VH	HF	U.S	Med	Gov	NFP	Com
www.bowen.org (Pain/Stress Mgt)		X	X	X			X								X		X		X	
www.bulkmsm.com (MSM Info)				X			X						X	X			X			X
www.cbshealthwatch.com		X		X	X		Mult	X	X			X	X	X	X		X			X
www.cdc.gov (Disease Control & Statistics)	X	S		X			X											X		
www.chronicneurotoxins.com	X	X	X	X		Fee	X		X		X						X			X
www.clinicaltrials.gov (Trials Dbase)	X	X		X	X		Lnk										X	X		
www.cyberanalysis.com (Psychologists)						Fee				X	X						X			X
www.drmirkin.com (Radio Host)	X	X		X	X	X	Mult	X				X	X	X	X		X			
www.drweil.com (Author's site)		X		X	X	X	Mult	X	X			X			X	X	X			
www.edstrom.com (Water Qual., Biofilms)			X				X													X
www.erc.montana.edu (Biofilms)	X						Lnk	X								X				
www.fda.gov (Food & Drug Agency)	X	X		X	X		X	X					X	X	X		X	X		
www.gene-chips.com (Multi-Tests)			X				X										X			X
Web-site URL Address / (Comment)	Txx	Dis	LT	Med	Qry	DrQ	FAQ	NL	HB	Sprt	PL	Alt	ND	VH	HF	U.S	Med	Gov	NFP	Com
www.genomicsnews.com			X		FAC		X	X					X							X
www.google.com (Best Web Queries)	X	X	X	X	X		X		X		X	X	X	X	X					X
www.healingwell.com (Books)		X		X	X		X	X	X	X		X								X
www.healingwithnutrition.com Vitamins		X		X	X		Mult					X	X	X	X	X				
www.healthfinder.gov (Practitioners)		X	X	X	Lnk		X				Lnk	X			X			X		
www.healthgrader.com (Locator)							X				X	X								
www.healthwell.com (Herbs)		X			X		X			X		X	X	X	X					X
www.healthy.net (Medline)		X			X		X	X	X			X		X	X					X
www.herbalgram.org (Am Bot. Counc'l)				X	X		X		X			X		X					X	

Web-site URL Address / (Comment)	Txx	Dis	LT	Med	Qry	DrQ	FAQ	NL	HB	Sprt	PL	Alt	ND	VH	HF	U.S	Med	Gov	NFP	Com
www.herbmed.com (Herbals Dbase)					X		Herb					X		X	X				X	
www.hopkins-arthritis.org (Clinic)		X		X	X		X							X		X	X			
www.igenex.com (LD Blood Tests)		X	X				Lnk				X						X			X
www.ilads.org (Int'nl Lyme Dis.Assn)		X	X		X		X			X	X						X			X
www.immed.org (Molecular Med)		X	X		X		X				X						X			X
www.immuno-sci-lab.com (Multi-PCR)		X	X		X		X				X						X			X
www.intelihealth.com (Harvard Medical School)		X	X	X	X	X	X		X				X	X	X		X			X
http://jama.ama-assn.org		X		X	X		x	X			X						X		X	
www.lib.uiowa.edu/hardin/md (Links to Meta Directory)	X	X	X		X		Libr		X						X	X	X			
www.lymealliance.org		X		X	X		X	X											X	
www.lymenet.org (Library Abstracts)		X		X	X		Arch	X		X							X		X	
Web-site URL Address / (Comment)	Txx	Dis	LT	Med	Qry	DrQ	FAQ	NL	HB	Sprt	PL	Alt	ND	VH	HF	U.S	Med	Gov	NFP	Com
www.mayoclinic.com (Authoritative Info)	X	X	X	X	X	X	Arch	X							X		X			
www.mdlab.com (Multi-PCR Tests)		X	X	X	X		Lnk				X						X			
www.medscape.com (NLM Portal)	X	X		X	X		Multi	X		X	X		X				X	X		
www.merckhomeedition.com		X		X	Lnk		Mult		X		X						X			X
www.mercola.com (Great Medical Site)	X	X	X	X	X	X	Arch	X	X		X	X	X	X	X		X			
www.miningco.com/health (Herbs)				X	X		Nut.					X	X	X	X					X
www.muhealth.org/~arthritis (Dbase)		X	X	X	X		Lnk		X					X	X	X				
www.naet.com (AllergyTreatments)		X	X		Lnk		X	X	X	X	X	X	X	X	X		X			X
www.navigator.tufts.edu (Diet Nutr Sites)					Lnk		Lnk					X	X	X	X	X				
www.ncf.carleton.ca (Gen.Topic Srch)					X					X						X				

Web-site URL Address / (Comment)	Txx	Dis	LT	Med	Qry	DrQ	FAQ	NL	HB	Sprt	PL	Alt	ND	VH	HF	U.S	Med	Gov	NFP	Com
www.niaid.nih.gov (Allergy & Infectious Diseases)		X		X	X		X										X	X		
http://nccam.nih.gov (FAQ, Dbase, Drug Trials)		X		X	X		FAQ										X	X		
www.nlm.nih.gov (Archiv. Dbases, Abstr., Journals @ N'l Library of Medicine)	X	X		X	X		FAQ	X	X			X		X	X		X	X		
www.nutriteam.com (Mold, Parasites)	X	X		X	X		FAQ	X				X	X	X						X
www.nutritionreporter.com (Vitamins)		X		X			Arch	X				X	X	X	X		X			
www.pdr.net (Physician's Desk Referen.)	X	X		X	Lnk		Mult		X						X		X			X
www.pilates-studio.com (Dance) Mind-Body Training : Like Tai Chi							X					X			X				X	X
www.pittsburgh.com (Gen Srch Eng.)					X		Topic													X
www.puritan.com (Drugs vs Vitamin Interactions)		X			X		X	X				X	X	X						X
Web-site URL Address / (Comment)	Txx	Dis	LT	Med	Qry	DrQ	FAQ	NL	HB	Sprt	PL	Alt	ND	VH	HF	U.S	Med	Gov	NFP	Com
http://repro-med.net (Infertility)			X								X					X	X			
www.rheumatic.org (Antibiotic Treatment)		X		X			X		X	X				X			X		X	
www.rheumatology.org (Rheumatologists)		X			Lnk		X	X	X		X					X	X		X	
www.roadback.org (Dr Brown's heritage)		X		X			X		X	X							X		X	
www.rxlist.com (Drug Data base)				X	Db	X	X													
www.scleroderma.org (Help Site)		X		X	FAQ		X	X		X							X		X	
www.seniors.gov (Soc. Sec. Admin, Lnks)		X		X	X		X	X			X	X		X	X			X		
www.shasta.com/cybermom (CFS/GWI)	Lnk	X	Lnk	X	FAQ		X			X							X		X	
www.stanford.edu (Medical Library)		X	X	X	X		Lnk				X		X	X	X	X	X			

Web-site URL Address / (Comment)	Txx	Dis	LT	Med	Qry	DrQ	FAQ	NL	HB	Sprt	PL	Alt	ND	VH	HF	U.S	Med	Gov	NFP	Com
http://store.springnet.com (Drug Ref.)	X	X		X					X								X			X
www.thearthritiscenter.com (Clinic)	X	X	X	X		X	X				X	X	X				X			
www.thecanadiandrugstore.com				X			X													X
www.the-thyroid-society.org	X	X		X			X		X	X							X		X	
http://thyroid.about.com (Comprehensive)	X	X	X	X	X		X				X		X	X			X			X
www.toxnet.nlm.nih.gov (Toxin Dbase)	X				X		x													
www.tldp.com (Townsend Letter)		X	X	X			Arts	X				X	X	X	X		X			
www.uams.edu (Medical Library)		X	X	X	X		Lnk				X		X	X	X	X				
www.usda.gov (Veterinary, Food)		X	X		X		Lnk						X					X		
www.yahoo.com (Web Search Engine)	X	X	X	X	X		Multi		X			X	X	X	X					X

Appendix V:

OUTLINE OF AN EATING PROGRAM FOR OPTIMAL WELLNESS

The following information took me over 8 years to compile and is still evolving. I have used it successfully for tens of thousands of patients in my office and hundreds of thousands of people on the Internet.

What appears below is a very brief outline of my proven Eating Program. The longer, detailed version of the Program can be found at www.mercola.com/forms/wellness_condensed.htm. If you follow all the hyperlinks (blue underlines) on this site you will find the equivalent of a 300-page book. Nearly half of the detailed guidelines are based on the collected experiences of the people I have cared for. The program evolves as new information is obtained and added.

This nutritional program does produce immediate benefit in everyone. I have found that it is necessary, but not necessarily sufficient for everyone. Healing is frequently quite complicated. I find that there are four pillars of healing: Biochemical (i.e., Nutritional), Structural, Spiritual, and Emotional. If the nutritional program is not working then the other pillars need to be addressed.

My nutritional program is a challenge to follow and requires a firm commitment. Frequently you will initially be a social outcast with most of your family and friends.

Conscientiously follow the program with all its cautions and most of you will see miracles occur within two weeks. The chronic health problems that you have suffered with for so long will be gone, as will be the need for the medications you have taken to control the symptoms.

Additionally, to help you follow the nutritional recommendations, my staff has compiled a 257-page cookbook that you can purchase for $15 over your computer. Download *The Low Grain, No Sugar Cookbook* to your computer from www.mercola.com. You receive the book immediately and there are no shipping or handling charges.

Dr. Joseph Mercola, D.O.

Eating Program (Outline)

GENERAL GUIDELINES:

AVOID:

Sugar: Limiting sugar is CRITICAL
Aspartame (NutraSweet or Equal)
Sucralose (Splenda)
Trans-fatty acids (all fried foods and margarine)
MSG (caution: may not be listed in ingredients)
All artificial preservatives and chemicals, if possible
Most all grains:
if you have indications of high insulin levels, such as overweight, high blood pressure, high cholesterol or diabetes, you should avoid ALL GRAINS, including rice, millet, spelt, oats, quinoa, teft, amaranth and grain-like foods like potatoes
Chewing gum:
- wastes digestive enzymes
- source of sugar or artificial sweetener
- Bananas and oranges: can be highly allergenic and high in sugars

Dried fruits, especially raisins; do not have more than three servings of fruit per day

VEGETABLES

Eat more vegetables -- the greener the better: kale, Swiss chard, collards, spinach, dandelion greens, green and red cabbage, broccoli, red and green leaf lettuce, romaine lettuce, endive, Chinese cabbage, bok choy, fennel, celery, cucumbers, cauliflower, zucchini, Brussels sprouts.

AVOID:

Iceberg lettuce (low nutritional value)
Carrots and underground (root) vegetables
Potatoes, beets (root vegetables that are high in sugar)
Corn, popcorn, corn chips/tortillas
recall that corn is a grain, not a vegetable
avoid any food that has corn in its top five ingredients

BEVERAGES

Water: spring water or filtered; well water is generally OK
Drink water at room temperature, not chilled or iced

Lemon juice can be added occasionally for flavor change
Amount needed: one quart for every 50 pounds of body weight
Juice: only freshly processed vegetable juice
Green tea (in limited amounts as high fluoride content may cause problems)

AVOID:
Tap water
Softened or distilled water
Coffee, tea, colas, diet drinks, store bought fruit juices
Milk (all forms, especially skim milk), cheese, ice cream)
Get vitamin D from supplements or sun exposure
Get calcium from green vegetables or supplements
No need for children to drink any milk after age of 2 years

PROTEIN

Meats:
Grass Fed
Poultry: chicken, turkey, ostrich
Game meats: venison, buffalo, lamb
Eggs: organic only (but only 3-4 times per week)
Seeds: (raw only) sunflower, pumpkin, sesame, flax
Nuts: (raw only) cashews, Brazil nuts, almonds, pecans, but in limited quantities

AVOID:
Pork: ham, most bacon, pork roast and chops
Shellfish: shrimp, lobster, crabs, clams
Peanuts

BEANS AND LEGUMES

Generally excellent but not a complete protein source
Soak beans (not lentils) for 48-72 hours, rinsing every 12 hours
Cook them for 8-12 hours in a crockpot

AVOID:
All soy unless fermented or sprouted
Tofu, soy protein
Only miso, tempeh and soy sprouts are acceptable

WARNING! The above diet outline will generally cause you to lose weight. If you do not want or need to lose weight you can increase the following foods: beans, squash, fruits, nuts, brown (not white) rice, millet and yams. Stop the rice and yams if original symptoms worsen.

Listen To Your Body

Stop consuming any food or supplement that makes you sick in some way. You may have an allergy to that substance. Use the reaction as a guide to determine what is right for YOUR body.

INDEX

RHEUMATOID ARTHRITIS: THE INFECTION CONNECTION

Conventional Rheumatoid Arthritis (RA) treatments include toxic drugs that reduce painful symptoms but do not treat the root cause—bacterial infection. An immune system weakened by addictive drugs (such as antidepressants or antihistamines), improper diet, stress, and multiple infections is unable to produce the quantity and quality of natural antibodies to stave off new attacks.

Infection by pathogenic microbes has been proven to be the cause of many chronic illnesses, including RA. This book describes the steps necessary to:

- Identify, attack, and remove the cause(s) of the infection(s);
- Neutralize wastes (toxins and other harmful enzymes) generated by pathogens;
- Flush these wastes from the body; and
- Restore the body's systems to normal, healthy function.

Until recently, testing methods to identify these micro-organisms precisely and to prescribe effective treatments have not been available. Traditional treatments with immuno-suppressing drugs often breed stronger, more resistant bacterial organisms, which mutate and grow, over-whelming the immune system's resources. Undiagnosed food and chemical allergies can also amplify the severity of arthritis symptoms.

In this book, both the lay reader and physician will find an effective course of treatment possibly leading to a cure for RA and other chronic illnesses with arthritis-like symptoms.

Please address all correspondence, including requests for quantity discounts to:

K. Poehlmann
RA Infection Connection
P.O. Box 7009
Torrance, CA 90504

Order Form

<u>Mail Orders</u>: Please send ____ copies of

Rheumatoid Arthritis: The Infection Connection to:

Name: ______________________________

Address: ______________________________

City: ______________________________

State, zip: ______________________________

(sorry, shipping to U.S. destinations only)

___ copies @ $ 14.95 ______

Sales Tax (California residents only) ______

First copy shipping: $4.00 ______

Additional shipping: $2.00 per copy ______

Total: ______

Send this Mail Order Form with check/money order (payable to K. Poehlmann) to:

RA Infection Connection
P.O. Box 7009
Torrance, CA 90504

Please allow ten days for checks to clear.
Bulk & special discounts available on request

To buy via the Internet, use GOOGLE query to locate a site selling this book:

GOOGLE [*Arthritis Poehlmann Infection Connection*]

Available on www.Amazon.com
and www.RA-Infection-Connection.com
Order in quantity via
Orders@RA-Infection-Connection.com

RHEUMATOID ARTHRITIS: THE INFECTION CONNECTION

Conventional Rheumatoid Arthritis (RA) treatments include toxic drugs that reduce painful symptoms but do not treat the root cause—bacterial infection. An immune system weakened by addictive drugs (such as antidepressants or antihistamines), improper diet, stress, and multiple infections is unable to produce the quantity and quality of natural antibodies to stave off new attacks.

Infection by pathogenic microbes has been proven to be the cause of many chronic illnesses, including RA. This book describes the steps necessary to:

- Identify, attack, and remove the cause(s) of the infection(s);
- Neutralize wastes (toxins and other harmful enzymes) generated by pathogens;
- Flush these wastes from the body; and
- Restore the body's systems to normal, healthy function.

Until recently, testing methods to identify these micro-organisms precisely and to prescribe effective treatments have not been available. Traditional treatments with immuno-suppressing drugs often breed stronger, more resistant bacterial organisms, which mutate and grow, over-whelming the immune system's resources. Undiagnosed food and chemical allergies can also amplify the severity of arthritis symptoms.

In this book, both the lay reader and physician will find an effective course of treatment possibly leading to a cure for RA and other chronic illnesses with arthritis-like symptoms.

Please address all correspondence, including requests for quantity discounts to: K. Poehlmann
RA Infection Connection
P.O. Box 7009
Torrance, CA 90504

Order Form

Mail Orders: Please send ____ copies of

Rheumatoid Arthritis: The Infection Connection to:

Name: ______________________________

Address: ______________________________

City: ______________________________

State, zip: ______________________________

(sorry, shipping to U.S. destinations only)

___ copies @ $ 14.95	______
Sales Tax (California residents only)	______
First copy shipping: $4.00	______
Additional shipping: $2.00 per copy	______
Total:	______

Send this Mail Order Form with check/money order (payable to K. Poehlmann) to:

RA Infection Connection
P.O. Box 7009
Torrance, CA 90504

Please allow ten days for checks to clear.
Bulk & special discounts available on request

To buy via the Internet, use GOOGLE query to locate a site selling this book:

GOOGLE [*Arthritis Poehlmann Infection Connection*]

Available on www.Amazon.com
and www.RA-Infection-Connection.com
Order in quantity via
Orders@RA-Infection-Connection.com